IMMUNOLOGICAL PARAMETERS OF HOST-TUMOR RELATIONSHIPS

Edited by
DAVID W. WEISS, Ph.D.

Head, Department of Immunology, Hebrew University—
Hadassah Medical School, Jerusalem

Academic Press   New York / London

Academic Press, Inc.
111 Fifth Avenue
New York, N. Y. 10003

Distributed in the United Kingdom by

Academic Press (London), Ltd.
Berkeley Square House
London WIX 6BA

Library of Congress Catalogue Card No. 76–142182

ISBN 0–12–743550–6

Printed in Israel at Central Press, Jerusalem

CONTENTS

PERSPECTIVES OF HOST-TUMOR RELATIONSHIPS

PREFACE AND INTRODUCTION

The ISRAEL JOURNAL OF MEDICAL SCIENCES occasionally undertakes to bring out, as special issues, collections of invited communications on particular aspects of medical science. By presenting under the same cover the most recent findings and views of leading workers in the international scientific community, these special symposia-in-print intend to create ready opportunities for a critical evaluation of the current status, and the likely avenues of development, of topics of unusual interest and immediacy.

The present issue focuses on a subject which has come to be recognized only within the past several years as of cardinal significance to the clinician as well as to the biologist, the immunology of the host-parasite relationship in neoplasia. No attempt was made to obtain an inclusive review of this area, and, indeed, the magnitude and scope of research which now suddenly marks the field would forbid the endeavor. Instead, contributions were invited selectively with the aim of presenting an overview of new information and thought on a number of the facets which delimit its central questions and dilemmas. To attain the broadest perspective, we sought the participation both of recognized leaders in the field and of investigators who have entered it more recently and whose approaches appear to hold special promise, and both reports of original research and discursive considerations are represented. To all those who joined in this undertaking, I express my sincere gratitude and appreciation.

To speak of neoplasia as a host-parasite relationship no longer requires justification. It is today apparent that neoplastic disease is the pathological manifestation of an ongoing confrontation between two significantly distinct populations of cells, the normal constituents of the host organism and the neoplastic variants. It is equally clear that these obviously pathogenic variants possess a sufficient degree of independence to force us to view them as no less "autonomous" than many of the classical microbial and viral parasites. It follows that the same labile interplay of host, parasite and environmental variables which governs the dynamics of host-parasite associations in infectious diseases is also determinant of the interaction of host and neoplastic cell. A biologically correct approach to the study of the natural history of neoplasia has indeed become impossible without this frame of reference (1, 2), and a major task of the tumor biologist today is to underline the necessity and the implications of this conceptual framework to the clinician and to laboratory investigators who address themselves to oncological problems.

A convocation of information and opinion on host factors in neoplasia in 1970 is thus no longer bedevilled by doubts as to its relevancy. The underlying question "Does the host react against his own cancer cells?" (3) has been replaced by others, no less difficult to answer, but questions which proceed from a realistic assessment of the nature of neoplastic processes. Cardinal among these are

1

two: "How does the host react to his own tumor cells?" and "Why is the potential reactiveness of the host at times aborted, and why at other times—the instances of progressive, destructive neoplastic disease—is host reactivity too limited to destroy the neoplastic parasite?"

At a period when immunology represents a focal point of experimental biology and medicine, the terms "host," "parasite" and "reaction" bear almost automatically in an immunological direction. It may be necessary, therefore, to emphasize in the context of any discussion on host-tumor relationships that immunological homeostasis is by no means the only control mechanism by which the organism attempts to preserve its integrity. Immunological reactions may, in fact, serve as importantly in an auxilliary manner to phagocytic, hormonal and other physiological control systems as they do in providing a specific means of destruction of antigenic invaders. Nonetheless, the focus today is on the immune response in its own right, as a paramount determinant of the outcome of an oncogenic event. Provided that it does not obscure the existence of other means and of other, collaborative functions of the immunological apparatus, this inclination would appear to be justified.

Because the very nature of immunological responsiveness lies in its qualitative specificity and precision, immune reactions hold a special promise of providing a vehicle through the layers of overlapping similarities between host and neoplastic cells which make these relationships so uniquely difficult to untangle, or to interfere with therapeutically. There is increasing reason to believe that the very evolution of the immune mechanism in the vertebrates, very possibly preempting, at least in existing species, a considerable portion of the organism's genome (4), has been largely in the direction of creating an effective surveillance mechanism (5) against neoplastic mutants. And, it may well be that this specific immunological surveillance is totally effective, and perhaps to a large extent independent of other means, in the vast majority of instances where a stem cell acquires neoplastic properties, progressive neoplasia constituting a small minority of exceptions.

If this is true, then the dilemma of the experimentalist in this area, to which George Klein alludes in the title of his present paper, is only too real, and in more than one respect. Neoplastic disease may have to be seen not as the cumulative end result of a number of contributory events of pathogenic potential, but rather negatively, as the rare exception to the consequence of a series of events which normally lead to nothing grossly detectable. To analyze, and to try to reverse, the failure of what most commonly is a highly efficient, fundamental and specifically evolved defence is in itself a task of frustration: We have learned that even the most artifactual means of highly effective therapy, such as the antibiotics, are often limited in their efficacy when the inherent host defenses are very low. Here, then, we may be trying to understand and correct a fault by which a single or a very few antigenic variants succeeded in establishing themselves against the very processes developed to cope with this situation, processes efficacious to a degree which forbids in the overwhelming number of instances the prolonged survival of alien cells, even despite heroic efforts to facilitate this where such survival would be beneficial. This task is the more frustrating in light of the fact that all other means of effecting the destruction of the neoplastic variant (invader is not the proper term in neoplasia, "traitor" would be more appropriate!) have so far been limited, and, because of the intimate biological proximity of host and parasite in these systems, are likely to remain so. Today, it is the possibility of immunological intervention in malignancy which seems to many to hold new

2

promise—and yet we may have to say at one and the same time that there is justification for this promise, and that it may be absurd against the background of an already demonstrated and massive failure.

The dilemma of the tumor immunologist is even more elementary, however. This entire facet of oncology is built on the cornerstone of the actual antigenicity of neoplastic cells. The history of what three or four years ago appeared to be the final and firm establishment of this concept has been a very stormy one. From a beginning of exaggerated optimism in the early years of experimental cancer biology, based to a considerable extent on the then recent successes of immunological attack on infectious disease agents, the climate of opinion shifted to the opposite extreme. With the recognition that transplantation experiments in non-inbred animals may have revealed only homograft, not tumor-specific, reactions, and that the formidable technical difficulties of serological studies designed to demonstrate such specificity in these systems caused these, too, to remain inconclusive, investigations in the area of tumor immunology came to be considered maverick from the start. It was only in the late 1950s and early 1960s, following the demonstrations by Foley, Prehn, the Kleins and others, that neoplastic cells can evoke specific immune reactions in proven isogenic systems that tumor immunology was restored to the status of a respectable field of investigation. A flood of communications following these reports showed the existence of what appeared to be tumor-specific antigens in virtually every animal model examined, and subsequently in an increasing number of different human neoplasms as well. And then, several years ago, it became apparent that the picture is nowhere near as consistent and clear as this impressive body of evidence suggested at first.

Disturbing reports began to appear that not all tumors necessarily possess specific immunogenicity; the paper in this volume contributed by Baldwin and Embleton makes this point well. It may perhaps still be argued that such supposedly nonimmunogenic tumors are, in fact, antigenic but induce enhancing, tolerogenic and resistance factors in such proportions as to cancel each other out. If this is the case, neoplastic transformation may continue to signify, universally, qualitative changes recognizable as such by the immunological apparatus. Even so, it becomes evident that some tumors may lack the properties requisite for inciting a protective immune response, and this possibility in turn raises the likelihood of effective selection of variants of many tumor cell populations which are operatively, if not intrinsically, nonimmunogenic.

A more subtly disturbing dilemma arises from the gathering doubt as to whether many of the tumors which do behave immunogenically really owe this property to truly tumor-specific antigens, or only to antigens displaced in time and place from normal, that is to say, antigens appearing normally on different cells of the same organism, or at different ontogenic stages, or in very different quantities. Even such "time and place" surface antigens may well confer *de facto* immunogenicity on a cell, but the chances of selection against them during the course of a given tumor process are probably greater than against antigens which appear *de novo* in and on a cell at the point of its departure from normal. Moreover, if tumor immunogens are only time and place antigens, a major argument for the qualitative uniqueness of the neoplastic state is destroyed. The firm demonstration of the embryonic or organ-specific nature of tumor antigens may open different insights into the nature of the crucial neoplastic event, and into problems of differentiation at large, but this new uncertainty cannot be obviated: What precisely is the relationship between tumor-associated antigenic changes and the neoplastic condition, and what are the implications of the manifestation of these antigens for the biologist and for the therapist?

There is a still more protean quandary, and one which marks all facets of immunology which pertain to the interaction of host organisms with antigenically foreign substances. This is the inherently dualistic, double-edged-sword nature of immunological recognition. Depending on a variety of parameters of host and environmental origin, the same chemical determinant may induce resistance or enhancement, reactivity or specific unresponsiveness, and it has been clearly shown that even changes in the physical nature of the determinant can shift the expression of the immune response from one manifestation to the other. It is especially disconcerting to note, as Phyllis Blair points out in her review, that specific immunological tolerance consequent to neonatal antigenic exposure may be more readily manifested in an inhibition of cellular than of humoral reactivity. If this is true as well for other circumstances which lead to specific unresponsiveness, host animals may frequently find themselves impaired in that compartment of the immune response which is primarily associated with the rejection of solid foreign tissues, and still capable of responding with precisely the "wrong" means.

The recent findings reported here from our laboratory with hormonally-induced, mammary tumor virus-free preneoplastic and neoplastic mammary tissues of BALB/c mice have another disturbing implication, to the same final effect: It appears that a strongly expressed, and perhaps dominant, antigen of these tumor cells is mammary tissue related, and that the immune response directed against it is commonly manifested by enhancement. As reviewed by Dr. Blair, this is not the only observation as to the presence of organ-specific antigens on the surface of such cancer cells. It is not known whether organ-specific antigens somehow have a particular predilection for evoking the formation of antibodies with strong enhancing potential in the autochthonous and isogenic host, but the possibility may not be farfetched: Such antibodies can be envisaged as playing a very necessary role in protecting auto-antigenic organs and tissues from the "horror autotoxicus" of self-destruction. A function of the immune response vital to the normal existence of multitissue organisms may thus conceivably backfire when normal growth equilibria are disrupted by a neoplastic event.

The lability of the equilibria which lead to the opposite phenotypic expressions of immunological potential is such that the outcome of the presentation of a new antigen to an animal under a given set of conditions cannot be predicted at the outset. This may mean, as George Klein also emphasizes in his contribution, that the nature of each patient's reactivity against his own neoplastic cells must be determined individually, as must be the effects on that particular immunological microcosm of any planned immunological intervention or, for that matter, of all therapeutic measures which could conceivably impinge on the immune response. Compared to this, the difficulties inherent in therapeutic interventions in infectious disease relationships by means of antibiotics or active and passive immunization seem very small indeed.

This special issue of the Journal centers on these dilemmas, and on the possible avenues of circumventing, if not solving, them. Reports in the first section analyze the nature of the relationship between immunological reactivity and susceptibility to progressive neoplasia in a number of different systems, and discuss the influence of immunological depression and immunological activation in oncogenesis and tumor development. The emphasis in the second section is on current findings on the nature of tumor-associated antigens and of the immune responses against them. Here, too, several distinct models are discussed, and the problem of the bimodality of the results of immunological recognition of cell antigens is a recurrent theme. A number of communications deal specifically with host-tumor relationships in man, but even in the reports based on animal work, the extensions of observations to the clinic are stressed throughout. It is of interest that mammary carcinomas of mice, the animal model which proved at first to be the most refractory to an immunological approach, and which was for some years cited as illustrating the nonantigenicity of spontaneous neoplasms, appears today as a system of choice for many investigators, despite, or perhaps because of, the very great complexity of interacting host and tumor factors.

It must be said, finally, that the term dilemma would not correctly epitomize the current status of tumor immunology unless we stress that this is also a dilemma of hope. For all the predicaments which face the investigator of tumor immune phenomena, it must not be forgotten that it is, in fact, possible to heighten considerably the refractoriness of host animals to neoplastic isografts and autografts, and even to the development and progression of spontaneously arising tumors. This has been accomplished in a number of host-tumor systems by both specific and nonspecific immunological means, and, as Sir Macfarlane Burnet points out in his discussion, nonspecific stimulation of low immunological responsiveness appears today a particularly rewarding avenue of investigation. For instance, recent studies by Diane Yashphe, Shlomo Ben-Ephraim and myself with a tumor-protective methanol-insoluble fraction of BCG organisms have shown that pretreatment with this material, termed MER, renders guinea pigs capable of responding with pronounced delayed hypersensitivity reactions to haptens which do not sensitize

in the absence of complete Freund's adjuvant. In parallel experiments, MER also rendered mice reactive to antigens presented in a physical state, or in quantities, insufficient to elicit responsiveness in normal control animals; and, the substance could counteract the effects of immunosuppressive agents, as has also been reported by other workers for intact, living BCG. Low host responsiveness, inherent in the tumor relationship or induced by chemotherapy or radiation, is thus not necessarily an uncorrectable condition. Neither may it be beyond our reach to so affect the immunological apparatus, afferently or centrally, as to reduce those components which most readily lead to enhancement, even if attempts in this direction must, for the time being, remain largely empirical and even centered on the individual instance.

Whereas the transition to the clinic of immunological approaches to the control of neoplastic cells represents today a very difficult and hazardous step, there also exists, therefore, a starting point of founded optimism. The basic predicament of those working in the area of host-tumor relationships today is, consequently, how to find the appropriate stance between the extremes of hope and dismay, for each of which there is considerable ground. If I may be permitted to conclude this introductory discussion on a purely personal note, I would wish to resort to a dictum, from Mishnah Aboth, chapter 2, which I have found helpful when caught in such a polarity: "It is not thy duty to complete the work, but neither art thou free to desist from it."

DAVID W. WEISS

I owe a dept of gratitude for the initiative and frequent advice of the Editor of the Israel Journal of Medical Sciences, Dr. Moshe Prywes, and I wish also to express my great appreciation to the Editorial Secretaries, Rebekah Soifer and Audrey Young, for their patient help and large contribution in editing this issue.

Jerusalem, 1 Elul 5730 (2 September, 1970)

REFERENCES

1. Weiss, D. W. Immunological parameters of host-parasite relationships in neoplasia. *Ann. N.Y. Acad. Sci* **164**: 431, 1969.
2. Weiss, D. W. Immunological parameters of host-tumor relationships: Spontaneous mammary neoplasia of the inbred mouse as a model. *Cancer Res.* **29**: 2368, 1969.
3. Kidd, J. G. Does the host react against his own cancer cells? *Cancer Res.* **21**: 1170, 1961.
4. Trentin, J. J., Wolf, N., Cheng, V., Fahlberg, W., Weiss, D. and Bonhag, R. Antibody production by mice repopulated with limited numbers of clones of lymphoid cell precursors. *J. Immunol.* **98**: 1326, 1967.
5. Burnet, F. M. "Cellular immunology." Cambridge, Cambridge University Press, 1969, p. 286.

THE IMMUNE MECHANISM
AND SUSCEPTIBILITY
TO PROGRESSIVE NEOPLASIA

IMPLICATIONS OF IMMUNOLOGICAL SURVEILLANCE FOR CANCER THERAPY

F. M. BURNET

School of Microbiology, University of Melbourne, Victoria, Australia

The stimulus to write this paper probably had three components: 1) For a number of years I have been developing the concept of immunological surveillance as an important factor in the natural history of malignant disease (1–3). 2) In recent years there has been much soul-searching in regard to the best treatment of the commonest form of human cancer, breast carcinoma in women. A *Lancet* annotation (4) late in 1969 said that there is no approach to unanimity in regard to the appropriate treatment of early carcinoma of the breast. 3) Perhaps as a reaction against the current interest in nonspecific inhibitors of immune responses such as 6-mercaptopurine and cyclophosphamide, X-irradiation, cortisone and antilymphocytic serum, there is some revival of interest in nonspecific enhancers of immune response, with bacterial endotoxins, unrelated antigens and perhaps estrogens and androgens in mind.

THE PRESENT POSITION OF CANCER THERAPY

For many years the standard approach to the treatment of early cancer of the breast has been a Halsted type radical mastectomy with removal of the pectoralis muscles and the contents of the axilla. Some operators also removed the supraclavicular and internal mammary lymph nodes. Postoperative irradiation of the relevant areas has also been part of the standard treatment in most centers.

The prognosis following such treatment depends on various clinical factors including the size and histological character of the tumor, presence of palpable nodes, histological demonstration of tumor cells within the nodes removed at operation, and the degree of attachment of the tumor to skin and underlying tissues. Success is never 100% but with early treatment, 90% of five-year survivals and around 75% of 10-year survivals can be expected. It can almost be guaranteed that there will be no local recurrence of tumor with ulceration. When death from cancer occurs it is from internal metastases. In this discussion we have no concern with anything but the primary tumor and local lymphatic spread. The palliative treatment of metastases introduces a new set of considerations. The primary objective of therapy when the diagnosis is first made is to secure such effective control at this phase that distant metastasis does not occur.

Controversy—and opportunity—centers on the treatment of the lymph nodes. If immune responses of the type known to be demonstrable in many experimental situations and assumed to provide a basis for immunological surveillance in man, can play a significant part in the effective elimination of residual cancer cells after surgery, the draining lymph nodes could be important. X-irradiation is a potent immunosuppressive and is liable to leave unpleasant local fibrosis as well; there is clearly a growing opinion that it should be used only where it is demonstrably needed. There are similar objections to the unnecessary surgical ablation of draining lymph nodes.

Judging from an authoritative British symposium (5) some points that were clear in 1967 were a) that preoperative X-irradiation was undesirable; b) that with large local tumors the presence of palpable lymph nodes not subsequently found to contain tumor, gave a better prognosis than if no palpable nodes were present; c) that simple mastectomy with postoperative irradiation gave the same results as the radical operation also with postoperative radiation; d) that after radical mastectomy, routine irradiation gave no better results than irradiation used to deal with clinical recurrence when it occurs. It was clear that S. J. Cutler's remark that there may be "a need for increased attention to the possibility of enhancing host responses" was acceptable to many of those present at the symposium.

One could perhaps summarize the situation by saying that the conventional treatment of breast cancer has reached a plateau of basically satisfactory results that has not been altered by various changes in detail of the standard surgery plus radiotherapy approach. Any improvement seems likely to come only by reinforcing, in some way, the biological resistance to tumor growth. There are two visible approaches, at the immunological level with which this paper is mainly concerned, and by hormone therapy which conceivably may also act through an immunological link.

IMMUNOLOGICAL SURVEILLANCE

For reasons that have been fully expounded in recent reviews of cancer immunity (6–8), the immunological position in relation to the common forms of human cancer as exemplified by our prototype of breast cancer can never be known with certainty, but the following interpretation would probably be accepted as reasonable by most of those interested in the field:

• Each clone of malignant cells has its own individuality and each is likely to carry at least some antigenic determinants new to the individual in whom it has arisen. It is equally probable that new antigenic determinants in any collection of tumor clones from different individuals will cover a wide range of patterns. At the practical level it is necessary to assume that each tumor is antigenically distinct from every other as far as its new antigens are concerned. These, of course, are the only ones that could be involved in immunological responses by the body.

Unless unexpected new developments arise, there is no visible approach to specific immunization against an operable cancer. The only immunological opening is some form of nonspecific stimulation of antigenic responses in general. In the literature, one finds a good deal of work on this general theme. There are agents which facilitate antibody production, which activate the phagocytic function of the reticuloendothelial system and which can allow an experimental animal to resist a bacterial challenge which would otherwise be lethal. For historical rather than logical reasons, most such work has been concerned with the use of adjuvants added to an inoculum to increase the antibody response, but for many years, possibly for centuries, there have been records that an acute local or general infection appears to have been beneficial to some chronic preexisting disability including occasionally cancer. This led to the clinical use of "Coley's toxin" in cancer therapy and once the laboratory study of bacterial endotoxins was initiated, an interesting field for investigation with many unexpected ramifications was opened up. Much of the present discussion will be related to the effects of bacterial endotoxins.

HOMOGRAFT IMMUNITY

The process of elimination of tumor cells is essentially equivalent to homograft rejection. It requires 1) that adequate amounts of the new antigenic determinant pass to the local lymph nodes; 2) that reactive immunocytes of the thymus-dependent type are present and react by proliferation to contact with the tumor specific TS antigen; 3) that such reactive immunocytes pass to the interface between normal and abnormal tissue and initiate a process, involving other "nonsensitized" cells as well, which is cytotoxic for the tumor cells; 4) that the damaged or necrotic tumor cells be eliminated and the tissue repaired by standard processes.

Clearly the achievement of this result may be prevented for many reasons: 1) The new antigen may be unable to reach the draining lymph nodes or other lymphoid tissue in which thymus-dependent (TD) cells of appropriate reactivity are present. 2) So much of the new antigen is liberated that available immunocytes are paralyzed (eliminated) instead of proliferating. 3) Circumstances are such that the main immune response is one of antibody production (IgG) against the new antigen, giving rise to the enhancement effect, which is equivalent to the inhibition of processes mediated by TD immunocytes. 4) The tumor cells may have sufficient proliferative capacity to overcome any attack by cytotoxic immunocytes. This may be associated with loss of the primary TS antigen or production of locally paralyzing amounts of antigen. Both could be manifestations of "progression," i.e., sequential somatic mutation with selective proliferation of the mutant.

If we are to seek possibilities of "enhancing host responses," each of these points may need to be kept in mind.

DIFFICULTIES OF THE CLINICAL APPROACH

There will probably always be insuperable difficulties in gaining a satisfactory understanding of the part being played by immune responses in human cancer. If the accepted teaching is correct, virtually every tumor is initiated from a single cell whose own individuality is generated both in the course of normal differentiation and as a result of somatic mutation either independent of or associated with the neoplastic change. The antigenic determinants made available to evoke immune responses by the development of the primary malignant clone and any secondary clones, will be variable in number and in quality. The immune responses may be analogous to those provoked by the diversity of new antigens observed in chemically induced sarcomas and hepatomas in mice, rats and guinea pigs. There may be normally "inaccessible" tissue antigens released or genetic anomalies associated with malignant change may allow the synthesis of antigens that are appropriate not to the cell of origin but to cells in the fetal state or some quite different type of adult somatic cell. The possibilities of variation between tumors are clearly almost unlimited even when we are concerned only with their potential immunogenicity.

On the side of the host there is the still largely unexplored question as to the extent of genetic or acquired variation in immunological effectiveness which is relevant to the subsequent appearance of clinical malignancy. It is well known that most of the serious congenital deficiencies in the immune system are associated with an abnormally high incidence of neoplastic disease, particularly of the lymphoid system (see ref. 9). In addition, there is significant concordance of lymphoproliferative disease in identical twins, and there has been much recent concern at the undue incidence of such conditions in recipients of transplanted organs under prolonged immunosuppressive therapy.

11

There was once interest in the possibility that a person's "constitution" or "diathesis" helped to determine whether he would or would not suffer from cancer in later life. Ungar (10) in 1953, for instance, stated that a comparison of cancer patients with comparable noncancer patients showed that only 27% of the former showed an "inflammatory diathesis" as against 61% of controls. One gathers that the term, inflammatory diathesis, referred to a tendency to show active symptoms in childhood infections or to suffer from allergic manifestations.

Three more recent studies all point in the same direction. Fisherman (11) found 3.2% of some 1,200 cancer patients giving a history of allergic conditions (eczema, hay fever or asthma) as against 11 to 13% in a control series. Mackay and Baum (12) found both groups two to three times higher but in the same approximate ratio, cancer patients 9%, controls 21%.

Ure (13) comparing cancer and noncancer patients in a gynecological service, obtained an even more striking difference in a rather small series i.e., ⟨ 4% as against 28% in controls.

BACTERIAL ENDOTOXINS

Interest in bacterial endotoxins goes back to the 19th century when Coley gained the impression from earlier records and from his own experience that associated bacterial infection sometimes had a strikingly beneficial effect on the malignant process. He subsequently claimed that a mixed toxin of streptococci and *Bacillus prodigiosus* could be a useful adjunct to surgery in cancer treatment. The method was never generally adopted nor, on the other hand, has it ever become extinct. Monographs on end results have recently been published from the New York Cancer Research Institute (14).

The interest of academic immunologists in endotoxin springs largely from Rowley's (15) finding that the cell walls of *Salmonella typhosa* had an easily demonstrable effect in increasing the resistance of mice to a variety of bacteria. Several reviews dealing with pharmacological and immunological aspects are available (16–21).

Virtually all gram-negative bacteria produce endotoxin and following the work of Westphal's school (19), we can accept all those endotoxins which have been used in the last 20 years, derived from *Escherichia coli* or various salmonellas for the most part, as equivalent to the lipopolysaccharide O-antigens of the corresponding bacterium.

There is near consensus that the pharmacological reactions of endotoxin (i.e., purified bacterial lipopolysaccharide) are to a very large extent immunological in origin. The evidence for this is necessarily almost all indirect since all normal mammals contain large numbers of endotoxin-producing bacteria in the gut. It is particularly relevant that Schaedler and Dubos (20) found that a pathogen-free stock of mice which had no *E. coli* and very few gram-negative bacteria of any sort in the predominantly lactobacillary intestinal flora, was almost wholly insusceptible to endotoxin shock. Such animals became susceptible if they were a) given a heat-killed vaccine of gram-negative bacteria, b) foster suckled as infants by a mouse of a conventional stock with plentiful coliform bacteria in the gut. Less direct evidence is seen in the relative insusceptibility of newborn rabbits which, in terms of dose/kg, are many thousandfold more resistant to the lethal action of endotoxin than are adult animals (18). Then there is the finding that all normal animals contain a range of natural antibodies bactericidal for gram-negative organisms in the blood (21). These are always IgM in type and, except in animals which allow passage of IgM to the fetus, such as the rabbit, they are absent at birth.

In man and other mammals, purified endotoxin produces a reaction on intradermal injection which is, in many ways, intermediate between an Arthus-type reaction and a typical delayed hypersensitivity response. In man, for instance, erythema appears within 5 hr and is gone by 48, which in both respects differs sharply from a tuberculin reaction. There is a general resemblance in the fever and leukopenic-leukocytosis response to endotoxin in a normal animal and that of a soluble antigen given i.v. to a sensitized one. In all comparisons with standard immunological reactions, the endotoxic reactions are more acute and are provoked with very much smaller amounts of material than are needed of any of the soluble antigens (22).

From the point of view of any relevance to cancer therapy the most important capacity of endotoxin is to facilitate the production of antibody and, by implication, of delayed hypersensitivity immunocytes against other antigens. There is abundant evidence of the capacity to facilitate antibody production, e.g., against bovine γ-globulin in mice and rabbits (23) and there is equally extensive evidence for its protective effect against a wide variety of bacterial infections in mice (15, 24). It is of course by no means implied that the two phenomena are necessarily related. There is much less evidence in regard to the direct influence of endotoxin on homograft rejection and other reactions based on cellular immunity. It has been shown by Al-Askari et al. (25) that endotoxin given i.v. accelerates the rejection of first set skin homografts in rabbits. I can find no reference to any experiments in which endotoxin or analogous agents were tested for any capacity to inhibit the induction of tumors in experimental animals by any of the standard methods. It would obviously be unreasonable to expect any influence on a standard transplantable tumor, but Donaldson et al. (26) were able to demonstrate that X-ray therapy of a highly malignant transplantable melanoma in golden hamsters gave better results when it was combined with endotoxin administration. Endotoxin alone had no effect.

It makes a reasonable working hypothesis, susceptible in principle to experimental test, to assume that appropriate immunological stimulation by bacterial endotoxin would improve the results of conventional surgical-irradiation treatment of operable cancer.

POSSIBLE USE OF ENDOTOXIN
AS AN ACCESSORY TO THERAPY

If the principle of nonspecific immunological stimulation as an accessory to standard cancer treatment is to be explored experimentally, the use of bacterial endotoxin seems to be the logical starting point. Assuming that Stetson, Dubos and others are correct in ascribing the characteristic actions of endotoxin to an unusual type of sensitization and tolerance resulting from constant low-grade entry of endotoxin from the bowel, it would seem desirable to prepare endotoxin for therapeutic use from coliform organisms commonly present in the human bowel during childhood. It should be in the form of at least semi-purified lipopolysaccharide and show typical pyrogenic and Shwartzman-type activity in rabbits and protection against bacterial infection in mice. It would clearly also be desirable to have some appropriate laboratory test to establish its capacity to accelerate homograft rejection, particularly of very small grafts. It is doubtful whether there is any satisfactory laboratory model for the wide variety of autochthonous human tumors that the cancer surgeon and radiotherapist is called on to treat. One wonders, however, whether careful search might not provide some suitable example of chemically provoked tumor, perhaps Huggins' dimethylbenz-anthracene induced breast tumors in rats (27). It is of interest that Huggins (28) indicated that rats needed to be in good health and free of chronic respiratory infection if a high proportion of breast cancers were to be obtained.

It is well known that cancer patients show a sharply diminished capacity to reject skin or human tissue culture cell grafts (29), and show an abnormally low percentage of tuberculin, streptococcal (VARIDASE®) and other skin hypersensitivities as well as resisting sensitization to chemicals like dinitrochlorobenzene (30). It is not clear whether this nonreactivity in part precedes the appearance of cancer or is wholly a manifestation of processes related to the malignancy. Irrespective of this, if endotoxin therapy were to be effective it should be capable of reevoking skin reactivity to tuberculin or other appropriate skin test reagents in nonreactive patients not too far advanced in secondary malignant disease. Without going into detail, this should provide a preliminary approach at the clinical level.

It is quite possible that I am unduly impressed with the claims that individuals who have suffered from allergic disease are *ipso facto* less liable to cancer than others. It fits well into the developing picture of immunological surveillance that recurrent episodes of immunological activity, including, as Brostoff and Roitt (31) have recently shown, an element of delayed hypersensitivity, should as it were, keep the surveillance mechanism "up to the mark." An authoritative confirmation of such findings, preferably using prospective rather than retrospective statistical data, would greatly strengthen the case for serious experimental tests of appropriate immunological stimulation as an adjuvant to cancer therapy or even as a partial prophylaxis against neoplasia.

THE BEARING OF PERSONALITY AND
HORMONAL BALANCE ON
IMMUNOLOGICAL SURVEILLANCE AND CANCER

Each human individual is unique and immensely complex and for many years physicians have tried to sort their patients into constitutional or personality types and to seek correlation of type with disease, particularly cancer. If immunological factors are of importance in determining the onset of cancer and, as I am suggesting in this paper, have potential for improving therapy, it may be legitimate to conclude with a brief survey of possible relationships between the two fields of interest.

From fairly wide casual reading in regard to relationships between personality type and disease, two significant features seem to emerge. The first is that there is a considerable concordance that a personality type can be recognized which has been variously labeled introvert (Jung, Eysenck), schizo-thymic (Kritschmer), super-stable (Jobring), and cerebrotonic (Sheldon), and the second, that within this group there is a diminished incidence of cancer and of most major abdominal disease but an excess of minor respiratory infections, of allergic conditions and of neurodermatitis (32). The evidence that a history of allergic disease is much less frequent in cancer patients than in equivalent noncancer controls has already been discussed. This provides a clear suggestion that the personality-cancer relationship may be mediated immunologically. Specific studies of the point seem called for.

Personality, general health and capacity to handle bodily emergencies, all obviously depend on the hormonal balance of the body. There are indications from recent experimental work that pituitary somatotrophic and thyrotrophic hormones are needed if immune responses are to be normal (33). As in pituitary dwarf mice, there may be forms of human disease in which hormonal imbalance is manifested by immunological deficiency. There is also an obvious possibility that hormonal deficiencies, particularly of estrogens, may play a part in senescence, including the rising incidence of cancer with age, and it is natural in the present context to wonder whether hormonal deficiencies produce deleterious effects in part by weakening the efficiency of immunological surveillance and other immunological responses. Particularly in relation to postmenopausal difficulties in women, there has been considerable study of the possibility of reducing the incidence of cancer by continued administration of estrogens. Several groups of treated women have been observed whose cancer experience was lower than that to be expected from figures for the whole population (34–36) but in the absence of specifically designated control groups the findings cannot be accepted as significant. They may, however, well be adequate to justify properly planned and adequately controlled trials on a sufficiently large scale to give unequivocal results.

CONCLUSION

This paper is an attempt to look at the possible implications of modern work on cancer immunity, for the handling of cancer at the clinical level. I have written it as a biologist rather than a physician and I have made no attempt to do more than suggest lines of thought which might stimulate those directly concerned with cancer treatment to undertake responsible clinical experimentation which might improve their end results.

My other objective is to draw attention to the real possibility that personality and hormonal balance are related to susceptibility to malignant disease by their influence on the effectiveness of immunological surveillance. There is important work to be done on the degree of correlation between allergic conditions, body build and personality type in adolescence or young adult life and the pattern of degenerative and malignant disease in later life. Important possibilities of prophylaxis and even for therapy might result from such investigations.

REFERENCES

1. BURNET, F. M. Immunological factors in the process of carcinogenesis. *Brit. med. Bull.* **20**: 154, 1964.

2. BURNET, F. M. The concept of immunological surveillance. *Progr. exp. Tumor Res.* (*Basel*) (in press).

3. BURNET, F. M. "Immunological surveillance." Sydney, Pergamon Press, 1970.

4. EDITORIAL. Treatment of early cancer of the breast. *Lancet* **ii**: 1175, 1969.

5. FORREST, A. P. M. and KUNKLER, P. B. (Eds.) "Prognostic factors in breast cancer." Edinburgh, E. & S. Livingstone, 1968.

6. OLD, L. J. and BOYSE, E. A. Immunology of experimental tumors. *Ann. Rev. Med.* **15**: 167, 1964.

7. KLEIN, G. Tumor antigens. *Ann. Rev. Microbiol.* **20**: 223, 1966.

8. SCHLESINGER, M. and AMOS, B. Antigenic alterations of host tissues during tumor growth, in: Rapaport, F. T. and Dausset, J. (Eds.), "Human transplantation." New York, Grune and Stratton, 1968, p. 601.

9. MILLER, D. G. The immunologic capability of patients with lymphoma. *Cancer Res.* **28**: 1441, 1968.

10. UNGAR, F. H. Problem of allergy and malignant tumors. *Acta Un. int. Cancr.* **9**: 213, 1953.

11. FISHERMAN, E. W. Does the allergic diathesis influence malignancy? *J. Allergy* **31**: 74, 1960.

12. MACKAY, W. D. and BAUM, M. The role of immune factors in breast cancer, in: Forrest, A. P. M. and Kunkler, P. B. (Eds.), "Prognostic factors in breast cancer." Edinburgh, E. & S. Livingstone, 1968, p. 319.

13. URE, D. M. J. Negative association between allergy and cancer. *Scot. med. J.* **14**: 51, 1969.

14. FOWLER, G. A. Beneficial effects of acute bacterial infections on bacterial toxin therapy on cancer of the colon or rectum. New York, New York Cancer Research Institute, 1969, Monograph 10.

15. ROWLEY, D. Endotoxin-induced changes in susceptibility to infections, in: Landy, M. and Braun, W. (Eds.), "Bacterial endotoxins." New Brunswick, N. J., Rutgers Univ. Press, 1964, p. 359.

16. THOMAS, L. The physiological disturbances produced by endotoxins. *Ann. Rev. Physiol.* **16**: 467, 1954.

17. LANDY, M. and BRAUN, W. "Bacterial endotoxins." New Brunswick, N. J., Rutgers Univ. Press, 1964.

18. LEE, L. and STETSON, C. A. The local and generalized Shwartzman reactions, in: Zweifach, B. W., Grant, L. and McCluskey, R. T. (Eds.), "The inflammatory process." New York, Academic Press, 1965, p. 791.

19. LÜDERITZ, O., STAUB, A. M. and WESTPHAL, O. Immunochemistry of O and R antigens of Salmonella and related enterobacteriaceae. *Bact. Rev.* **30**: 192, 1966.

20. SCHAEDLER, R. W. and DUBOS, R. Relationship of intestinal flora to resistance, in: Landy, M. and Braun, W. (Eds.), "Bacterial endotoxins." New Brunswick, N. J., Rutgers Univ. Press, 1964, p. 390.

21. LANDY, M. and WEIDANZ, W. P. Natural antibodies against gram-negative bacteria, in: Landy, M. and Braun, W. (Eds.), "Bacterial

endotoxins." New Brunswick, N. J., Rutgers Univ. Press, 1964, p. 275.

22. STETSON, C. A. Symposium on bacterial endotoxins. IV. Immunological aspects of the host reaction to endotoxins. *Bact. Rev.* **25**: 457, 1961.

23. WARD, P. A., JOHNSON, A. G. and ABELL, M. R. Studies on the adjuvant action of bacterial endotoxins on antibody formation. III. Histologic response of rabbit spleen to a single injection of a purified protein antigen. *J. exp. Med.* **109**: 463, 1959.

24. BOEHME, D. and DUBOS, R. J. The effect of bacterial constituents on the resistance of mice to heterologous infection and on the activity of their reticulo-endothelial system. *J. exp. Med.* **107**: 523, 1958.

25. AL-ASKARI, S., ZWEIMAN, B., LAWRENCE, H. S. and THOMAS, L. The effect of endotoxin on skin homografts in rabbits. *J. Immunol.* **93**: 742, 1964.

26. DONALDSON, S. S., COOPER, JR., R. A. and FLETCHER, W. S. Effect of Coley's toxins and irradiation on the A. Melanoma 3 tumor in the golden hamster. *Cancer (Phila.)* **21**: 805, 1968.

27. HUGGINS, C., GRAND, L. C. and BRILLANTES, F. P. Mammary cancer induced by a single feeding of polynuclear hydrocarbons, and its suppression. *Nature (Lond.)* **189**: 204, 1961.

28. HUGGINS, C. Methodology of selective induction of cancers in adult rats, in: Forrest, A. P. M. and Kunkler, P. B. (Eds.), "Prognostic factors in breast cancer." Edinburgh, E. & S. Livingstone, 1968, p. 465.

29. SOUTHAM, C. M., MOORE, A. E. and RHOADS, C. P. Homotransplantation of human cell lines. *Science* **125**: 158, 1957.

30. LEVIN, A. G., McDONOUGH, JR., E. F., MILLER, D. G. and SOUTHAM, C. M. Delayed hypersensitivity response to DNFB in sick and healthy persons. *Ann. N. Y. Acad. Sci.* **120**: 400, 1964.

31. BROSTOFF, J. and ROITT, I. M. Cell-mediated (delayed) hypersensitivity in patients with summer hay-fever. *Lancet* **ii**: 1269, 1969.

32. SHELDON, W. H. "The varieties of temperament." New York, Harper, 1942.

33. PIERPAOLI, W., BARONI, C., FABRIS, N. and SORKIN, E. Hormones and immunological capacity. II. Reconstitution of antibody production in hormonally deficient mice by somatotropic hormone, thyrotropic hormone and thyroxin. *Immunology* **16**: 217, 1969.

34. WALLACH, S. and HENNEMAN, P. H. Prolonged estrogen therapy in postmenopausal women. *J. Amer. med. Ass.* **171**: 1637, 1959.

35. WILSON, R. A. The roles of estrogen and progesterone in breast and genital cancer. *J. Amer. med. Ass.* **182**: 327, 1962.

36. WILSON, R. A., BREVETTI, R. E. and WILSON, T. A. Specific procedures for the elimination of the menopause. *West. J. Surg.* **71**: 110, 1963.

INFLUENCE OF HOST FACTORS ON LEUKEMOGENESIS BY THE RADIATION LEUKEMIA VIRUS

NECHAMA HARAN-GHERA

Department of Experimental Biology, Weizmann Institute of Science, Rehovot, Israel

ABSTRACT

The leukemogenic activity of the radiation leukemia virus could be effectively evaluated by injecting the virus directly into the thymus of adult C57BL/6 mice, provided these hosts were further exposed to transient immune impairment within a few days after virus inoculation. In the present study, the immunosuppressive agents used as coleukemogenic factors were: whole-body irradiation (its effect being compared with local thymus irradiation), heterologous antithymocyte serum, or urethane. The combined "virus-host" treatment induced an 80 to 100% lymphoid leukemia incidence at an average latent period of 80 to 100 days, whereas omitting further treatment of the host reduced the incidence to 15 to 25%. Delaying host immune impairment for 30 or 60 days after virus inoculation resulted in a reduction in the lymphoid tumor incidence (70 vs. 20 and 5% respectively, in the radiation-treated mice). This decrease in leukemia development was found to be unrelated to the amount of virus present in the host, and could be attributed to an immunization phenomenon.

The leukemogenic activity of the radiation leukemia virus isolated from radiogenic lymphoid tumors of the C57BL strain of mice was first demonstrated by its tumorigenic effect when injected into isologous newborn mice (1). A more sensitive technique for showing the leukemogenic activity of this agent was later described, namely, injecting the virus directly into a several-day-old thymus grafted under the kidney capsule in an adult thymectomized irradiated host (2). The age of the thymus at the time of virus inoculation seemed at first of importance, on the basis of the proposal (3, 4) that the susceptible cells for leukemic neoplastic transformation are the large and medium lymphocytes present in abundance in a several-day-old growing thymus. However, further observations on the focal thymolytic effect of the radiation leukemia virus leading to active regeneration (5), which is an important permissive factor in leukemogenesis (6), suggested that thymus age might not, after all, be crucial in this induction system. Indeed, recent studies have demonstrated that the age of the thymus at the time of virus inoculation did not affect the rate of tumor induction (7). We have therefore adopted the alternative technique of injecting the leukemogenic virus directly into the intact thymus of an adult mouse, instead of into the thymus graft as in the previous studies (2). The present experiments provide a comparison of the different test systems used to demonstrate the leukemogenic activity of the radiation leukemia virus.

Although the virus exerts its leukemogenic effect locally and directly on the thymus (8), host treatment affecting the immunological integrity of the animals alters the tumor incidence. The aim of the present work was to analyze the tumor-host relationship in leukemogenesis by the radiation leukemia virus, by determining host effects that cause an increase or decrease in the tumor induction yield.

MATERIALS AND METHODS

Animals. Male mice of the C57BL/6 strain, from our inbred mouse colony were used when newborn, or five to eight weeks old. They were housed in an air-conditioned room at 21 to 24 C, and fed Purina Laboratory Chow and water ad lib.

All dead mice were autopsied routinely; unless lymphoid leukemia could be diagnosed unequivocally, the relevant tissues were examined histologically (fixation in Bouin's fluid and staining with hematoxylin and eosin).

X-irradiation. The physical conditions for irradiation were: 1) For whole-body irradiation, Maximar 250-III General Electric, 230 kv, 15 ma, with 1 mm Al and 0.5 mm Cu filters; dose rate, 45 R/min. 2) For cell-free centrifugates, Rich & Seifert Dermovolt, 56 kv, 15 ma, with 0.5 Al filter; focal skin distance, 6 cm; field diameter, 60 mm; dose rate, 1,200 R/min.

Thymus graft: The thymus was removed from male or female C57BL/6 mice aged 12 to 24 hr, and transferred to chilled phosphate-buffered saline. One thymus lobe was promptly grafted, by means of a trocar made out of an 18-gauge stainless steel hypodermic needle, under the left kidney capsule near the adrenal.

Thymectomy. The operation was performed under ether anesthesia. The thymus was removed by suction through an incision in the neck and thoracic wall extending to the level of the second rib.

Preparation and inoculation of virus and cell-free centrifugates (CFC). Preparations of CFC or virus were made from fresh normal tissues, or from thymic lymphoid leukemias induced by a serial passage line of the radiation leukemia virus, originally isolated from irradiated nonleukemic tissues (2). The different tissues were homogenized in 5 vol of chilled phosphate-buffered saline (PBS). The homogenate was centrifuged at $10,000 \times g$, three times for 15 min each, the pellet being discarded each time, and the final supernatant fluid was exposed to a single dose of 10,000 R irradiation, and thereafter used for inoculation. The entire process was carried out at 4 C. According to the purpose of the experiment, 0.02 ml quantities of virus, CFC or PBS were injected directly (using a 30 gauge needle) into one thymus lobe, which was exposed by a mid-line, anteroposterior incision through the sternum from the manubrium halfway to the diaphragm and carefully exteriorized by gentle traction with forceps; 0.1 ml quantities of virus, CFC, or PBS were injected into the exposed kidney or spleen.

Preparation and administration of heterogeneic antithymocyte serum (ATS). Random-bred rabbits received two i.v. injections, 14 days apart, of a cell suspension of 750×10^6 thymocytes from two-month-old male C57BL/6 mice. One hour prior to the two injections of thymocytes, each rabbit received 1,600 units of heparin i.m. They were bled seven days after the second injection of thymocytes, and the serum was decomplemented at 56 C for 30 min, filtered, and stored at −15 C. Control serum from normal rabbits (NRS) was prepared similarly. The antisera were injected twice (0.5 ml/injection), at a five-day interval, by the subcutaneous route. The activity of the ATS was evaluated by a homograft reaction test, as previously described (9).

RESULTS

Different routes of virus administration. The leukemogenic activity of a CFC, prepared from a radiation leukemia virus induced lymphoma, was tested by administration of the virus preparation via different routes: 1) injecting 0.05 ml i.p. into mice aged 24 hr or less; 2) injecting 0.02 ml into an eight-day-old isogenic thymus grafted under the kidney capsule of thymectomized young adult hosts, with or without exposure three days thereafter to a single dose of 400 R whole-body irradiation; 3) injecting 0.02 ml into one lobe of the intact thymus of young adult animals, and three days thereafter exposing one group of these hosts to 400 R whole-body irradiation.

TABLE 1. *Lymphoid leukemia induction in C57BL/6 mice by the radiation leukemia virus*

Treatment of host[a]	Leukemia incidence	Average latent period (days)
Newborn + virus i.p.	11/20 (55%)	175
Thx → 7d → th. gr → 8d → virus	3/20 (15%)	130
Thx → 7d → th. gr → 8d → virus → 3d → 400 R WB	18/20 (90%)	95
Thx → 7d → th. gr → 8d → PBS → 3d → 400 R WB	1/20 (5%)	170
Intact thymus + virus	5/20 (25%)	142
Intact thymus + virus ———→ 3d ———→ 400 R WB	33/34 (97%)	84
Intact thymus + PBS ———→ 3d ———→ 400 R WB	2/25 (8%)	210

[a] The animals, except for the newborn, were five to six weeks old when experimental procedure was begun.

Virus = A 5% cell-free centrifugate (CFC) in phosphate buffered saline (PBS) was prepared from a lymphoid leukemia induced by passage material from the radiation leukemia virus; 0.05 ml CFC was injected i.p. into newborns, or 0.02 ml into the thymus graft or into the intact thymus.

Thx = Thymectomy.

th. gr = One lobe of an isologous newborn thymus grafted under the kidney capsule.

WB = Whole-body irradiation.

TABLE 2. *Enhancement of lymphoid leukemia induction by different host treatments*

Treatment of host[a]	Leukemia incidence	Average latent period (days)
Intact thymus + virus	11/40 (27%)	174
Intact thymus + virus → 2d → 400 R WB	36/40 (90%)	90
Intact thymus + virus → 2d → 400 R on thymus only	10/31 (32%)	160
Intact thymus + virus → 2d → ATS × 2	31/40 (77%)	116
Intact thymus + virus → 2d → NRS × 2	13/30 (43%)	158
Intact thymus + virus → 2d → urethane × 5	29/40 (72%)	183
Intact thymus + PBS → 2d → urethane × 5	8/26 (30%)	41
Intact thymus + PBS → 2d → ATS × 2	0/30 (0%)	—
Intact thymus + PBS → 2d → NRS × 2	0/20 (0%)	—

[a] The animals were two-month-old males.

Virus = A 5% CFC prepared from a radiation leukemia virus induced lymphoid leukemia, and 0.02 ml was injected into one thymus lobe.

WB = Whole-body irradiation.

ATS = Antithymocyte rabbit serum; 0.5 ml injected s.c. twice at a five-day interval.

NRS = Normal rabbit serum; 0.5 ml injected s.c. twice at a five-day interval.

Urethane = One mg/g body weight in saline, injected i.p. once weekly for five consecutive weeks.

The leukemogenic activity of 400 R whole-body irradiation alone was tested in a control group by injecting PBS, instead of the virus preparation, into the thymus graft or into the intact thymus before irradiation.

The lymphoid leukemia incidence in the differently treated groups is summarized in Table 1. The leukemogenic agent, when injected i.p. into newborn mice, induced 55% lymphoid tumors at an average latent period of 175 days, compared to a 90 or 97% incidence, respectively, when the agent was injected directly into a thymus graft or into an intact thymus of young adult hosts (at an average latent period of 84 to 95 days), provided these animals were exposed within a few days after virus inoculation to whole-body irradiation. Omitting the irradiation reduced the lymphoid leukemia incidence in such inoculated young adults to 15 to 25%.

Whole body irradiation of 400 R, by itself, had a low leukemogenic activity (inducing 5 to 8 % lymphoid leukemia at an average latent period of 200 days).

Effect of host treatment on lymphoid leukemia induction. As demonstrated in the previous experiments (Table 1), inoculation of the leukemogenic virus directly into the thymus of young adult mice caused only a low incidence of tumor development, whereas exposure of the animals thereafter to irradiation increased the yield. The present experiment was aimed at testing whether further treatment of such inoculated mice with agents other than irradiation which cause similar defects in the immune integrity of the host would also enhance leukemia development. The agents chosen for this experiment were: Whole body irradiation vs. local irradiation of the thymus (shielding the rest of the body), ATS as compared to NRS and urethane (1 mg/g body wt dissolved in saline, injected i.p. once weekly for five consecutive weeks).

As shown in Table 2, leukemia induction could be increased from a 27 % incidence in mice that received only inoculation of the virus into the thymus (male C57BL/6 mice, two months old), to 90 % with further treatment of whole-body irradiation, 77 % when the animals were administered ATS and 80 % with urethane treatment following virus inoculation. Although the disease develops first in the thymus, inoculation of the virus directly into this organ, followed by local irradiation of the thymus (with the same dose used for whole-body irradiation), did not enhance tumor development. NRS had a slight coleukemogenic effect. ATS or NRS treatment alone did not cause lymphoid tumor development, whereas five weekly injections of urethane induced 30 % lymphoid leukemia after a long mean latent period of 410 days (compared to 183 days in mice treated first with the virus and thereafter with urethane).

Host treatment at different time intervals after virus inoculation. Is the coleukemogenic effect exerted by further host immunosuppressive treatment after virus inoculation into the

TABLE 3. *Reduction in lymphoid leukemic incidence by delaying further host treatment after virus inoculation into the thymus*

| Further host treatment[a] | Leukemia incidence in mice after virus inoculation into thymus and further host treatment started at the following time intervals[b] | | | |
	2 days	7 days	20 days	30 days
None	3/20 (15%) (132 days)[b]	—	—	5/20 (25%) (112 days)
400 R WB	19/20 (95%) (92 days)	16/20 (80%) (108 days)	13/20 (65%) (142 days)	5/21 (24%) (148 days)
ATS	14/20 (70%) (136 days)	11/20 (55%) (120 days)	6/20 (30%) (122 days)	6/20 (30%) (130 days)
NRS	6/20 (30%) (120 days)	4/20 (20%) (152 days)	5/20 (25%) (110 days)	3/20 (15%) (125 days)
Urethane	16/20 (80%) (183 days)	—	—	10/22 (45%) (264 days)

[a] The initial host treatment of all the mice included injection of 0.02 ml virus preparation directly into one thymus lobe of six- to eight-week old male mice.
[b] Average latent period of tumor development.
WB = Whole-body irradiation.
ATS = Antithymocyte rabbit serum; 0.5 ml injected s.c. twice at a five-day interval.
NRS = Normal rabbit serum; same treatment schedule as for ATS.
Urethane = One mg/g body weight (in saline) injected i.p. five times at weekly intervals.

thymus affected by the time interval between these two procedures? The present experiment was devised to clarify this question. Virus was inoculated into the thymus, and further treatment with 400 R whole-body irradiation, ATS, NRS or urethane was started at two, seven, 20 or 30 days after virus injection.

Delaying host treatment after inoculation of the leukemogenic virus into the thymus reduced the leukemia incidence in the different groups. In the present experiment (Table 3), the tumor incidence following virus injection into the thymus was 15 to 25%. An 80 to 95% leukemia induction rate was obtained when the interval between virus injection and irradiation was two to seven days, compared with 24% after 30 days. A similar decrease was noted in the ATS-treated group: 70% tumors when ATS was injected two days after virus administration, vs. 30% after a 30-day interval. In the urethane-treated group, there was also a difference, both in tumor incidence and in the average latent period for tumor development, depending on when the urethane was given. An 80% incidence at an average latent period of 183 days was recorded when urethane was administered two days after virus injection, compared with 45% at an average latent period of 264 days when

the treatment was delayed for 30 days. The coleukemogenic effect of NRS was too slight to evaluate any reduction in tumor incidence as a result of delaying its administration for 30 days.

Virus viability in the thymus. It is thus evident that virus injection into an adult thymus induces only a low incidence of lymphoid leukemia, whereas further treatment of these mice with irradiation, ATS or urethane increased the tumor yield, provided that further host treatment was carried out within a few days after virus inoculation. Delaying the coleukemogenic treatment to 30 days diminished the leukemia incidence. These results could perhaps be attributed to a decrease in virus titer during this prolonged interval. Experiments were therefore designed to test the viability and amount of virus at different time intervals after its introduction into the thymus. This evaluation was made by testing the leukemogenic activity of CFC (and their serial dilutions) prepared from intact thymuses, in which "thymus-virus" interaction lasted for different time intervals.

One hundred and twenty male C57BL/6 mice were used for the initial treatment, all receiving a single injection of 0.02 ml virus directly into one thymus lobe. The mice were thereafter divided into six groups. Three of

TABLE 4. *Persistence of virus viability in the thymus*

Experimental procedure	Leukemia incidence	Average latent period (days)
Intact thymus + virus[a] ⟶ 7d → 400 R WB	14/20 (70%)	100
Intact thymus + virus[a] ⟶ 30d → 400 R WB	4/20 (20%)	230
Intact thymus + virus ⟶ 60d → 400 R WB	1/20 (5%)	190
Intact thymus + CFC I → 7d → 400 R WB	20/20 (100%)	112
Intact thymus + CFC II → 7d → 400 R WB	18/20 (90%)	87
Intact thymus + CFC III → 7d → 400 R WB	15/20 (75%)	115

[a] Five-week-old male mice were used; 0.02 ml of virus preparation (a 5% CFC) was injected directly into one thymus lobe of 120 mice. These mice were then either exposed to 400 R whole-body irradiation at different time intervals, or their thymus was removed at different time intervals and the 5% CFC prepared from these thymuses tested for leukemogenic activity.
WB = Whole-body irradiation.
CFC I = 5% cell-free filtrate prepared from thymuses seven days after virus injection.
CFC II = 5% cell-free filtrate prepared from thymuses 30 days after virus injection.
CFC III = 5% cell-free filtrate prepared from thymuses 60 days after virus injection.

TABLE 5. *Lymphoid leukemic induction by virus and CFC serial dilutions*

Leukemogenic agent	Leukemogenic activity of dilutions[a]			
	10^{-2}	10^{-3}	10^{-4}	10^{-5}
CFC I	9/10 (90%) (102 days)	11/12 (91%) (110 days)	8/12 (66%) (120 days)	1/12 (8%) (160 days)
CFC II	10/10 (100%) (95 days)	10/12 (82%) (102 days)	9/12 (75%) (92 days)	—
CFC III	9/10 (90%) (120 days)	10/10 (100%) (114 days)	7/10 (70%) (98 days)	2/10 (20%) (168 days)
Virus	10/10 (100%) (100 days)	8/10 (80%) (130 days)	6/10 (60%) (114 days)	1/10 (10%) (135 days)

[a] The leukemogenic activity was tested by injecting 0.02 ml of the virus dilution into one thymus lobe of two-month-old male mice and after two days exposing the animals to 400 R whole-body irradiation.
Virus = The virus preparation used in the experiment described in Table 4.
CFC I, CFC II, and CFC III = Cell-free centrifugates prepared as described in Table 4.

the groups were exposed to 400 R whole-body irradiation seven, 30 or 60 days after virus injection, and the leukemia incidence in relation to time of irradiation compared. The amount and viability of the virus in the thymus of these hosts shortly before exposure to irradiation was determined by removing the thymus of the remaining three groups of un-irradiated hosts seven, 30 or 60 days after virus injection into the thymus. CFC was prepared from thymuses pooled at each time interval, and their leukemogenic activity was tested by injecting 0.02 ml CFC into the intact thymus of a normal host, and seven days thereafter exposing the animals to 400 R whole-body irradiation. Virus titration was performed by testing the leukemogenic activity of serial dilutions in PBS of the thymus extracts and of the original virus preparation used for host injection at the start of the experiment.

A 70% leukemia induction rate was obtained when the interval between virus inoculation and irradiation was seven days, compared to 20% when the interval was 30 days, and 5% after 60 days. An increase in the average latent period was also recorded in these three groups (Table 4). The leukemogenic activity of CFC prepared from thymuses "harboring" the virus for seven, 30 or 60 days was similar, ranging from a 70 to 100% tumor induction potency within 87 to 115 days (Table 4). The different serial dilutions of the three thymus extracts and of the original virus passage, when tested for leukemogenic activity, showed a similar potency (Table 5). Up to a dilution of 10^{-4}, the tumor incidence in the four test dilutions was 60 to 100%, whereas a dilution of 10^{-5} gave only borderline activity (Table 5).

These experiments revealed that there was no decrease in virus titer within several weeks after its introduction into the thymus, and therefore suggest that the decrease in tumor incidence was not related to the amount of virus present in the thymus at the time of irradiation.

Immunization. Another plausible explanation for the observed decrease in tumor incidence occurring with the postponement of irradiation after virus inoculation into the thymus is that the animals were rendered resistant to lymphoid tumor development due to some "virus-thymus" interaction in the normal, unirradiated host. The present experiment was designed to test this assumption. Immunization of C57BL/6 mice by the radiation leukemia virus was evaluated by testing host resistance against isotransplantation of lymphoid leukemic cells induced by the same

TABLE 6. *Transplantation resistance to lymphoid leukemic cells induced in adult C57BL/6 mice by the radiation leukemia virus*

Treatment of host[a]	Takes after s.c. inoculation of cell doses[b]		
	10^6	5×10^5	10^5
Intact thymus + leukemic thymus CFC	2/11 (18%)	2/10 (20%)	0/10 (0%)
Intact thymus + normal thymus CFC	8/10 (80%)	4/10 (40%)	2/10 (20%)
Intact thymus + normal spleen CFC	8/11 (72%)	4/10 (42%)	1/10 (10%)
Intact thymus + normal kidney CFC	9/10 (90%)	5/10 (50%)	2/10 (20%)
Intact thymus + PBS	10/10 (100%)	5/10 (50%)	2/10 (20%)
Intact spleen + leukemic thymus CFC	10/10 (100%)	6/10 (60%)	3/10 (30%)
Intact spleen + PBS	10/10 (100%)	6/10 (60%)	3/10 (30%)
Intact kidney + leukemic thymus CFC	10/10 (100%)	6/10 (60%)	3/10 (30%)
Intact kidney + PBS	9/9 (100%)	6/10 (60%)	3/10 (30%)

[a] Six- to eight-week-old male mice were used.
[b] Subcutaneous challenge with leukemic cells was performed 30 days after CFC or PBS injection into the thymus, kidney or spleen.
CFC = 5% cell-free centrifugate; 0.02 ml was injected directly into the thymus, or 0.1 ml into the spleen or kidney.

virus. CFC were prepared from radiation virus induced lymphoid leukemic thymus, normal thymus, normal spleen and normal kidney. The ability of each of these extracts to immunize was tested by injecting 0.02 ml of CFC or PBS directly into one thymus lobe of normal mice, and challenging these injected mice with 10^6, 5×10^5 or 10^5 leukemic cells. Tumor cell takes were recorded in these differently treated mice. As seen in Table 6, only those mice that received an injection of leukemic thymus CFC into their thymus rejected 10^6 leukemic cells: the tumor take incidence in this group was 18%, compared to 80 to 100% takes in mice that were injected with other CFC preparations or PBS into the thymus.

The route of leukemic CFC introduction for eliciting host immunization seems of importance. The mice were rendered resistant to further leukemic cell challenge only when the leukemic CFC was injected directly into the thymus. Inoculation of the leukemic CFC into the spleen or kidney failed to immunize, and such treated mice showed 100% tumor cell takes (the same incidence as in the control groups), compared to 18% takes when the same agent was injected directly into the thymus (Table 6).

DISCUSSION

An alternative sensitive method to the conventional procedure for testing the leukemogenic activity of a cell-free extract (by injection into newborns) was established by introducing the leukemogenic agent directly into the thymus of adult mice and inducing transient immune impairment of the host shortly thereafter. Previous studies undertaken in our laboratory have already indicated the role and type of immune impairment involved in leukemogenesis by the radiation leukemia virus (10). In the present work it is shown that three different agents—radiation, ATS, and urethane—which are known to exert transient immune deficiencies (11–13) significantly enhance lymphoid leukemia development. Host exposure to 400 R whole-body irradiation after inoculation of the leukemogenic virus into the thymus increased the tumor incidence to 90%, compared to 27% in nonirradiated mice and 32% in similarly treated mice receiving 400 R irradiation only locally on the thymus. These results clearly indicate that although the disease develops first in the thymus, virus inoculation into the thymus and further local irradiation of this target organ do not provide the necessary optimal conditions for tumor development. Only whole-body irradiation, which causes transient immune impairment, is capable of enhancing tumor development, and immune reactivation of this deficit does indeed prevent further tumor development (10). ATS, the potent immunodepressive agent, served effectively as a coleukemogenic factor, although it does not exert any marked damaging effect on the thymus or bone marrow—features considered to be of importance in radiation leukemogenesis (14). In mice more than one to two months of age, urethane—a known coleukemogenic agent (15)—is considered to cause thymus injury, but is ineffective with respect to bone marrow damage (16). It was shown to be an immunosuppressive substance (13), and this capacity, rather than its local damaging effect on the thymus (as in the case of local injury produced by local thymus irradiation, which did not, however, markedly affect the tumor incidence), seems a more plausible explanation for its being a causative factor in the enhancement of leukemia development by the radiation leukemia virus.

The remarkable decrease in the lymphoid leukemia incidence due to delaying transient immune impairment following virus inoculation (by treating the mice with X-rays, ATS or urethane at two, seven, 20, 30 or 60 days after inoculation of the virus into the thymus) could have been attributed either to a decrease in virus titer during the prolonged interval between virus inoculation and further host treatment, or to an immunization phenomenon. Experimental evidence provided in the present communication, showed that there was, in fact, no decrease in virus titer. Hosts inoculated with virus exhibited a similar virus activity in their thymuses seven, 30 or 60 days

after virus inoculation, whereas similarly treated hosts in the same experiment had a lower tumor incidence when 30 or 60 days elapsed between virus injection and immunosuppressive treatment. It seemed plausible therefore, to assume that "thymus-virus" interaction might contribute to a build-up of resistance in the host. This interaction could lead to the neoplastic transformation of some thymus cells, and, it is reasoned, such transformed cells would be abolished by the integrity of the host's immune reaction. These hosts would not become leukemic, but rather be immunized by such tumor cells, whereas transient immunological deficiency would enhance the proliferation of the transformed neoplastic cells. Indeed, experimental evidence indicated that C57BL/6 mice would be immunized by introducing the radiation leukemia virus directly into the thymus of normal hosts (17). Immunization of C57BL/6 mice by the radiation leukemia virus was evaluated by testing host resistance against isotransplantation of lymphoid leukemias induced by the same virus: Only those mice which received virus injection directly into the thymus rejected challenge with 10^6 leukemic cells, the tumor-take incidence in such treated mice being 18% as compared to 80 to 100% in the control groups. The site of virus inoculation is apparently of importance, for virus injection into the spleen or kidney, instead of the thymus, was ineffective.

It is of interest to note that a decrease in tumor cell challenge of normal young C57BL/6 mice to a dose of 5×10^5 or 10^5 cells gave a limited tumor cell take—50 to 60% with the higher cell dose, and 10 to 30% with 10^5 cells. This decrease might perhaps be due to a natural build-up of resistance in the C57BL/6 strain of mice, arising from the fact that the virus is present during postnatal life in nonirradiated C57BL mice. Whether the immunization is caused by the virion or by the neoplastic cell is unclear, but the same course of events that takes place by introducing the virus into the thymus could happen, to a lesser degree, in normal untreated mice, which show an increase in virus titer with age (18).

REFERENCES

1. LIEBERMAN, M. and KAPLAN, H. S. Leukemogenic activity of filtrates from radiation-induced lymphoid tumors of mice. *Science* **130**: 387, 1959.
2. HARAN-GHERA, N. Leukemogenic activity of centrifugates from irradiated mouse thymus and bone marrow. *Int. J. Cancer* **1**: 81, 1966.
3. AXELRAD, A. A. and VAN DER GAAG, H. C. Susceptibility to lymphoma induction by Gross's passage A virus in C3H/f Bi mice of different ages: Relation to thymic cell multiplication and differentiation. *J. nat. Cancer Inst.* **28**: 1065, 1962.
4. KAPLAN, H. S. The role of cell differentiation as a determinant of susceptibility to virus carcinogenesis. *Cancer Res.* **21**: 981, 1961.
5. HARAN-GHERA, N. The mechanism of radiation action in leukemogenesis. III. Thymolytic effect induced by the leukemogenic agent. *Israel J. med. Sci.* **4**: 1169, 1968.
6. KAPLAN, H. S. The role of radiation in experimental leukemogenesis *Nat. Cancer Inst. Monogr.* **14**: 207, 1964.
7. HARAN-GHERA, N. The role of immune impairment in viral leukemogenesis, in: Severi, L. (Ed.) "Immunity and tolerance in oncogenesis," *IV Perugia Quadrennial International Conference.* 1970, p. 585.
8. HARAN-GHERA, N., LIEBERMAN, M. and KAPLAN, H. S. Direct action of a leukemogenic virus on the thymus. *Cancer Res.* **26**: 438, 1966.
9. HARAN-GHERA, N. and PELED, A. The mechanism of radiation action in leukemogenesis. IV. Immune impairment as a coleukemogenic factor. *Israel J. med. Sci.* **4**: 1181, 1968.
10. HARAN-GHERA, N. The mechanism of radiation action in leukemogenesis. II. The role of radiation in leukemia development. *Brit. J. Cancer* **21**: 739, 1967.
11. TALIAFERRO, W. H., TALIAFERRO, L. G. and JARASLOW, B. M. "Radiation and immune mechanism." New York, Academic Press, 1964, p. 31.
12. MONACO, A. P., WOOD, M. L., VAN DER WERF, B. A. and RUSSELL, P. S. Effects of antilymphocyte serum in mice, dogs and man, in: Wolstenholme, G. E. W. and O'Connor, U. (Eds.) "Antilymphocytic serum," Ciba Foundation Study Group no. 29. London, J. and A. Churchill, Ltd., 1967, p. 111.
13. MALMGREN, R. A., BENNISON, B. E. and McKINLEY, T. W. Reduced antibody titers in mice treated with carcinogenic and cancer chemotherapeutic agents. *Proc. Soc. exp. Biol. (N.Y.)* **79**: 484, 1952.
14. KAPLAN, H. S. and BROWN, M. B. Radiation injury and regeneration in lymphoid tissues, in: Rebuck, J. (Ed.), "The leukemias: Etiology, pathophysiology, and treatment." New York, Academic Press, 1957, p. 163.
15. KAWAMOTO, S., IDA, M., KIRSCHBAUM, A. and TAYLOR, G. Urethane and leukemogenesis in mice. *Cancer Res.* **18**: 725, 1958.
16. HARAN-GHERA, N. and KAPLAN, H. S. Significance of thymus and marrow injury in urethane leukemogenesis. *Cancer Res.* **24**: 1926, 1964.
17. HARAN-GHERA, N. Host resistance against isotransplantation of lymphomas induced by the radiation leukemia virus. *Nature (Lond.)* **222**: 992, 1969.
18. HARAN-GHERA, N. and PELED, A. Isolation of a leukemogenic filterable agent from tissues of irradiated and normal C57BL mice. *Brit. J. Cancer* **21**: 730, 1967.

MOUSE MAMMARY TUMORIGENESIS BY MAMMARY TUMOR VIRUS IN THE ABSENCE OF THYMUS, SPLEEN OR BOTH ORGANS

FRANCESCO SQUARTINI

Institute of Pathological Anatomy and Histology, Medical School, University of Pisa, Italy

ABSTRACT

Neonatal thymectomy caused a drastic reduction in the occurrence of hyperplastic premalignant changes, such as alveolar nodules and ductular plaques, in the mammary glands of mammary tumor virus infected mice. In BALB/cf(C3H) virgin females, thymectomy decreased mammary tumor incidence from 82 to 46% and delayed tumor onset by about five months. In BALB/cf(RIII) force-bred females, thymectomy delayed tumor onset by about two months but did not significantly affect the final mammary tumor incidence. In RIII females, either virgins or breeders (normal and force-bred), thymectomy had no effect on frequency and onset of mammary tumors. In BALB/cf(C3H) females, neonatal splenectomy decreased both incidence and age of onset of mammary tumors. In females of the same strain previously thymectomized, splenectomy partially suppressed the depressive effect of thymectomy on mammary tumorigenesis and restored to a large extent the pattern of intact controls. In RIII females, neonatal splenectomy alone or associated with thymectomy, like thymectomy alone, did not significantly affect mammary tumorigenesis.

INTRODUCTION

Mammary tumors occurring in mature female mice usually represent the end point of a viral infection which takes place at birth. In this respect, the "neoplastic disease" of mouse mammary gland (i.e. from virus infection to animal death by the resulting tumor) is unusually long, covering the entire life span of the animal. This makes the mouse mammary tumor system one of the most complex and also one of the most complete experimental models for studies on virus-tumor-host relationships.

Much interest has recently been focused on the relationships between mammary tumor virus (MTV) and the immunological system of the host mice. This communication summarizes our recent data (1–3) derived from the study of mammary tumorigenesis in the absence of thymus, or spleen, or both.

MATERIALS AND METHODS

Strains. The following mouse substrains were used: BALB/c/Cb/Se (BALB/c), BALB/cf(C3H)/Cb/Se [BALB/cf(C3H], RIII/Dm/Se (RIII) and BALB/cf(RIII). The last was established in Perugia by foster-nursing BALB/c mice on RIII mother (4).

Viruses. With the exception of BALB/c mice,

supposedly MTV-free, all strains carry spontaneous (milk-transmitted) MTV infection. BALB/cf (RIII) mice also carry spontaneous, milk-transmitted leukemia virus infection (5, 6). BALB/c mice were artificially infected at two to four days of age with a single i.p. injection of 25 mg equivalent (0.05 ml) of lactating mammary tissue extract in saline from BALB/cf(C3H) multiparous females.

Operations. Thymectomy was performed by the method of Miller (7) during the first day of life. Splenectomy was performed through a left lateral incision during the second day of life. Postmortem examinations of the mediastinal and abdominal regions were carried out in operated mice. The animals with thymus remnants were excluded from consideration; animals with large remnants of spleen were also discarded. Often the splenectomized mice showed a small node of splenic or scar tissue, corresponding to about one-tenth or less of the normal spleen size, at the site of operation; these animals were considered as splenectomized.

Breeding. At 28 days of age, the females were weaned and either kept as virgins or mated, normal or force-bred, according to the experiment. Normally bred females were separated from males at each pregnancy and allowed to nurse their offspring. Forcibly bred females were kept continuously with males and not allowed to nurse their offspring, which were killed on the day of birth.

Observation. Weanling mice were housed in metal cages and fed a diet of pellets and tap water. The females carrying spontaneous MTV infection were observed each week throughout their lives for the occurrence of tumors. At the time a tumor appeared, the age of the mouse was recorded. The mammary tumors occurring in BALB/cf (RIII) force-bred females were measured once a week with calipers at the two largest diameters,

and the average of these values was used as a weekly measure of the neoplastic process. The nature of the tumors was confirmed by histological examination.

Noduligenic test. The BALB/c females, artificially infected with MTV by injection, were subjected to the standard noduligenic assay (8): daily s.c. injections of 1 μg of estradiol 17 β + 500 μg of deoxycorticosterone acetate in aqueous suspension for 90 days. This treatment was started at the 36th day of life, and the animals were killed 36 days after the last injection. The mammary glands were prepared as whole mounts and the hyperplastic alveolar nodules present in them were counted under a dissecting microscope.

RESULTS
Mammary tumorigenesis in thymectomized mice

Viral tumorigenesis in the mouse mammary gland proceeds by steps, from the normal gland to preneoplastic lesions, usually in the form of hyperplastic alveolar nodules or in the form of plaques, and from these lesions to overt mammary cancer.

Hyperplastic alveolar nodules. In order to investigate the effect of thymectomy on hyperplastic alveolar nodules, a group of BALB/c virgin females was subjected to thymectomy shortly after birth, injected with MTV at two to four days of age, and then subjected to the noduligenic assay. The results of nodule count are reported in Table 1. In control BALB/c mice which were neither operated on nor infected with MTV, there were 20% of nodule-bearing animals and 0.2 nodules per mouse. In both intact and sham-operated

TABLE 1. *Effect of thymectomy on mammary noduligenesis by MTV in BALB/c virgin female mice (noduligenic test)*

Operations at day 1	Treatment at days 2 to 4	No. of mice	Mice with nodules (%)	Nodules counted	Nodules/ mouse	Range
—	—	20	4 (20)	4	0.2	0 to 1
—	MTV	21	21 (100)	277	13.2	1 to 41
Thymectomy	MTV	18	7 (39)	49	2.7	0 to 13
Sham-thymectomy	MTV	5	5 (100)	60	12.0	5 to 23

TABLE 2. Effect of thymectomy on the appearance of different types of mammary tumors in force-bred BALB/cf (RIII) female mice

Animals	No. of mice	Mean no. of pregnancies/ mouse	No. of mice with tumors	Total no. of tumors	Mean no. of tumors/ tumor-bearing mouse	No. of tumors occurring out of pregnancy	Tumors occurring during pregnancy					
							No.	No. of pregnancy-independent tumors	No. of pregnancy-dependent tumors			
									Type 1	Type 2	Type 3	Total
Controls	150	6.2	124 (82.7)	205	1.65	64	141	26 (18.4)	54 (38.3)	39 (27.6)	22 (15.6)	115 (81.5)
Thymectomized	72	5.6	54 (75)	84	1.55	58	26	20 (77)	1[a] (3.8)	5 (19.2)	0	6 (23)

Figures in parentheses are percentages.
[a] χ^2 11.797; $P < 0.001$.

BALB/c controls infected with MTV the percentage of mice with nodules was 100, and the average number of nodules per mouse was 13.2 and 12 respectively. In contrast, the group of thymectomized females infected with MTV showed a marked reduction in the number of nodule-bearing mice (39% instead of 100) (χ^2 5.586; $P < 0.02$) and in the number of nodules per mouse (2.7 instead of 12 to 13).

Plaques. BALB/cf (RIII) female mice, like other hybrid (9, 10) or inbred mice (11, 12), develop pregnancy-dependent mammary tumors endowed with very slow progression towards autonomous growth (13). Pregnancy-dependence of BALB/cf (RIII) mammary tumors may be of three different types. Dependent tumors of type I grow only during pregnancy and regress completely after parturition. Dependent tumors of type II undergo only a partial regression after delivery and grow to a larger extent during the subsequent pregnancy. Dependent tumors of type III are stationary or slow-growing for long periods of time, and show slight fluctuations in their growth trends at each pregnancy. During their natural history, the pregnancy-dependent tumors either may change the type of dependence from total to partial, or they may become independent by progression. Totally dependent tumors, or type I, are premalignant "plaques" showing an organoid tubular structure. Under the microscope, disappearance of these tumors after pregnancy is accompanied by a small plaque-shaped scar of fibrous tissue with remnants of epithelial structures. When progression occurs in plaques, this usually assumes the aspect of a focal area of different structure which infiltrates the entire lesion, showing the typical varied morphology of cystic and hemorrhagic mammary adenocarcinoma. Plaques and hyperplastic alveolar nodules are considered to be alternative steps in mouse mammary tumorigenesis (10).

In order to determine the effect of thymectomy on the occurrence of pregnancy-dependent mammary tumors, or plaques, a number of BALB/cf(RIII) females were thymectomized at birth and force-bred. The behavior of their mammary lesions was followed through several pregnancies and is reported in Table 2. In intact BALB/cf(RIII) control females, 38.3% of the mammary tumors occurring during pregnancies were totally dependent and 81.5% showed some type of pregnancy-dependence. These figures were very much lower in thymectomized females, where only one out of 26 mammary tumors, or 3.8%, was totally dependent and only six, or 23%, were in some way dependent. This means that thymectomy hampers the formation of the wholly dependent plaques, or that it expedites the progression of the tumors (1).

Mammary tumors. The effect of neonatal thymectomy on the occurrence of mammary tumors has been studied in various strains of mice and under different host conditions. In BALB/cf(C3H) female mice kept as virgins, that is, under a basal state of endogenous hormonal stimulation, neonatal thymectomy had a pronounced effect on mammary tumorigenesis, causing a decrease in the mammary tumor incidence from 82 to 46% and a delay of about five months in the appearance of the first palpable tumor (Table 3). The difference in the occurrence of mammary tumors between the thymectomized and control females was highly significant (χ^2 9.38; $P < 0.01$), and was not dependent on a possibly shorter survival of the thymectomized females, as these lived, on the average, 47 days longer than control animals (3).

Effect of breeding stimulation. Forced breeding can apparently modify the pattern of tumor incidence. In BALB/cf(RIII) female force-bred mice, the final mammary tumor incidence of thymectomized animals (75%) was close to that of the controls (82.7%), and there was no difference in the time of appear-

TABLE 3. *Effect of thymectomy on mammary tumorigenesis in BALB/cf(C3H) virgin female mice*

										Age in months											Total	Mean age at onset (days)	Mean age at death (days)
	8	9	10	11	12	13	14	15	16	17	18	19	20	21	22	23	24	25	26			
Control females: 39																						
Developing mammary tumors	1	0	0	4	3	6	2	1	7	1	3	0	1	1	1	1	0	0	0	32	434	487
Dying without mammary tumors	0	0	0	0	0	0	0	0	0	0	1	0	1	0	2	2	0	0	1	7	—	660
Cumulative percentage	3			13	20	36	41	44	61	64	72	74	77	79	82					82.0		
Thymectomized females: 28																						
Developing mammary tumors	0	0	0	0	0	1	1	1	2	2	1	0	0	1	1	3	0	0	0	13[a]	536	538
Dying without mammary tumors	0	0	0	0	0	1	0	2	3	1	0	0	0	0	1	5	2	0	0	15	—	549
Cumulative percentage						4	7	11	18	25	28			32	36	46				46.4		

[a] χ^2 9.378; $P < 0.01$.

TABLE 4. *Effect of thymectomy on mammary tumorigenesis in BALB/cf(RIII) force-bred female mice*

	Age in months																				Total	Mean age at onset (days)	Mean age at death (days)
---	3	4	5	6	7	8	9	10	11	12	13	14	15	16	17	18	19	20	21	22	---	---	---
Control females: 150																							
Developing mammary tumors	0	6	19	29	25	19	9	5	3	3	3	1	1	1	0	0	2	1	0	0	124	237	337
Dying without mammary tumors	0	3	1	0	3	3	3	2	2	2	2	0	1	1	0	2	0	0	0	1	26	—	328
Cumulative percentage		4	17	36	53	65	71	75	77	78	79	80		81		82	82				82.7		
Thymectomized females: 72																							
Developing mammary tumors	1	5	5	4	7	5	3	4	3	4	0	3	6	1	2	0	0	1	0	0	54[a]	296	381
Dying without mammary tumors	0	0	0	0	0	1	0	1	1	1	3	3	1	1	2	3	0	1	0	0	18	—	437
Cumulative percentage	1	8	15	21	31	37	42	47	51	57	61	69	71	74				75			75.0		

[a] x^2 1.799; $P < 0.20$.

TABLE 5. *Effect of thymectomy on mammary tumorigenesis in RIII virgin female mice*

	Age in months																					Total	Mean age at onset (days)	Mean age at death (days)
---	10	11	12	13	14	15	16	17	18	19	20	21	22	23	24	25	26	27	28	29	30	---	---	---
Control females: 38																								
Developing mammary tumors	1	0	1	1	0	1	1	2	0	2	2	1	0	3	0	0	0	1	0	0	0	16	539	578
Dying without mammary tumors	1	1	0	1	0	0	0	0	0	0	2	0	2	1	0	2	3	3	2	2	1	22	—	680
Cumulative percentage	3		8			10	13	18		24	29	31		33			39	42				42.1		
Thymectomized females: 24																								
Developing mammary tumors	0	0	0	0	1	0	1	0	0	2	0	0	0	1	3	0	2	0	0	0	0	8[a]	498	549
Dying without mammary tumors	0	0	0	0	0	0	0	0	0	0	1	3	3	1	3	4	3	2	0	0	1	16	—	697
Cumulative percentage			4		8		12			21				29	33							33.3		

[a] x^2 0.477; $P < 0.50$.

ance of the first palpable tumors (Table 4). This indicates that the depressive effect of thymectomy on mammary tumorigenesis may be overcome in part by forced breeding. Nevertheless, the appearance of most mammary tumors in thymectomized females was delayed: the average age at tumor onset was 296 days in the thymectomized females, as compared with 237 days in the control animals. Because of this delay, the difference in mammary tumorigenesis between thymectomized and control females was statistically significant after the first year of observation (χ^2 11.29; $P < 0.001$), although significance was lacking at the end of the experiment.

BALB/cf (RIII) force-bred females have an incidence of lymphatic leukemia, which is thymic dependent (4), and suppression of leukemia by thymectomy might have influenced these results. There were 21 cases of leukemia (six in hosts with mammary tumors) in the control females and only three (one in an animal with mammary tumor) in those thymectomized (3).

Significance of mouse strain. The effect of thymectomy on mammary tumorigenesis was also dependent on the strain used. In RIII female mice kept as virgins, neonatal thymectomy had no effect on mammary tumorigenesis (Table 5). It neither caused a significant decrease of mammary tumor incidence nor delayed their appearance. The average age at onset of mammary tumors in thymectomized

RIII females was somewhat less than in the controls, although the average life-span was the same in both groups.

This apparent refractoriness of RIII female mice to the effect of thymectomy on mammary tumorigenesis was further investigated and confirmed under different host conditions (Table 6). In virgins, normally bred and force-bred animals, no significant differences were observed between thymectomized and control mice. The increase in endogenous hormonal stimulation resulted in a comparable stimulatory effect on mammary tumorigenesis in thymectomized and control RIII females (3).

Comment. It appears that neonatal thymectomy hampers the formation of hyperplastic alveolar nodules and plaques in the mammary glands of some but not all MTV-carrying mice. Thymus removal causes a decrease of, and delay in, the occurrence of mammary tumors, dependent on the strain tested and on breeding stimulation (1, 2). These data are generally in agreement with the findings of other workers (14–18).

To explain the depressive effect of early thymectomy on mammary tumorigenesis in MTV-carrying mice, three hypotheses were originally proposed: a) that thymectomy alters the hormonal milieu necessary for mammary tumor development; b) that the thymus is essential early in life for the development and multiplication of MTV; and c) that the development of mammary tumors

TABLE 6. *Effect of thymectomy on mammary tumorigenesis in RIII female mice under different host conditions*

Host condition	Controls				Thymectomized					
		With mammary tumors				With mammary tumors				
	No. of mice	No.	%	Age at onset (days)	No. of mice	No.	%	Age at onset (days)	χ^2	P
Virgins	38	16	42.1	539	24	8	33.3	498	0.477	< 0.50
Normally bred	38	30	78.9	301	13	11	84.6	305	0.197	< 0.70
Force-bred	37	35	94.6	245	53	48	90.5	271	0.493	< 0.50

is related to the immunological responsiveness of the host animal to the virus (14). Recent experiments (19, 20) seem to favor the latter hypothesis since they suggest that host immune responses may indeed contribute to the development and establishment of the mammary cancer cells.

Mammary tumorigenesis in splenectomized mice

The spleen, which comprises approximately 60% of the mouse lymphoreticular cells (21), represents the largest organ involved in immune responsiveness of this animal. A significant, though transient increase in the weight of the spleen occurs in suckling mice receiving MTV via the mother's milk, compared with MTV-free controls of the same genotype (4, 22). Splenic enlargement is frequently observed even in adult mice carrying spontaneous MTV infection, especially when they develop mammary tumors (23). The following experiments were devised to investigate whether removal of the spleen has any effect on mammary tumorigenesis by MTV of otherwise normal or thymectomized mice. The purpose was to find out whether the function of the thymus on mouse mammary tumorigenesis is in some way mediated by the spleen. Virgin female mice of strains BALB/cf (C3H) and RIII were used since the former is responsive and the latter unresponsive to the depressive effect of thymectomy on mammary tumorigenesis. The results are presented in Table 7.

Mice responsive to thymectomy: BALB/cf (C3H). As also reported above, in BALB/cf (C3H) virgin females thymectomy delayed the appearance of mammary tumors, and significantly decreased the final tumor incidence (from 82 to 46.4%). Splenectomy caused a decrease in the average age of mammary tumor onset, due both to acceleration of early tumorigenesis and suppression of late tumorigenesis. Final tumor incidence in

TABLE 7. *Mammary tumorigenesis in BALB/cf(C3H) and RIII virgin female mice intact, thymectomized, splenectomized, or thymectomized and splenectomized*

Strain and operation	No. of mice	With mammary tumors				Without tumors			x^2	P
		No.	%	Age at onset[a] (range)	Age at death[a]	No.	Mean age at death[a]	Total age at death[a]		
BALB/cf(C3H) virgin females										
No operation	39	32	82.0	434 (232 to 666)	487	7	660	518	—	—
Thymectomy	28	13	46.4	536 (372 to 686)	583	15	549	565	9.378	<0.01
Splenectomy	25	13	52.0	380 (168 to 552)	456	12	574	514	6.590	<0.02
Thymectomy and splenectomy	31	22	71.0	474 (282 to 620)	501	9	653	545	1.203	<0.30
RIII virgin females										
No operation	38	16	42.1	539 (284 to 689)	578	22	680	637	—	—
Thymectomy	24	8	33.3	498 (370 to 622)	549	16	697	648	0.477	<0.05
Splenectomy	27	9	33.3	466 (343 to 593)	506	18	655	605	0.513	<0.50
Thymectomy and splenectomy	21	4	19.0	447 (307 to 600)	495	17	653	623	3.209	<0.10

[a] Days.

the splenectomized females was significantly reduced, from 82 to 52% (x^2 6.59; $P < 0.02$). In contrast, splenectomy performed in thymectomized females suppressed most of the effect of thymectomy on mammary tumorigenesis and largely restored the situation observed in the intact controls.

Mice unresponsive to thymectomy: RIII. In RIII virgin females, neither thymectomy, as also reported above, nor splenectomy had a significant effect on the mammary tumor incidence. The same also applied to animals subjected to thymectomy as well as splenectomy, although in these mice the incidence of mammary tumors was lower at the borderline of significance than in the other groups. The average age of mammary tumor onset in the RIII females (539 days) was reduced after thymectomy (498 days), splenectomy (466 days), and thymectomy plus splenectomy (447 days). This was due to a moderate reduction of late developing tumors in the females on whom operations were performed.

Comment. None of these observations is attributable to great differences in the life span of the animals, since the average survival was approximately the same in each strain in all four groups of mice. In BALB/cf (C3H) females, both thymus and spleen are apparently involved in mammary tumorigenesis, whereas in RIII females neither thymus nor spleen seems to play a major role. This may suggest relations between thymic and splenic functions in mammary tumorigenesis in some genotypes. It also appeared that combined thymectomy and splenectomy rendered the animals fully susceptible again to tumor development. Whether this may indicate that some equilibrium between humoral and cellular immune factors plays a part in mouse mammary tumorigenesis by MTV is at present a matter of conjecture.

DISCUSSION

Removal of the thymus prevents, to a large extent, nodule and plaque formation in the mammary glands of some MTV-carrying mice. The depression exerted by thymectomy on occurrence of mouse mammary tumors has also been confirmed. In addition, the results presented clearly indicate that the effects of thymectomy on mammary tumorigenesis in MTV-carrying mice depend to a large extent on mouse strain and breeding condition. Personal data and those available from previous work in this field may be summarized as follows. In C3H virgin and breeding females, thymectomy caused a decrease and delay of mammary tumorigenesis (14, 15). The same effect has been observed here in BALB/cf(C3H) virgin females. However, in BALB/cf(C3H) force-bred females, there was only a delay of mammary tumorigenesis after long periods of observation (18). This applied also to BALB/cf(RIII) force-bred females (1, 17). On the other hand, no effects of thymectomy on mammary tumorigenesis were seen in either virgin or breeder, normal or force-bred, RIII females.

It was thus shown that the depressive effect of thymectomy on mammary tumorigenesis in high-cancer-strain mice may be overcome in part by forced breeding. Force-bred females bear several litters and multiple pregnancy, according to recent investigations (24), should have restored, at least in part, the immunological functions in the thymectomized mothers, including the formation of enhancing antibodies. On the other hand, forced breeding increases or accelerates mammary tumorigenesis even in intact mice, probably because of the increased hormonal stimuli that this procedure provides to the mammary glands. Therefore, the partial suppression of the thymectomy effect by forced breeding might also be merely due to hormonal factors. This is in line with recent data showing that mice thymectomized shortly after birth or weaning develop ovarian, uterine and mammary-hypoplasia probably due to endocrine defects (25).

Another interesting finding of this investigation is the apparent refractoriness of RIII female mice to the depressive effect of thymectomy on mammary tumorigenesis. An explanation for this fact is lacking at present, but several possibilities may be envisaged. For one, RIII mice may possess accessory thymic tissue somewhere in the body. Ectopic thymic tissue has been demonstrated in BALB/c animals (15, 26) in which, however, it is unable to suppress the effect of neonatal thymectomy on MTV-induced mammary tumorigenesis (1, 18). Another possibility is that the immune response against MTV or MTV-infected cells in RIII mice is different from that of other strains of mice carrying spontaneous MTV infection, or that the MTV agent itself carried by RIII mice is different from that of other strains. A number of differences in genesis and behavior of mammary tumors between RIII and other high-mammary-tumor strains [C3H, BALB/cf (C3H)] have previously been reported (27–31). Such differences involve both the RIII genotype (4, 32, 33) and the MTV which it harbors (13, 34).

Removal of the spleen in thymectomized females suppressed most of the effect of thymectomy on mammary tumorigenesis and restored to a large extent the situation observed in intact controls. This finding still demands explanation. It has been shown for other virus induced murine tumor systems that depression of cellular immunity (by thymectomy) or stimulation of humoral immunity (by complete Freund's adjuvant) can have the same stimulating effect on tumorigenesis (15, 35). Removal of the spleen, thymus or both organs could readily be envisaged to radically alter crucial aspects of the normal equilibrium between cellular and humoral immunity as well as of hormonal components of the host milieu.

Supported by a grant from the Jane Coffin Childs Memorial Fund for Medical Research (Fund's Project No. 206), New Haven, Connecticut, USA.

REFERENCES

1. Squartini, F., Olivi, M. and Bolis, G. B. Thymic dependence of mouse mammary tumor virus and mouse mammary tumors, in: Severi, L. (Ed.), "Immunity and tolerance in oncogenesis," *IV Perugia Quadrennial International Conference, 1969* (in press).
2. Squartini, F. and Bolis, G. B. Mammary tumorigenesis in splenectomized mice. *Texas Rep. Biol. Med.* (in press).
3. Squartini, F., Olivi, M. and Bolis, G. B. Mouse strain and breeding stimulation as factors influencing the effect of thymectomy on mammary tumorigenesis. *Cancer Res.* (in press).
4. Squartini, F. Relationship between mammary tumor virus and other oncogenic viruses in mouse mammary tumorigenesis, in: "Carcinogenesis: A broad critique." Baltimore, Williams & Wilkins Co., 1967, p. 257.
5. Squartini, F. and Rossi, G. Detection of a leukaemogenic agent in BALB/c mice foster-nursed by RIII. *Lav. Ist. Anat. Univ. Perugia* **22**: 185, 1962.
6. Squartini, F., Bolis, G. B. and Rossi, G. BALB/c[f(RIII)]f(C57 black). *Lav. Ist. Anat. Univ. Perugia* **27**: 137, 1967.
7. Miller, J. F. A. P. Role of the thymus in transplantation tolerance and immunity, in: Wolstenholme, G. E. W. and Cameron, M. P. (Eds.), "Ciba Foundation Symposium on Transplantation." London, J & A. Churchill Ltd., 1962, p. 384.
8. Nandi, S. New method for detection of mouse mammary tumor virus. II. Effect of administration of lactating mammary tissue extracts on incidence of hyperplastic mammary nodules in BALB/cCrgl mice. *J. nat. Cancer Inst.* **31**: 75, 1963.
9. Foulds, L. Mammary tumours in hybrid mice: Growth and progression of spontaneous tumours. *Brit. J. Cancer* **3**: 345, 1949.
10. Foulds, L. The histologic analysis of mammary tumors of mice. II. The histology of responsiveness and progression. The origins of tumors. *J. nat. Cancer Inst.* **17**: 713, 1956.
11. Squartini, F. and Rossi, G. Accrescimento e progressione dei tumori mammari nei topi femmina del substrain RIII/Dm/Se. *Lav. Ist. Anat. Univ. Perugia* **19**: 105, 1959.
12. Squartini, F. and Rossi, G. Analisi morfologica della "responsiveness" e della progressione nei tumori mammari del "substrain" RIII/Dm/Se. *Lav. Ist. Anat. Univ. Perugia* **19**: 165, 1959.
13. Squartini, F., Rossi, G. and Paoletti, I. Characters of mammary tumours in BALB/c female mice foster-nursed by C3H and RIII mothers. *Nature (Lond.)* **197**: 505, 1963.
14. Martinez, C. Effect of early thymectomy on development of mammary tumors in mice. *Nature (Lond.)* **203**: 1188, 1964.
15. Law, L. W. Studies of thymic function with

emphasis on the role of the thymus in oncogenesis. *Cancer Res.* **26**: 551, 1966.

16. OLIVI, M. and BOLIS, G. B. Tumorigenesi spontanea nei topi timectomizzati (BALB/cf/RIII/Se substrain). *Lav. Ist. Anat. Univ. Perugia* **27**: 77, 1967.

17. OLIVI, M., BARBIERI, G., BUCCIARELLI, E. and BOLIS G. B. Primi dati sulla tumorigenesi spontanea nei topi timectomizzati (RIII/Dm/Se e BALB/cf/Cb/Se substrains). *Lav. Anat. Ist. Univ. Perugia* **25**: 29, 1965.

18. HEPPNER, G. H., WOOD, P. C. and WEISS, D. W. Studies on the role of the thymus in viral tumorigenesis. I. Effect of thymectomy on induction of hyperplastic alveolar nodules and mammary tumors in BALB/cfC3H mice. *Israel J. med. Sci.* **4**: 1195, 1968.

19. HEPPNER, G. H. Neonatal thymectomy and mouse mammary tumorigenesis, in: Severi, L. (Ed.), "Immunity and tolerance in oncogenesis." *IV Perugia Quadrennial International Conference, 1969* (in press).

20. YUNIS, E. J., MARTINEZ, C., SMITH, J., STUTMAN, O. and GOOD, R. A. Spontaneous mammary adenocarcinoma in mice: Influence of thymectomy and reconstitution with thymus grafts or spleen cells. *Cancer Res.* **29**: 174, 1969.

21. BARD, D. S. and PILCH, Y. H. The role of the spleen in the immunity to a chemically induced sarcoma in C3H mice. *Cancer Res.* **29**: 1125, 1969.

22. SQUARTINI F., OLIVI, M., BOLIS, G. B., RIBACCHI, R. and GIRALDO, G. Reciprocal interference between mouse mammary tumor virus and leukemia virus. *Nature (Lond.)* **214**: 730, 1967.

23. REID, W. Splenic enlargement in association with mammary tumours in mice, in: Currie, A. R. (Ed.), "Endocrine aspects of breast cancer." Edinburgh, E. & S. Livingstone Ltd., 1958, p. 321.

24. OSOBA, D. Immune reactivity in mice thymectomized soon after birth: normal response after pregnancy. *Science* **147**: 298, 1965.

25. SAKAKURA, T. and NISHIZUKE, Y. Effect of thymectomy on mammary tumorigenesis, noduligenesis and mammogenesis in the mouse. *Gann* **58**: 441, 1967.

26. DUNN, T. B. Questions of immunity and tolerance in reticulum cell neoplasms in mice, in: Severi, L. (Ed.), "Immunity and tolerance in oncogenesis," *IV Perugial Quadrennial International Conference, 1969* (in press).

27. SQUARTINI, F. Strain differences in growth of mouse mammary tumors. *J. nat. Cancer Inst.* **26**: 813, 1961.

28. SQUARTINI, F. Responsiveness and progression of mammary tumors in high-cancer-strain mice. *J. nat. Cancer Inst.* **28**: 911, 1962.

29. SQUARTINI, F. and RIBACCHI, R. Irregolarità nella propagazione del "mammary tumor agent" attraverso i topi RIII. *Lav. Ist. Anat. Univ. Perugia* **20**: 5, 1960.

30. SQUARTINI, F. and ROSSI, G. Responsiveness and progression of the morphological precursors of breast cancer in inbred mice: A review, in: Severi, L. (Ed.), "The morphological precursors of cancer." Perugia, Division of Cancer Research, 1962, p. 319.

31. SQUARTINI, F. and SEVERI, L. Strain differences in the mammary tumour-inducing virus as detected by the characters and behaviour of neoplasms, in: Wolstenholme, G. E. W. and O'Connor, M. (Eds.), "Ciba Foundation Symposium on Tumour Viruses of Murine Origin." London, J. & A. Churchill Ltd., 1962, p. 82.

32. ANDERVONT, H. B. and DUNN, T. B. Studies on the mammary-tumor agent of strain RIII mice. *J. nat. Cancer Inst.* **28**: 159, 1962.

33. ANDERVONT, H. B. and DUNN, T. B. Further studies on the mammary tumor agent of strain RIII mice. *J. nat. Cancer Inst.* **35**: 38, 1965.

34. SQUARTINI, F., ROSSI, G. and PAOLETTI, I. Trasmissione extracromosomica dei caratteri tumorali: effetto del "foster-nursing" sul comportamento biologico e morfologico dei tumori mammari del topo. *Lav. Ist. Anat. Univ. Perugia* **22**: 203, 1962.

35. TER-GRIËGOV, V. S. and IRLIN, I. S. The stimulating effect of complete Freund's adjuvant on tumour induction by polyoma virus in mice and by Rous sarcoma virus in rats. *Int. J. Cancer* **3**: 760, 1968.

INCREASED INCIDENCE OF SPONTANEOUS LUNG ADENOMAS IN MICE FOLLOWING NEONATAL THYMECTOMY*

N. TRAININ and M. LINKER-ISRAELI

Department of Experimental Biology, Weizmann Institute of Science, Rehovot, Israel

ABSTRACT

The aim of the present study was to investigate the role of immunologic impairment provoked by neonatal thymectomy in the appearance of spontaneous lung adenomas in mice. Inbred SWR mice and random-bred Swiss mice were thymectomized at three days of age, normal nonthymectomized litters being used as controls. The thymectomized animals showed a normal pattern of development, although their immunologic competence was impaired, as measured by the level of hemolysins and hemagglutinins to sheep red blood cells following specific immunization and by their tumor homograft response. Groups of intact and neonatally thymectomized SWR and Swiss mice were killed at the age of seven and 13 months. Significantly higher incidences of spontaneous lung adenomas were observed in the thymectomized than in the intact animals.

Thymectomy in young mice is followed, under certain experimental conditions, by impairment of their immunocompetence and enhancement of their neoplastic response to chemical carcinogens (1, 2). We have demonstrated that in random-bred Swiss or inbred SWR mice thymectomized at three days of age and treated with a single dose of 7, 12-dimethylbenz(a)anthracene or urethan, the formation of induced lung adenomas was enhanced as compared to nonoperated controls (3). Similarly, injections of antilymphocytic serum into SWR or Swiss mice were followed by an impairment of their immuno-

logic functions and an increased incidence of urethan-induced lung adenomas, as compared to controls injected with normal rabbit serum (4). In addition, we have recently shown that neonatally thymectomized mice undergoing a mild graft-vs.-host reaction when injected with nonsyngeneic lymphoid cells, manifest a further impairment of immunologic functions; in parallel, it was found that their neoplastic response was higher than in the thymectomized controls (5). It appears, therefore, that immunosuppression and enhancement of the neoplastic response are closely interrelated. This hypothesis has recently been further supported by experiments in which the increased neoplastic susceptibility of thymectomized SWR mice to urethan could be

---

* Part of this work was presented at the Xth International Cancer Congress, Houston, Texas, May 1970.

abolished when restoration of immunologic capacity was achieved by grafting syngeneic thymus tissue into the thymus-deprived animals (4).

Our previous work dealt with tumor induction by small doses of carcinogens (3–5), and the interference with the immunologic defenses of the host by higher doses of chemical carcinogens has been well documented (6, 7). The present experiments were aimed, therefore, at testing whether the immunosuppression caused by neonatal thymectomy alone might modify the incidence of spontaneous lung adenomas that occur in certain strains of mice (8). For this purpose, mice were neonatally thymectomized, and the spontaneous incidence of lung adenomas checked at different intervals.

MATERIALS AND METHODS

Mice. Inbred SWR/Jax mice, bred at the Weizmann Institute of Science by sibling mating, and albino Swiss mice originally obtained from Royalhart Laboratory Animals (New Hampton, N.Y.) and since maintained in our laboratory by random breeding, were used throughout these experiments. The animals were housed in plastic cages in air-conditioned rooms kept at 21 to 25 C. After weaning at 30 days of age and being separated according to sex, they were fed Purina Laboratory Chow pellets and tap water ad lib.

Thymectomy. The mice were thymectomized at the age of three days, under ether anesthesia, by an adaptation of Miller's technique (9). At the end of the experiment, or after death, they were autopsied, and the absence of mediastinal thymic tissue was ascertained by gross inspection or, where indicated, by sectioning and microscopic examination. Any thymectomized animal found to contain a thymic remnant was discarded. Whole litters of mice of the same strain and age were left intact as controls.

Peripheral blood cell counts. Absolute and differential white cell counts were performed on blood from the caudal vein. Absolute counts were made using human white cell diluting pipettes and hemocytometers. Differential white cell counts were made on blood smears stained with May-Grünwald-Giemsa.

Circulating antibodies. Mice were injected i.p. with 0.2 ml of a 10% saline suspension of sheep erythrocytes. For the hemolysin and hemagglutinin tests, the mice were bled from the tail five and 10 days, respectively, after challenge with the antigen. The sera were incubated for 30 min at 56 C for complement inactivation, and then divided into 14 tubes of serial twofold dilutions. In the hemolysin test, guinea pig complement (Bacto complement, Difco Laboratories, Detroit, Mich.), diluted 1:20 in Kolmer's saline, and an equal volume of sheep erythrocytes from a 1% saline suspension, were added to each tube. The tubes were incubated for 30 min at 37 C, left overnight at room temperature, and then read. The endpoint was the highest dilution showing a 100% lysis. For the agglutinin test, equal volumes of serum and erythrocytes in a 1% saline suspension were incubated for 1 hr at 37 C, and then left overnight at room temperature. The endpoint was the last tube in which agglutination was detected with the naked eye.

Origin of tumors. SBL tumor is a solid fibrosarcoma, originally induced by a s.c. injection of benzo(a)pyrene into a C57Bl/6 mouse (H-2^b histocompatibility locus) and kept in our laboratory by serial transfer through six generations of syngeneic recipients.

C tumor is a solid fibrosarcoma primarily induced into a C3H/eb mouse (H-2^k) by a s.c. injection of benzo(a)pyrene, and subsequently serially transferred through syngeneic recipients.

Tumor grafting. The tumors were cut into small fragments of about equal size (1 to 2 mm^3) and inoculated i.m. by trocar into the right hind leg of the Swiss and SWR recipients. The mice were palpated daily at the site of implantation to detect the appearance of the neoplastic graft, and the death rate of the tumor-bearing animals was registered.

Recording of lung adenoma incidence. At the specified intervals, mice were killed and autopsied. The lungs were examined with a low-power dissecting microscope, and the number of lung adenomas recorded.

Statistical analysis. Differences between groups of mice with various indexes of lung adenomas were tested for significance by the χ^2 test.

The 95% confidence interval for peripheral blood lymphocytes was evaluated by the Student's "t" test.

RESULTS

Enhancement of spontaneous lung adenoma

TABLE 1. *Influence of neonatal thymectomy[a] on spontaneous lung adenoma formation in SWR and Swiss mice*

Strain	Group	Age (months)	Mice bearing lung adenomas/total	% of animals with tumors	Average no. of tumors/animal	Individual incidences of tumors[b]
SWR	Thymectomized	7	12/28	42	0.54	0(16), 1(10), 2(1), 3(1)
	Intact	7	12/88	14	0.15	0(76), 1(11), 2(1)
SWR	Thymectomized	13	16/36	44	0.64	0(20), 1(12), 2(3), 5(1)
	Intact	13	5/27	18	0.26	0(22), 1(4), 2(1)
Swiss	Thymectomized	7	5/21	24	0.29	0(16), 1(4), 2(1)
	Intact	7	2/21	10	0.09	0(19), 1(2)
Swiss	Thymectomized	13	35/73	48	0.88	0(38), 1(23), 2(8), 3(2), 5(1), 14(1)
	Intact	13	22/97	23	0.27	0(75), 1(18), 2(4)

[a] Thymectomy performed at three days of age.
[b] Figures in parentheses represent number of animals.

TABLE 2. *Influence of neonatal thymectomy[a] on number of peripheral lymphocytes[b], primary hemolysins[c] and hemagglutinins[c], and homograft response[d] in SWR mice[e]*

Group	Average no. of lymphocytes (95% C.I.)[f]	Log₂ of titer hemolysins (mean)	Log₂ of titer hemagglutinins (mean)	Mice with lethal takes of SBL tumor (H-2[b])
Thymectomized	6,800 [8] (4,200 to 9,300)	5 [7]	7 [8]	6/7 (86%)
Intact	8,740 [16] (6,840 to 10,600)	9 [6]	11 [7]	0/10

[a] Thymectomy performed at three days of age.
[b] Peripheral blood lymphocytes counted at termination of experiment.
[c] Hemolysins and hemagglutinins tested five and 10 days respectively after challenge with sheep erythrocytes.
[d] SBL (H-2[b]) tumor grafted s.c.
[e] SWR mice killed at the age of seven months.
[f] 95% confidence interval as evaluated by Student's "t" test.
Figures in square brackets represent number of animals tested.

TABLE 3. *Influence of neonatal thymectomy[a] on number of peripheral lymphocytes[b], primary hemolysins[c] and hemagglutinins[c], and homograft response[d] in Swiss mice[e]*

Group	Average no. of lymphocytes (95% C.I.)[f]	Log₂ of titer hemolysins (mean)	Log₂ of titer hemagglutinins (mean)	Mice with lethal takes of a tumor SBL(H-2[b])	C(H-2[k])
Thymectomized	2,180 [18] (1,600 to 2,700)	4 [10]	6 [10]	5/7 (71%)	3/13 (23%)
Intact	2,690 [15] (1,900 to 3,500)	7 [6]	9 [7]	2/6 (33%)	0/19

[a] Thymectomy performed at three days of age.
[b] Peripheral blood lymphocytes counted at termination of experiment.
[c] Hemolysins and hemagglutinins tested five and 10 days respectively after challenge with sheep erythrocytes.
[d] SBL (H-2[b]) and C (H-2[k]) tumors grafted s.c.
[e] Swiss mice killed at the age of 13 months.
[f] 95% confidence interval as evaluated by Student's "t" test.
Figures in square brackets represent number of animals tested.

formation in neonatally thymectomized SWR and Swiss mice. Groups of intact and neo-natally thymectomized SWR and Swiss mice were killed at the age of seven and 13 months.

As can be seen in Table 1, 42% (12/28) of the thymectomized SWR mice bore lung ade-nomas as compared with 14% (12/88) in the controls, this difference being highly signifi-cant ($P < 0.001$). In the group of SWR mice killed at the age of 13 months, 44% (16/36) of the thymectomized mice bore lung tumors, as compared to 18% (5/27) in the controls, this difference also being significant but less so than at the first interval ($0.05 < P < 0.02$).

Swiss mice also displayed a difference in the spontaneous incidence of lung tumors (Table 1). At the age of seven months, 24% (5/21) of the thymectomized animals, as com-pared with 10% (2/21) in the nonoperated controls, bore tumors. This difference was more striking when the Swiss mice were checked at the age of 13 months: 48% (35/73) of the thymectomized animals bore lung ade-nomas, as compared with 23% (22/97) in the intact controls ($0.005 < P < 0.001$). As shown in Table 1, not only the percentage of ani-mals bearing lung adenomas, but also the individual incidence of tumors was higher in the thymectomized than in the control mice.

Impairment of immunocompetence in SWR and Swiss mice by neonatal thymectomy. The immunologic competence of the mice was evaluated by the number of lymphocytes in the peripheral blood, the level of circulating antibodies to sheep red blood cells, and the homograft response to tumor implants.

As can be seen in Tables 2 and 3, the number of peripheral blood lymphocytes was not significantly decreased after thymectomy either in the SWR or in the Swiss mice. This consistency in the level of lymphocytes after thymectomy has already been observed in SWR mice (3). On the other hand, primary responses to sheep red blood cells were much

lower in the thymectomized SWR and Swiss mice than in their respective intact controls. In the seven-month-old SWR mice, mean titers of hemolysins were decreased after thy-mectomy from nine to five, and of hemag-glutinins from 11 to seven. This decrease was also striking in the 13-month-old thymecto-mized Swiss mice: from seven to four for hemolysins and from nine to six for hemag-glutinins. The homograft response, evaluated by the number of lethal takes in recipient mice, was also seriously impaired after thy-mectomy, both the SBL and C fibrosarcomas being more accepted by thymectomized than normal recipients. The SBL tumor gave lethal takes in 86% of the thymectomized SWR mice, but in none of the intact controls. The respective incidences of lethal takes for Swiss mice were 71% in the thymectomized animals and 33% in the intact controls. The same pattern was obtained when Swiss mice were challenged with the C tumor, the incidences of lethal takes being 23 and 0%, respectively, for the thymectomized and intact mice.

DISCUSSION

The hypothesis that malignant transforma-tion involves a change in the antigenic struc-ture of the transformed cell was confirmed by the finding of specific tumor antigens (TSTA) (10) in tumors induced experimentally by chemical carcinogens (11–13) and by vi-ruses (14–16). Whereas virus-induced tumors appear to have a TSTA specific for each causal virus, most of the chemically-induced tumors do not show cross reactions when tested against tumors induced by the same carcinogen (17, 18).

The antigenicity of spontaneous tumors, which mostly arise late in life, would seem to be especially interesting for investigation because of the similarity of such systems to human neoplasms. Although early results were contradictory (19), the antigenicity of spontaneous mammary tumors in mice has been demonstrated both *in vivo* (20–24) and *in vitro* (25). The existence of specific antigens in other animal and human spontaneous tumors also has been observed under various conditions (26, 27), and methods for purification of the soluble antigens have been devised (28, 29).

Whereas some of the so-called "spontaneous tumors" used in these reported experiments, such as mammary adenocarcinomas and lymphomas, have been shown to be of viral etiology (30, 31), lung adenomas are considered to be of nonviral origin. By studying the influence of heredity on the pulmonary tumor incidence in mice, Heston and Deringer long ago established the linkage between susceptibility to lung adenoma formation and various known mouse genes (32, 33).

Antigenic specificity in urethan-induced lung adenomas was demonstrated *in vivo* by Prehn (34), and recently with *in vitro* methods by Della Porta and Colnaghi (personal communication). We further assumed that although TSTA in spontaneous lung adenomas has not yet been found, the antigenicity of these tumors could be indirectly demonstrated by impairing the immune functions of the animal, thus facilitating the escape of a neoplastic clone of cells from the "surveillance mechanism" (35) of the host. The results of the present experiments seem to be in agreement with these assumptions. Neonatal thymectomy impaired the immunologic competence of SWR and Swiss mice, as indicated by their lower titers of primary responses to sheep erythrocytes, and by their decreased resistance to tumor homografts. Under these conditions, a higher incidence of spontaneous lung adenomas was observed. Immune impairment thus apparently facilitates the development of a spontaneous nonviral tumor characteristic for the genetic system tested. Whether this is true as well for other spontaneous tumors, in other organs and in other strains, remains to be investigated.

The authors wish to express their thanks to Miss H. Hamami and Mr. I. Serussi for skillful technical assistance.

Supported in part by a grant from the Israel Cancer Association.

REFERENCES

1. Miller, J. F. A. P., Grant, G. A. and Roe, F. J. C. Effect of thymectomy on the induction of skin tumors by 3,4-benzopyrene. *Nature (Lond.)* **199**: 920, 1963.
2. Nishizuka, Y., Nakakuki, K. and Usui, M. Enhancing effect of thymectomy on hepatotumorigenesis in Swiss mice following neonatal injection of 20-methylcholanthrene. *Nature (Lond.)* **205**: 1236, 1965.
3. Trainin, N., Linker-Israeli, M., Small, M. and Boiato-Chen, L. Enhancement of lung adenoma formation by neonatal thymectomy in mice treated with 7, 12-dimethylbenz(a)anthracene or urethan. *Int. J. Cancer* **2**: 326, 1967.
4. Trainin, N. and Linker-Israeli, M. Influence of immunosuppression and immunorestoration on the formation of urethan-induced lung adenomas. *J. nat. Cancer Inst.* **44**: 893, 1970.
5. Trainin, N. and Linker-Israeli, M. Increased incidence of urethan-induced lung adenomas in neonatally thymectomized mice challenged with lymphoid cells. *Cancer Res.* **29**: 1840, 1969.
6. Malmgren, R. A., Bennison, B. E. and McKinley, T. W., Jr. Reduced antibody titers in mice treated with carcinogenic and cancer chemotherapeutic agents. *Proc. Soc. exp. Biol. (N.Y.)* **79**: 484, 1952.
7. Linder, O. E. A. Survival and skin homografts in methyl-cholanthrene treated mice with spontaneous mammary cancers. *Cancer Res.* **22**: 380, 1962.
8. Shimkin, M. B. Pulmonary tumors in experimental animals, in: Gruenstein, J. P. and Haddow, A. (Eds.), "Advances in cancer research." New York, Academic Press Inc., 1955, v. III, p. 223.
9. Miller, J. F. A. P. Studies on mouse leukemia. The role of thymus leukemogenesis by cell-free leukemic filtrates. *Brit. J. Cancer* **14**: 93, 1960.
10. Sjögren, H. O. Transplantation method as a tool for detection of tumor specific antigens. *Progr. exp. Tumor Res.* **6**: 289, 1964.
11. Foley, E. J. Attempts to induce immunity against mammary adenocarcinoma in inbred mice. *Cancer Res.* **13**: 578, 1953.
12. Prehn, R. T. and Main, J. M. Immunity to methylcholanthrene-induced sarcomas. *J. nat. Cancer Inst.* **18**: 769, 1957.
13. Old, L. J., Boyse, E. A., Clarke, D. A. and Carswell, E. Antigenic properties of chemically induced tumors. *Ann. N.Y. Acad. Sci.* **101**: 80, 1962.
14. Habel, K. Polyoma tumor antigen in cells transformed in vitro by polyoma virus. *Virology* **18**: 553, 1962.
15. Koch, M. A. and Sabin, A. B. Specificity of virus-induced resistance to transplantation of

polyoma and SV40 tumors in adult hamsters. *Proc. Soc. exp. Biol. (N.Y.)* **113**: 4, 1963.

16. Evans, C. A. and Ito, Y. Antitumor immunity in the Shope papilloma carcinoma complex of rabbits. *J. nat. Cancer Inst.* **36**: 1161, 1966.

17. Burnet, M. Immunological factors in the process of carcinogenesis. *Brit. med. Bull.* **20**: 154, 1964.

18. Defendi, V. Effect of SV40 virus immunization on growth of transplantable SV40 and polyoma virus tumors in hamsters. *Proc. Soc. exp. Biol. (N.Y.)* **113**: 12, 1963.

19. Hauschka, T. S. Immunological aspects of cancer: A review. *Cancer Res.* **12**: 615, 1952.

20. Hirsch, H. M., Bittner, J. J., Coley, H. and Iversen, I. Can the inbred mouse be immunized against its own tumor? *Cancer Res.* **18**: 344, 1958.

21. Prince, J. E., Fardon, J. C., Nutini, L. G. and Sperti, G. S. Induced resistance to an indigenous transplantable mouse tumor. *Cancer Res.* **17**: 312, 1957.

22. Revesz, L. Detection of antigenic differences in isologous host-tumor systems by pretreatment with heavily irradiated tumor cells. *Cancer Res.* **20**: 443, 1960.

23. Morton, D. L. Successful immunization against a spontaneous mammary tumor in C₃H/Hen mice. *Proc. Amer. Ass. Cancer Res.* **3**: 346, 1962.

24. Weiss, D. W., Faulkin, L. J. and De Ome, K. B. Acquisition of heightened resistance and susceptibility to spontaneous mouse mammary carcinomas in the original host. *Cancer Res.* **24**: 732, 1964.

25. Heppner, G. H. and Pierce, G. In vitro demonstration of tumor specific antigens in spontaneous mammary tumors of mice. *Int. J. Cancer* **4**: 212, 1969.

26. Old, L. J., Boyse, E. A., Geering, G. and Oettgen, H. F. Serologic approaches to the study of cancer in animals and in man. *Cancer Res.* **28**: 1288, 1968.

27. Klein, G. and Oettgen, H. F. Immunologic factors involved in the growth of primary tumors in human or animal hosts. *Cancer Res.* **29**: 1741, 1969.

28. Davies, D. A. L. Isolation and purification of transplantation and tumor-specific antigens. *Transplantation* **6**: 660, 1968.

29. McKenna, J. M. Demonstration and partial isolation and characterization of a specific soluble antigen in human tumors. *Transplantation* **6**: 648, 1968.

30. Barnum, C. P., Ball, Z. B. and Bittner, J. J. Partial separation of the mammary tumor milk agent and a comparison of various sources of the agent. *Cancer Res.* **7**: 522, 1947.

31. Gross, L. Pathogenic properties, and "vertical" transmission of the mouse leukemia agent. *Proc. Soc. exp. Biol. (N.Y.)* **78**: 342, 1951.

32. Heston, W. E. Inheritance of susceptibility to spontaneous pulmonary tumors in mice. *J. nat. Cancer Inst.* **3**: 79, 1942.

33. Heston, W. E. and Deringer, M. K. Relationship between the lethal yellow (A^y) gene of the mouse and susceptibility to spontaneous pulmonary tumors. *J. nat. Cancer Inst.* **7**: 463, 1947.

34. Prehn, R. T. Specific isoantigenicities among chemically induced tumors. *Ann. N.Y. Acad. Sci.* **101**: 107, 1962.

35. Klein, G. Recent trends in tumor immunology. *Israel J. Med. Sci.* **2**: 135, 1966.

EXPERIMENTAL MODELS FOR EVALUATION OF HOST DEFENSES IN CANCER

K. STERN* and A. GOLDFEDER

Department of Pathology, University of Illinois College of Medicine, Chicago, Illinois, and Cancer and Radiobiological Research Laboratory, New York University and Department of Hospitals, New York, New York, USA

ABSTRACT

X/Gf mice, resistant to induction of tumors by total body irradiation, were immunized with sheep red cells four, seven or 12 days after irradiation, in parallel with mice of the susceptible strains IBA and C57BL/S. Antibody levels were lower in irradiated than in nonirradiated mice of all strains. Changes in immune responses after irradiation did not discriminate between X/Gf mice and mice of the other two strains.

On the other hand, splenic phagocytosis of radiolabeled sheep red cells was not affected by presence of transplanted tumors in X/Gf mice whereas uptake of the radiolabel in the spleens of tumor-bearing C3H/S mice was significantly and consistently depressed.

These observations were interpreted in the light of previous experimental data obtained by the authors and other investigators. Immunocompetence and specific functions of the reticuloendothelial system may play decisive roles in the defense of the host against development and progression of malignant tumors.

During the last decade, a growing number of investigators have assigned a critical role to systemic host factors in development and progression of malignant tumors. Clinical observations have contributed an impressive body of circumstantial evidence concerning defense mechanisms which protect the host from cancer. For obvious reasons, controlled investigation of these phenomena requires animal experimentation, with success largely depending on the choice of adequate models. In this presentation, we propose to outline some critical problems in selection of experimental designs; describe some observations made recently in our laboratories; and relate our results and interpretations to relevant reports of other workers.

Definition and analysis of specific mechanisms of host resistance to cancer are complicated by three areas of uncertainty: 1) Even when consistent deviations from the norm are encountered in tumor hosts, a clearcut decision is rarely feasible as to whether these changes preceded the disease and are causally related to it, or are secondary effects of presence of tumors. 2) The majority of pertinent studies are based on induction, or transplantation, of tumors in basically healthy animals. It is at least problematic whether interpre-

---

* Present address: Department of Life Sciences, Bar Ilan University, Ramat Gan, Israel.

tations of results of such work can be meaningfully applied to cancer as it arises "in the natural course of events," i.e., in a host presumably already afflicted with some serious defect in defense mechanism(s). 3) Although several specific (e.g., genetic, metabolic, immunologic) mechanisms of host resistance have been considered and implicated, there is as yet no conclusive proof for the operation of any one of them.

In past work we have attempted to bypass some of these obstacles encumbering elucidation of host factors in neoplasia by using tumor-free, healthy mice of inbred strains with well-known propensity toward subsequent development of tumors. Large numbers of mice of ten inbred strains were tested for phagocytic activity of reticuloendothelial (RE) cells in liver and spleen (1–3), and for levels of natural and immune hemoantibodies for sheep red cells (SRC) and chicken red cells (CRC) (4–7). Both series of studies disclosed a close correlation between the biologic activities tested and resistance to cancer: RE phagocytosis as well as immune responses to hemoantigens were significantly higher in mice of strains with low incidence than in those with high incidence of various types of spontaneous tumors (mainly mammary carcinoma and leukemia). Analysis of natural hemagglutinins for SRC in mice of strains C57BL/S and C3H/S, and their F_1 hybrids and backcrosses, proved that the interstrain differences were genetically determined (8); analogous conclusions were derived from study of immune hemoantibodies for SRC carried out in parent strains, F_1 and backcrosses (unpublished observations).

Recently we reported that natural agglutinins for CRC and immune agglutinins and hemolysins for SRC determined in X/Gf mice exceeded, or were equal to, those found in comparable mice of strains C57BL/S and BALB/c/S (9). As demonstrated previously by Goldfeder et al. (10), X/Gf mice are characterized by high resistance to development of spontaneous tumors and induction of leukemia and solid tumors by X-irradiation or urethan or both. Thus, findings in this strain once more supported the hypothesis that potent immune responses may be linked with, or even be responsible for, resistance to cancer.

In order to further examine this phenomenon, we tested X/Gf mice and mice of other inbred strains by means of two experimental designs: a) immune responses to SRC were determined at specified intervals in control mice and mice given total body irradiation; b) RE phagocytosis of Cr^{51}-labeled SRC (Cr^{51}-SRC) was assayed in tumor-free and tumor-bearing mice.

MATERIALS AND METHODS

Animals. Three- to 6-month-old male mice, products of brother-to-sister matings of strains X/Gf, IBA, C57BL/S and C3H/S were used. Mice of the first two strains were raised in A. Goldfeder's New York laboratory. At appropriate times, they were shipped, by air express, to K. Stern's laboratory in Chicago.

X-irradiation. In A. Goldfeder's laboratory, mice were exposed to a total body dose of 300 R according to procedures previously described (10). C57BL/S mice, to be irradiated, were shipped to New York. At least one day elapsed between irradiation and shipment of mice to Chicago.

Immunization with SRC. Control and irradiated mice were injected i.p. with 0.5 ml of a 4% suspension in saline of SRC, either four, seven or 12 days after irradiation. Suitably matched nonirradiated mice were immunized at the same time.

Blood samples. Five and 10 days after immunization, blood was collected from the orbital plexus of all immunized mice. The experiments were terminated 14 days after immunization by exsanguination (cardiac puncture) of mice anesthetized with ether.

Autopsies. Weights of body, liver and spleen were determined. Livers and spleens were preserved in buffered formalin, and hematoxylin and eosin stained sections were prepared.

Determination of antibodies. Titers of agglutinins for SRC were determined by serial twofold dilutions of the sera, and hemolysins were measured as 50% units of hemolysis (H_{50} units/ml)

43

Table 1. *Immune responses to sheep red cells of inbred mice after whole body irradiation*

Interval between irradiation and immunization (days)	Group[a]	No. of mice	Agglutinin[b] ($\times$ or : SD) Days after immunization			Hemolysin[b] (H_{50} units/ml $\pm$ SD) Days after immunization		
			5	10	14	5	10	14
X/Gf								
4	C	10	34 (3.8)	18 (3.8)	111 (9.9)	172 (148)	25 (19)	54 (34)
	I	14	2 (2.4)[c]	6 (2.8)[d]	20 (3.8)	7 (4)[c]	12 (13)[d]	67 (47)
7	C	9	21 (4.3)	37 (8.1)	104 (3.7)	70 (37)	50 (34)	79 (49)
	I	18	5 (2.3)[c]	34 (3.0)	79 (4.1)	3 (5)[c]	35 (15)	57 (34)
12	C	9	55 (4.9)	59 (6.6)	75 (5.9)	90 (42)	86 (90)	67 (67)
	I	12	11 (3.1)[d]	55 (4.3)	108 (5.3)	6 (7)[d]	33 (18)[d]	19 (27)[d]
IBA								
4	C	6	23 (4.5)	40 (6.6)	161 (11.3)	47 (15)	53 (37)	33 (23)
	I	6	3 (2.6)[c]	14 (4.2)	46 (6.7)	1 (1)[d]	13 (19)[d]	9 (15)[d]
7	C	8	23 (3.8)	39 (5.4)	54 (6.5)	54 (46)	50 (32)	32 (22)
	I	19	2 (2.3)[c]	23 (3.3)	67 (3.8)	2 (2)[c]	24 (26)[d]	43 (33)
12	C	11	50 (4.3)	39 (3.5)	136 (5.9)	78 (53)	44 (37)	88 (52)
	I	12	8 (2.7)[c]	17 (2.7)	42 (3.5)	5 (9)[c]	15 (21)[d]	32 (32)[c]
C57BL/S								
4	C	8	23 (3.8)	25 (3.7)	64 (5.0)	47 (44)	59 (33)	15 (8)
	I	11	7 (2.1)[d]	13 (2.9)	47 (4.4)	1 (1)[c]	22 (21)[c]	21 (14)
12	C	16	83 (3.9)	50 (3.8)	28 (3.5)	78 (53)	42 (33)	14 (10)
	I	17	3 (1.8)[c]	26 (3.5)	26 (2.9)	1 (0)[c]	12 (24)[d]	8 (10)

[a] C = control; I = irradiated.
[b] Agglutinin values are geometric means, hemolysin values are arithmetic means
[c] $P < 0.01$.
[d] $P < 0.05 > 0.01$.

according to methods previously described (11). Resistance of antibodies to 2-mercaptoethanol (2-ME) was tested in some experiments.

Tumors. X/Gf and C3H/S mice were inoculated s.c. with 5 to 10×10^5 viable cells of isogeneic mammary carcinomas, contained in 0.5 ml of saline. Tumors were measured weekly with calipers in order to determine the proper time for assay of RE phagocytosis.

Assay of RE phagocytosis. On the day of use, SRC were labeled with $Na_2Cr^{51}O_4$ according to methods previously described (12, 13). Tumor-free and tumor-bearing mice in particular experiments received i.p. injections of 0.5 ml of a 10% suspension in saline of radiolabeled SRC, corresponding to a radioactivity of 0.3 to 0.5 μc per mouse, and the animals were killed 24 hr later. Weights of body, tumor, liver and spleen were determined and radioactivities of liver, spleen and remaining carcass were assayed in a total body counter (ARMAC, attached to Packard model 3002, Tri-Carb scintillation autogamma spectrophotometer). Percentages of total body radioactivity found in liver and spleen served as indicators of phagocytosis in these organs.

Calculation and evaluation of results. Mean values of data and their standard deviations were calculated for each group of individual experiments. Statistical significance of intergroup differences was evaluated by means of Student's "t" test.

RESULTS

Table 1 compares levels of agglutinins and hemolysins for SRC, as observed in mice immunized at designated intervals after irradiation, with findings in non-irradiated controls. These data also permit comparison of immune responses between mice immunized at three different time intervals after irradiation, and of the effects of irradiation on mice of three different strains. Significantly lower levels of antibodies than in controls were found

TABLE 2. *Autopsy findings in inbred mice after whole body irradiation*

Interval between irradiation and immunization (days)	Group[a]	No. of mice	Body weight (g) mean ± SD	% of body weight (mean ± SD) of	
				Liver	Spleen
X/Gf					
4	C	10	15.9 ± 2.2	5.7 ± 0.1	1.0 ± 0.3
	I	14	15.4 ± 2.2	5.7 ± 0.9	1.3 ± 0.3[c]
7	C	9	18.2 ± 3.6	5.7 ± 0.4	1.0 ± 0.3
	I	18	17.9 ± 3.3	6.0 ± 0.7	1.6 ± 0.5[b]
12	C	9	16.8 ± 2.5	5.6 ± 0.5	1.2 ± 0.2
	I	12	18.0 ± 3.0	6.1 ± 0.8	1.4 ± 0.4
IBA					
4	C	6	20.8 ± 1.3	5.6 ± 0.2	1.1 ± 0.2
	I	6	21.5 ± 1.5	5.7 ± 0.5	1.4 ± 0.3
7	C	8	20.0 ± 2.7	5.6 ± 0.6	0.9 ± 0.3
	I	19	18.3 ± 2.2	6.6 ± 0.7[b]	1.2 ± 0.4
12	C	11	22.7 ± 1.1	6.5 ± 0.5	1.0 ± 0.3
	I	12	21.3 ± 2.4	5.5 ± 0.6[b]	1.2 ± 0.2
C57BL/S					
4	C	8	25.6 ± 2.0	5.6 ± 0.5	0.6 ± 0.1
	I	11	25.9 ± 1.1	5.9 ± 0.4	0.5 ± 0.1
12	C	16	24.9 ± 2.2	4.9 ± 0.5	0.5 ± 0.1
	I	17	23.9 ± 1.5	4.9 ± 0.4	0.5 ± 0.1

[a] C = control; I = irradiated.   [b] $P < 0.01$.   [c] $P < 0.05 > 0.01$.

in all groups of irradiated mice, regardless of strain and timing of immunization. X/Gf mice immunized seven days after irradiation showed lesser interference with immune responses than X/Gf mice immunized four days after irradiation. When immunized 12 days after irradiation, X/Gf mice exhibited only moderate impairment of formation of agglutinins, while hemolysins were depressed to a greater extent than was noted in mice immunized four or seven days after irradiation. Mice of strain IBA and C57BL/S behaved similarly, except that C57BL/S mice were not tested seven days after irradiation. Thus, no clearcut strain-dependent differences were apparent in the effects on immune responses of preceding irradiation. Possibly, formation of agglutinins for SRC in irradiated X/Gf mice returned to control levels more readily than was the case in IBA mice. Sensitivity of an-

tibodies to 2-ME was tested in some serum samples collected at the end of the experiments in which mice were immunized 12 days after irradiation. Of seven sera of irradiated X/Gf mice tested, only two had 50% or more ME-resistant agglutinins, while this was the case in all five sera of IBA mice tested, and in three of four C57BL/S sera. Sera of non-irradiated mice showed similar strain-related differences. In no instance were sizable amounts of ME-resistant hemolysin detected.

Table 2 lists data obtained at the termination of experiments. X/Gf mice immunized four and seven days after irradiation exhibited significantly higher splenic weights than control mice. Such differences were not observed in the two other strains. As indicated by preliminary histologic survey, the rise in splenic weight of X/Gf mice was paralleled by the presence of increased lymphoid tissue in

Table 3. *Phagocytosis of Cr^{51}-labeled sheep red cells in tumor-free and tumor-bearing mice*

Strain and experiment no.	Group[a]	No. of mice	Tumor % of body wt ± SD	Liver % body wt ± SD	Liver % count/min ± SD per organ	Liver % count/min ± SD per g	Spleen % body wt ± SD	Spleen % count/min ± SD per organ	Spleen % count/min ± SD per 100 mg
X/Gf									
I	C	5	—	6.6 ± 0.6	60.4 ± 11.2	51.4 ± 14.8	0.8 ± 0.1	5.1 ± 1.1	3.4 ± 1.3
	T	5	6.5 ± 4.3	8.4 ± 2.0 (9.1 ± 2.1)[c]	63.8 ± 4.2	43.8 ± 11.3	1.4 ± 0.5[c] (1.5 ± 0.6)[c]	5.3 ± 2.5	2.2 ± 0.9
II	C	4	—	6.1 ± 0.2	74.2 ± 2.7	62.4 ± 6.3	1.1 ± 0.1	4.7 ± 2.4	2.2 ± 1.3
	T	5	8.1 ± 3.9	6.6 ± 0.7 (7.2 ± 1.0)	73.2 ± 6.6	52.3 ± 7.2	1.1 ± 0.1 (1.1 ± 0.3)	3.5 ± 2.2	1.6 ± 0.9
IIIa	C	5	—	6.3 ± 0.6	56.3 ± 17.3	54.3 ± 13.2	1.0 ± 0.3	7.0 ± 0.7	4.6 ± 1.1
	T	6	6.4 ± 2.2	7.4 ± 0.4[b] (8.0 ± 0.5)[b]	56.9 ± 7.1	43.4 ± 8.3	1.3 ± 0.5 (1.4 ± 0.5)	12.2 ± 6.5	5.2 ± 1.4
IIIb	C	4	—	5.3 ± 0.5	62.9 ± 7.2	67.7 ± 13.7	0.9 ± 0.3	11.0 ± 9.3	7.1 ± 6.2
	T	7	12.1 ± 3.8	6.2 ± 0.5[c] (7.0 ± 0.5)[c]	69.8 ± 15.6	58.7 ± 11.7	1.1 ± 0.3 (1.2 ± 0.3)	5.5 ± 4.5	3.3 ± 4.1
C3H/S									
I	C	5	—	6.0 ± 0.4	50.3 ± 14.5	40.2 ± 17.8	0.7 ± 0.3	9.2 ± 2.4	6.7 ± 2.1
	T	5	3.3 ± 1.4	7.2 ± 0.8[c] (7.5 ± 1.0)[c]	39.5 ± 13.4	23.6 ± 9.9	0.8 ± 0.1 (0.8 ± 0.1)	5.0 ± 2.5[c]	2.6 ± 1.3[b]
II	C	5	—	6.6 ± 0.5	49.9 ± 10.1	32.0 ± 8.4	0.6 ± 0.3	10.2 ± 3.2	7.3 ± 2.3
	T	6	16.4 ± 12.4	7.7 ± 1.5 (9.1 ± 0.7)[b]	62.6 ± 4.6[c]	30.3 ± 8.7	1.0 ± 0.2[c] (1.3 ± 0.1)[b]	5.1 ± 2.6[c]	1.6 ± 0.9[b]
III	C	5	—	6.6 ± 0.1	32.6 ± 11.7	18.6 ± 6.3	0.6 ± 0.3	9.8 ± 5.8	6.4 ± 3.9
	T	5	4.0 ± 1.6	8.2 ± 0.7[b] (8.5 ± 0.6)[b]	38.8 ± 10.2	20.4 ± 5.7	1.0 ± 0.1[b] (1.1 ± 0.1)[b]	7.7 ± 1.5	3.1 ± 0.6[c]

[a] C = control; T = tumor.
[b] $P < 0.01$.
[c] $P < 0.05 > 0.01$.
Figures in parentheses are percent of body weight minus tumor.

spleens of irradiated over that in control mice. In the IBA strain, hepatic weights of mice immunized seven days after irradiation exceeded those of controls significantly, while hepatic weights of mice immunized 12 days after irradiation were significantly lower than those of controls.

Table 3 summarizes the results of assay of RE phagocytosis in tumor-free and tumor-bearing mice. Experiments with X/Gf and C3H/S mice were carried out in parallel as indicated by corresponding numbers. In experiment III, X/Gf mice were divided into two subgroups: in IIIa, phagocytosis was assayed while the tumors were relatively small, while in IIIb tumors were permitted to grow to larger size. Experiment III with C3H/S mice was terminated at the same time as X/Gf, IIIa. The contrast between the behavior of tumor-bearing mice of the two strains is striking: whereas significant impairment of splenic phagocytosis occurred in all tumor-bearing C3H/S mice, this was not observed in X/Gf mice, in spite of the fact that in two of the three experiments tumor weights of C3H/S mice were smaller than those of X/Gf mice. Splenomegaly was less pronounced in tumor-bearing X/Gf than C3H/S animals.

Hepatomegaly occurred in tumor-bearing mice of both strains. Hepatic phagocytosis was not significantly affected, except for experiment II in which C3H/S mice had an increased uptake of radiolabel in the whole liver.

DISCUSSION

Analysis of humoral antibodies produced by mice of three inbred strains after total body irradiation did not permit separation of strains susceptible to radiation leukemogenesis (IBA, C57BL/S) from the resistant strain X/Gf. Conceivably, more discriminatory information might have been obtained by one or more modifications of the experimental design: assay of immune responses at more prolonged intervals after irradiation; use of different doses of antigen; and, study of cellular immune reactions.

On the other hand, phagocytic activity in the presence of transplanted tumors permitted clearcut differentiation between strains X/Gf and C3H/S. Splenic phagocytosis was consistently lower in tumor-bearing than in tumor-free C3H/S mice, paralleling findings previously observed in mice of four other inbred strains (13). By contrast, splenic phagocytosis of tumor-bearing X/Gf mice was not significantly depressed. Neoplasia and phagocytic activity of the RE system (RES) appear to interact with each other in a cyclic manner. Liability to development of tumors is associated with inferior phagocytic activity, as indicated by comparison of cancer-susceptible and cancer-resistant strains of mice (1–3). By the same token, presence of transplanted tumors in rats (14) and mice (13) specifically damaged splenic phagocytosis, while hepatic phagocytosis was markedly increased (14) or variably affected (13). Deterioration of splenic phagocytosis also resulted from induction in mice of tumors by means of chemical carcinogens (15). Finally, significant impairment of splenic phagocytosis was demonstrable in mice with spontaneous mammary carcinomas or spontaneous lymphomas, when compared with their tumor-free litter mates. Since tumor-free C3H/S female mice, of which close to 90% eventually develop mammary carcinoma, had lower splenic phagocytic activity than their brothers, the decrease in splenic phagocytosis preceded manifest tumor development (16). The findings observed in X/Gf mice add another facet to the interaction between the RES and malignant tumors: mice of this tumor-resistant strain appear to be less vulnerable than mice of other strains to the secondary damage inflicted on splenic phagocytosis by progressive tumor growth.

Several reviews have dealt with the large body of data recorded on the relationship between RES and neoplasia (3, 17–19). Before relating some more recent studies in this field to our work, some specific considerations must be pointed out in order to avoid misinterpretations. The widely used and valuable techniques of estimating clearance of i.v. injected colloidal carbon and other particulate substrates, cannot be expected to yield information on the general status of phagocytic activity of the RES. Results obtained with these methods primarily reflect the efficiency of Kupffer cells in the liver for removal from the circulation of particulate matter. Hence it is essential to determine localization of phagocytosed substrate in particular sites, such as liver and spleen. Increased clearance of i.v. injected particles, resulting from stimulation of hepatic phagocytosis, may well be associated with depressed splenic phagocytosis, as observed in some of our studies. Furthermore, different sites of RE activity probably differ functionally too. Thus, immune mechanisms depend to a larger extent on splenic macrophages than on RE elements in liver and other sites. In our work, rats with Lewis lymphomas showed increased hepatic and decreased splenic phagocytosis (14), accompanied by severe depression of formation of antibodies for SRC (unpublished observations). Finally, stimulation of phagocytic activity in hosts bearing nonisogeneic tumors may well reflect response to isoantigenic stimulation rather than to the tumor process per se.

In the light of these comments, the impairment in splenic phagocytosis documented in our work for tumor hosts does not necessarily conflict with reports of other authors describing increased total clearance rates of i.v. injected substrates. Kampschmidt and Upchurch (20) found significantly faster clearance rates of colloidal carbon in tumor-bearing than in control rats. This "stimulation of the RES" was more pronounced in non-inbred rats inoculated with Jensen or Walker tumors than in inbred Fischer rats with isogeneic tumors. Ringle and Thomson (21) noted normal carbon clearance in DBA/2 mice until six days after inoculation of L1210 ascites cells, while subsequently, clearance was markedly accelerated. Significantly, liver and spleen of the leukemic animals contained smaller amounts of carbon, and lungs larger amounts, than controls. Similar considerations may apply to the clinical studies of Salky et al. (22) who observed increased rates of clearance of a lipid emulsion in over 90% of 53 patients with malignant tumors. Differences in test substrates and type of neoplastic disease may account for the divergent findings of other workers. Groch and associates (23) noted delayed clearance of i.v. injected I^{131}-labeled aggregated serum albumin in most patients with acute leukemia, while this function of the RES was unaltered in patients with chronic leukemia or lymphoma. Accelerated clearance rates in leukemic patients were associated with increased red cell destruction or infection. Using much smaller doses of micro-aggregated serum albumin, Donovan (24) found impaired phagocytic activity in 22 cancer patients; he also noted that in nine patients favorable therapeutic response was accompanied by increase in clearance rates.

RE activity of the spleen may be responsible for some of its effects on carcinogenesis and growth of tumors. According to Pollard (25), splenectomy of germ-free rats, prior to administration of dimethylbenz-anthracene (DMBA), accelerated development of myelogenous leukemia, while DMBA induced mammary tumors more rapidly in splenectomized conventional rats. Kim (26) reported that mammary carcinomas induced in splenectomized rats by means of methylcholanthrene (MCH) were poorly antigenic and capable of metastasizing, properties not found in analogous tumors induced in intact rats. Easty (27) injected mouse tumor cells into chick embryos and observed a close parallelism between trapping ability of the organs and subsequent tumor growth. Two exceptions to this rule were the brain, in which poor trapping coincided with vigorous tumor growth, and the spleen in which there was poor tumor growth despite trapping of large numbers of neoplastic cells. The authors correlated the latter finding with the high RE activity of the spleen. More direct participation of RE cells may account for the differences described by Daniel (28) in carcinogenicity of i.m. injected suspensions of nickel sulfide in two strains of rats. Heavier local accumulation in phagocytes and lesser carcinogenicity of the compound distinguished Bethesda Black from hooded rats. The author proposed that this may reflect a diminished effective concentration of the carcinogen following phagocytosis, or more potent immune responses exerted by phagocytes of the resistant strain, or both.

Within recent years, the essential participation of macrophages in immune reactions has been thoroughly analyzed (29–31), and significant links between RE function, the immune response and carcinogenesis are further suggested by the observed immunosuppressive capabilities of all major classes of carcinogens. Stjernswärd (32) has reviewed pertinent work carried out with chemical carcinogens. Recently, Stutman (33) tested the formation of plaque forming cells (PFC) directed at SRC in I and C3H mice treated with MCH. Immunosuppression occurred only in C3H mice which are highly susceptible to MCH carcinogenesis, whereas this was not the case in strain I mice which are resistant to MCH.

Carcinogenesis, leukemogenesis and immunosuppression resulting from ionizing irradiation are well documented. Feldman and Nachtigal (34) interpreted the occurrence of metastases from carcinogen-induced mouse tumors after irradiation of the host as expression of damaged immune competence. Haran-Ghera and Peled (35, 36) demonstrated the significant contribution of immunosuppression to leukemogenesis mediated by radiation-connected viruses. In extension of this work, they reported that inoculation of C57BL mice with cell-free filtrates of irradiated nonleukemic C57BL tissue induced lymphomas in only 7 to 20% of animals with a long latent period, but incidence of lymphomas rose to 78 to 90% with shortened latent period when treatment was supplemented by injection of anti-mouse thymocyte serum (37).

Conclusive evidence on immunodepression exerted by oncogenic viruses has been surveyed by Salaman (38). Recently, Ceglowski and Friedman (39) found a close parallelism between the degree of immunodepression and susceptibility to leukemogenesis by Friend virus in six inbred strains of mice; e.g., the number of PFC in highly resistant C57BL mice immunized with SRC after infection with the virus remained higher than was the case in mice of other strains more susceptible to leukemogenesis.

Of particular relevance to the model used in the present work is the correlation postulated by Bentvelzen (40) between the failure of prolonged vertical transmission of the Bittner mammary tumor virus (MTV) in C57BL mice and the potent immune responses characterizing this strain. Thus, a vicious circle may operate in viral carcinogenesis: On the one hand, at least some viruses induce immunosuppression of the host, and, on the other, hosts with inherent (e.g., genetic) deficient immunocompetence are more likely to permit viral propagation. It is tempting to apply this interpretation also to observations of Goldfeder and Ghosh (41) on oncogenicity of the MTV transmitted to X/Gf from IBA mice. Whereas in the first generation of foster-nursed X/Gf mice mammary tumors arose in 46% of breeders and 14% of virgins, in the F_2 generation only 25% of breeders and 14% of virgins developed tumors. Progressive decrease in tumor incidence in subsequent generations reached a low of 4% in F_7. The probability that immune responses mounted by X/Gf mice were responsible for this inhibition of oncogenesis was raised to near certainty by the recent demonstration by Bentvelzen (personal communication) of natural antibodies for MTV in X/Gf mice.

In addition to its significant contribution to immunocompetence, the RES may also participate in homeostasis of growth. This possibility was suggested on the basis of significant increases in RE phagocytosis demonstrable during the period of rapid restoration of liver tissue after partial hepatectomy of rats (42–44). In experiments designed to explore this phenomenon, we found that administration to mice of isogeneic subcellular fractions inhibited hepatic and splenic phagocytosis of subsequently injected Cr^{51}-labeled SRC (45) or Au^{198} (46). Ribosomes proved to be particularly potent in interfering with phagocytosis of the test substrates. This suggests that macrophages may have some special task in dealing with these organelles responsible for protein synthesis. Significantly, subcellular fractions prepared from isogeneic mouse tumors were less capable of interacting with the

RES than fractions derived from normal tissues (46). Thus, one might speculate that a twofold disturbance of homeostasis affects hosts with malignant tumors: 1) some functional deterioration of the RES may precede development of neoplasia; 2) subcellular components of cancer may be deficient in providing the RES with stimuli required for regulation of growth.

What are the implications of the demonstrated or postulated role in host defense against cancer of immunologic mechanisms and functional activity of the RES? While direct applications of the experimental work described to clinical aspects of cancer are probably remote, the animal models employed may permit us to draw some guide lines of potential value for future efforts. Comparative investigation of carcinogenesis in animals of well defined genetic constitution facilitates assessment of the relative contribution to neoplasia of genetic and environmental factors. Such investigations may eventually help to identify the host at maximum risk from some specific carcinogens. Prolonged latent periods in development of malignant tumors can be utilized for study of mechanisms affecting the rate of carcinogenesis and exploit such knowledge, if possible, for reversing or arresting the process.

Supported in part by Grant U-1354 from the Health Research Council of the City of New York, and by General Research Support Grant of the National Institutes of Health to the University of Illinois College of Medicine.

REFERENCES

1. STERN, K. Storage of carmine in inbred mice. *Proc. Soc. exp. Biol.* (*N. Y.*) **67**: 315, 1948.
2. STERN, K. Uptake of colloidal radiogold by liver in mice of inbred strains. *Proc. Amer. Ass. Cancer Res.* **2**: 48, 1955.
3. STERN, K. The reticuloendothelial system and neoplasia, in: Heller, J. (Ed.), "Reticuloendothelial structure and function." New York, Ronald Press Co., 1960, p. 233.
4. DAVIDSOHN, I. and STERN, K. Natural and immune antibodies in mice of low and high tumor strains. *Cancer Res.* **9**: 426, 1949.
5. DAVIDSOHN, I. and STERN, K. Further studies on natural antisheep agglutinins in mice of inbred strains. *Cancer Res.* **10**: 571, 1950.
6. STERN, K. and DAVIDSOHN, I. Heterochemoantibodies in inbred strains of mice. I. Natural agglutinins for sheep and chicken red cells. *J. Immunol.* **72**: 209, 1954.
7. DAVIDSOHN, I. and STERN, K. Heterohemoantibodies in inbred strains of mice. II. Immune agglutinins and hemolysins for sheep and chicken red cells. *J. Immunol.* **72**: 216, 1954.
8. STERN, K., BROWN, K. S. and DAVIDSOHN, I. On the inheritance of natural antisheep agglutinins in mice of inbred strains. *Genetics* **41**: 517, 1956.
9. STERN, K. and GOLDFEDER, A. Radiation studies on mice of an inbred tumor-resistant strain. VI. Immune responses to heterologous red cells of non-irradiated and irradiated mice. *Int. Arch. Allergy* **35**: 504, 1969.
10. GOLDFEDER, A., KAUFFMAN, S. L. and GHOSH, A. K. Carcinogenesis in naturally tumor-resistant mice. *Brit. J. Cancer* **20**: 361, 1966.
11. STERN, K. Inhibition of immune responses to sheep red cells in rats pre-immunized with heterophilic antigen. *Clin. exp. Immunol.* **4**: 253, 1969.
12. STERN, K. Inhibition *in vivo* of reticuloendothelial phagocytosis of synthetic polyamino acids. *Proc. Soc. exp. Biol.* (*N. Y.*) **114**: 321, 1963.
13. STERN, K. Phagocytosis *in vivo* of heterologous red cells in mice with transplanted tumors. *Cancer Res.* **24**: 1063, 1964.
14. STERN, K. and DUWELIUS, A. Phagocytosis in liver and spleen of rats with Lewis lymphoma. *Cancer Res.* **20**: 587, 1960.
15. STERN, K. Host factors in resistance to cancer: Reticuloendothelial phagocytosis in mice with transplanted, spontaneous, and induced tumors. *Ninth Int. Cancer Cong., Tokyo*, 1966, p. 59.
16. STERN, K., BARTIZAL, C. A. and DIVSHONY, S. Changes in reticuloendothelial phagocytosis in mice with spontaneous tumors. *J. nat. Cancer Inst.* **38**: 469, 1967.
17. OLD, L. J., BENACERRAF, B., CLARKE, D. A., CARSWELL, E. A. and STOCKERT, E. The role of the reticuloendothelial system in the host reaction to neoplasia. *Cancer Res.* **21**: 1281, 1961.
18. STERN, K. Host factors in neoplastic disease. A review of current concepts and trends in cancer research. *Hebrew med. J.* **1**: 263; **2**: 280, 1962.
19. HALPERN, B. N., BIOZZI, G. and STIFFEL, C. Le système reticuloendothélial et l'invasion tumorale. In: Denoix, P. (Ed.) "Mechanisms of invasion of cancer." UICC monograph series, Berlin, Springer Verlag, 1967, v. 6, p. 149.
20. KAMPSCHMIDT, R. K. and UPCHURCH, H. F. Stimulation of the reticuloendothelial system in tumor-bearing rats. *J. Reticuloendothel. Soc.* **5**: 510, 1968.
21. RINGLE, D. A. and THOMSON, J. R. Effect of L-1210 leukemia on C/1431a carbon clearance in DBA/2 mice. *J. Reticuloendothel. Soc.* **4**: 151, 1967.
22. SALKY, N. K., DI LUZIO, N. R., LEVIN, A. G.

and GOLDSMITH, H. S. Phagocytic activity of the reticuloendothelial system in neoplastic disease. *J. Lab. clin. Med.* **70**: 393, 1967.

23. GROCH, G. S., PERILLE, P. E. and FINCH, S. C. Reticuloendothelial phagocytic function in patients with leukemia, lymphoma and multiple myeloma. *Blood* **26**: 489, 1965.

24. DONOVAN, A. J. Reticuloendothelial function in patients with cancer. *Amer. J. Surg.* **114**: 230, 1967.

25. POLLARD, M. Effect of splenectomy on the development of DMBA—induced myelogenous leukemia in rats. *Fed. Proc.* **27**: 608, 1968.

26. KIM, U. Role of spleen in metastasis of methylcholanthrene (MC) induced mammary carcinoma (MT) in rats. *Fed. Proc.* **27**: 608, 1968.

27. EASTY, G. C., EASTY, D. M. and TCHAO, R. The distribution of heterologous tumor cells in chick embryos following intravenous injection. *Europ. J. Cancer* **5**: 297, 1969.

28. DANIEL, R. Strain differences in the response of rats to the injection of nickel sulphide. *Brit. J. Cancer* **20**: 886, 1966.

29. FELDMAN, M. The immunogenic function of macrophages. *Symp. Intern. Soc. Cell Biol.* **7**: 43, 1968.

30. FELDMAN, M. Macrophages, lymphocytes and antibody formation. *Antibiot. and Chemother.* **15**: 56, 1969.

31. FISHMAN, M. Induction of antibodies *in vitro*. *Ann. Rev. Microbiol.* **23**: 199, 1969.

32. STJERNSWÄRD, J. Immunosuppression by carcinogens. *Antibiot. and Chemother.* **15**: 213, 1969.

33. STUTMAN, O. Carcinogen-induced immune depression: Absence in mice resistant to chemical oncogenesis. *Science* **166**: 620, 1969.

34. FELDMAN, M. and NACHTIGAL, D. Immunological tolerance and host-tumor relationship, in: Denoix, P. (Ed.), "Mechanisms of invasion of cancer." UICC monograph series, Berlin, Springer Verlag, 1967, v. 6, p. 118.

35. HARAN-GHERA, N. and PELED, A. Mechanism of radiation action in leukemogenesis: Isolation of a leukemogenic filtrable agent from tissues of irradiated and normal C57BL mice. *Brit. J. Cancer* **21**: 730, 1967.

36. HARAN-GHERA, N. Mechanism of radiation action in leukemogenesis: Role of radiation in leukemia development. *Brit. J. Cancer* **21**: 739, 1967.

37. HARAN-GHERA, N. and PELED, A. The mechanism of radiation action in leukemogenesis. IV. Immune impairment as a coleukemogenic factor. *Israel J. med. Sci.* **4**: 1181, 1969.

38. SALAMAN, M. H. Immunodepression by viruses. *Antibiot. and Chemother.* **15**: 393, 1969.

39. CEGLOWSKI, W. S. and FRIEDMAN, H. Murine virus leukemogenesis: Relationship between susceptibility and immunodepression. *Nature* (*Lond.*) **224**: 1318, 1969.

40. BENTVELZEN, P. Resistance to small amounts of Bittner mammary tumor virus in offspring of C57BL female mice with the virus. *J. Nat. Cancer Inst.* **41**: 757, 1968.

41. GOLDFEDER, A. and GHOSH, A. K. The incidence of mammary tumors in X/Gf mice foster-nursed by IBA/Gf females. *Proc. Amer. Ass. Cancer Res.* **10**: 31, 1969.

42. STERN, K. and DUWELIUS, A. Hepatic and splenic uptake of colloidal radiogold in rat after partial hepatectomy. *Proc. Soc. exp. Biol.* (*N.Y.*) **100**: 546, 1959.

43. LEONG, G. F., PESSOTTI, R. L. and BRAUER, R. W. Liver function in regenerating rat liver. $CrPO_4$ colloid uptake and bile flow. *Amer. J. Physiol.* **197**: 880, 1959.

44. STERN, K. Studies on reticuloendothelial function in relation to growth processes. *Ann. N. Y. Acad. Sci.* **88**: 252, 1960.

45. STERN, K. and MATSUMOTO, H. Phagocytosis of heterologous red cells in mice injected with isologous microsomes. *Proc. Soc. exp. Biol.* (*N. Y.*) **120**: 843, 1965.

46. STERN, K., TITCHENER, E. B. and DUWELIUS, A. Phagocytic activity in mice treated with isogeneic subcellular fractions. *Life Sci.* **8**. pt. II: 821, 1969.

EVIDENCE FOR IMMUNOLOGICAL SURVEILLANCE DURING SKIN CARCINOGENESIS

INFLAMMATORY FOCI IN IMMUNOLOGICALLY COMPETENT MICE

MARC A. LAPPÉ

Cancer Research Genetics Laboratory, University of California, Berkeley, California, USA

ABSTRACT

Histological evidence for immunological surveillance during skin carcinogenesis was sought by serially sectioning isografts of 3-methylcholanthrene treated skin transplanted to immunologically competent and incompetent mice. Focal microscopic lesions exhibiting mononuclear cell infiltration were commonly found only in immunologically competent hosts during the latent period of papilloma development. Sublethally irradiated or antilymphocyte serum treated hosts developed macroscopic papillomas without the appearance of microscopic lesions in all except one graft. The existence of histological criteria for the immunologic destruction of macroscopic papillomas provided a reference for assessing the significance of these microscopic lesions. Common histological features of microscopic inflammatory foci and known papilloma regression sites included dermal keratin debris, lymphocyte exocytosis, and mast cell degranulation associated with epithelial pyknosis. Coupled with the fact that foci were found preferentially in immunologically competent hosts where papilloma development is impaired, the histological evidence strongly suggests that the inflammatory foci represent the remnants of immunologically destroyed papillomas. As such, these observations provide evidence for the operation of immunological surveillance at the microscopic level.

INTRODUCTION

The term "immunological surveillance" was proposed by Burnet (1) to describe the immune elimination of microscopic foci of incipient tumors. Evidence for the operation of immunological surveillance during murine skin carcinogenesis has been largely inferred from studies which have demonstrated prolonged tumor latencies or reduced tumor incidences, or both, in immunologically competent, as compared to incompetent, hosts (2–4).

Such studies would be substantially reinforced if microscopic evidence for tumor destruction could be found during the period when the development of skin tumors is known to be impaired.

In a previous experimental series (5), the occurrence of inflammatory foci in the skin of immunologically competent mice in which there had been a lower than expected incidence of papillomas was reported. It was suggested that these foci represent the remnants of the "missing" papillomas, which had been immunologically destroyed. This possibility was subsequently reinforced by the absence of comparable lesions in a series of histological sections taken from immunologically depressed hosts (6). The purpose of the present study is to extend these observations and to determine if such inflammatory lesions actually represent the microscopic tumor destruction predicted by the theory of immunological surveillance (7, 8).

MATERIALS AND METHODS

Experimental design. The microscopic features of skin tumor formation and elimination were studied in isografts of 3-methylcholanthrene (MCA) treated skin transplanted to mice with varying degrees of immunologic competence. The procedures used here were essentially identical to those reported previously (5), except that the carcinogen treated skin isografts were sampled at fixed intervals during the latent period of papilloma development.

Skin papilloma initiation was accomplished by treating donors bilaterally with 10% disks of MCA for 10 days. After a five-day interval, the treated sites were excised, scraped and punched out to uniform circles of skin measuring approximately 18 mm OD. Each piece of carcinogen-treated skin was grafted by the method of Thoenes (9) to adult virgin female BALB/cCrgl mice in one of four groups: A) pretreated with 0.6 mg of methanol extraction residue of BCG (MER) injected in 0.1 ml saline 15 days before grafting; B) pretreated with a 0.1 ml injection of saline 15 days before grafting; C) Sublethally irradiated with 450 R of whole body X-irradiation one day before grafting; D) pretreated on seven consecutive days before grafting with an i.p. injection of 0.25 ml of antilymphocyte serum (ALS).

There were 28 to 36 mice in each group. Isogenicity of the BALB/cCrgl strain has been monitored by the success of second and third set isografts.

MER was kindly supplied by Dr. David Weiss, Hebrew University, Jerusalem. The protocol used has been found to increase the immunological competence of BALB/c female mice (5).

X-irradiation was administered under the following conditions: 150 kv, 10 ma, 1.0 mm Al filtration, at a target distance of 16 inches giving 175 R/min.

Antilymphocyte serum was prepared by the method of Levey and Medawar (10). The ALS pretreatment schedule was adjusted so that it produced an immunological depression in BALB/c mice comparable to that produced by X-irradiation. Skin allografts made from DBA/2 Crgl mice to ALS-treated BALB/c females survived three to six weeks after grafting (median survival time, 27 days): DBA/2 grafts made to X-irradiated females had a median survival time of 23 days.

Histology. Bandages were removed on day 9 after grafting the MCA-treated isografts. Three to four grafts in each group were randomly sampled for histological examination on days 9, 13, 17, 21, 25, 29, 34, 37 and 39 after grafting. These intervals encompass the latent period of papilloma development in this system [90 to 95% of the mice developing papillomas do so between days 13 and 30 after grafting (5)]. Animals bearing grafts were killed by cervical dislocation and the area occupied by the graft was dissected, fixed in Tellyesniczky's solution, sectioned serially, and stained with either hematoxylin and eosin or toluidine blue. Where possible, alternate sections from the same graft were stained with each dye. For staining mast cells, the procedure of Pearse (11) was followed.

RESULTS

Histology. Microscopic papillomas were commonly seen in sections taken from grafts transplanted to immunologically depressed hosts between two and four weeks after grafting. A typical submacroscopic papilloma developing in an X-irradiated host 17 days after grafting is shown in Fig. 1. The actual size of this papilloma was approximately 0.75 mm³. By the third week after grafting, papillomas appeared in about 20% of the immunologically depressed hosts which received either X-irradiation (Group C) or ALS treatment (Group D). Fig. 2 and 3 show papillomas on grafts made 21 and 25 days earlier than recipients in Group C. Typically, there is a dense collagen matrix and dermal fibroplasia beneath these lesions, but little or no stromal response.

Pre-papillomatous microscopic lesions

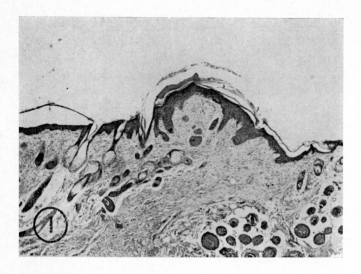

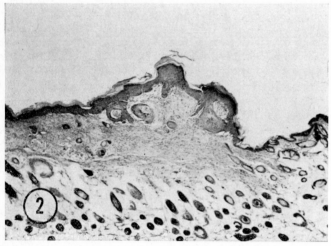

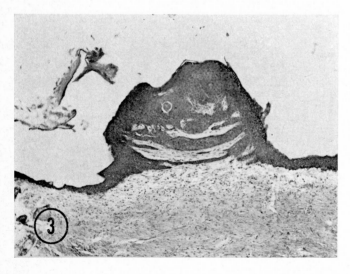

FIG. 1–3. Papilloma development in X-irradiated hosts (Group C) shown at 17, 21 and 25 days respectively after grafting MCA-treated skin. Hematoxylin and eosin. × 40.

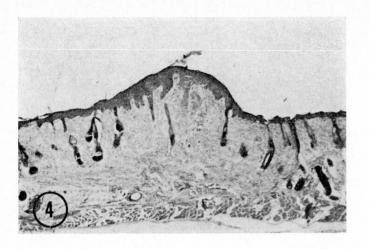

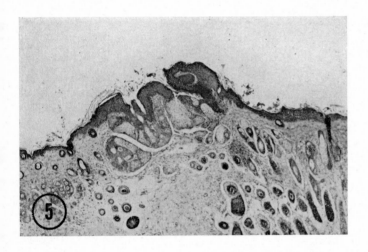

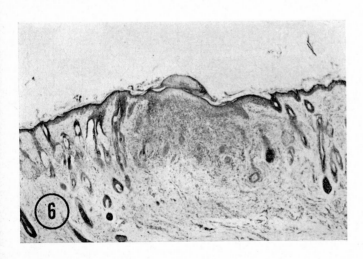

FIG. 4–6. Papilloma development in control hosts (Group B) shown at 17, 35 and 39 days respectively, after grafting MCA-treated skin. Hematoxylin and eosin. × 40.

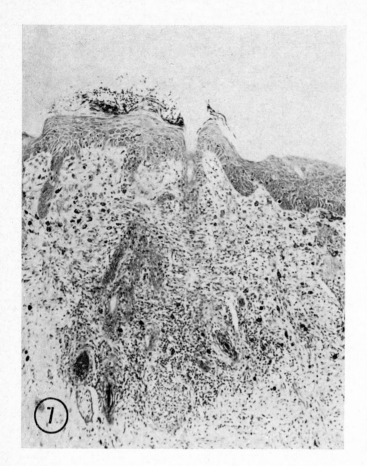

FIG. 7. High power view of section taken peripheral to the lesion shown in Fig. 6. Toluidine blue. × 90.

similar to those seen in immunologically depressed hosts were present by the 17th day after grafting in immunologically competent hosts (Group A or B). Fig. 4 shows a focal region of hyperplasia with possible peg formation in a control host grafted 17 days previously (compare to Fig. 1). In contrast to depressed hosts, macroscopic papillomas were not commonly seen in immunologically competent hosts until after the 4th week postgrafting. Fig. 5 shows a papilloma from a control host in Group B as it appeared 35 days after grafting. There is a small focus of mononuclear cells to the right of the picture. Focal areas of intense lymphocytic infiltration were found during the latent period of papilloma development in competent but not depressed hosts. One such lesion is shown in Fig. 6. A focal region of lymphocytes extends into the overlying hyperplastic epithelium. Note the presence of a parakeratotic cap and apparent obliteration of the dermal-epithelial junction.

A high-power view of an area peripheral to the lesion shown in Fig. 6 shows the characteristic infiltrate seen in similar inflammatory foci (Fig. 7). There is a dense cloud of lymphocytes peppered with plump, dark staining mast cells. Some lymphocytes can be found in the epithelium of the lesion. A comparable pattern of inflammation has previously been reported for macroscopic papillomas undergoing regression (5, 12).

This type of inflammatory response was found exclusively in grafts made to immunologically competent hosts. The stromal response to microscopic papillomas similar to those in Fig. 2 and 3 in X-irradiated or ALS-treated hosts is shown in Fig. 8 and 9, respectively. In contrast to the inflammatory response seen in grafts sectioned from Groups A and B, grafts in mice subjected to sublethal radiation or ALS (Groups C and D) exhibited essentially no mononuclear cells for the first three weeks after grafting. However, the presence of mast cells in the dermis around the bases of the papillomas was apparent. The pronounced dermal fibroplasia is characteristic of grafts made to both types of depressed hosts.

It has previously been established that the presence of a lymphocyte exocytosis (lymphocytes in skin epithelium) may signify a papilloma regression site, especially when such sites are found in conjunction with dermal keratin debris from former epithelial pearls (5). Two such sites found in MER-stimulated hosts 25 and 39 days after grafting are shown in Fig. 10 and 11. Only Fig. 10 can be identified with reasonable certainty as representing the residua of a former microscopic papilloma, because Fig. 11 lacks the keratin debris typical of papilloma regression sites.

Corroboration of this interpretation depends on the demonstration that such keratin is characteristically associated with the immunological destruction of micropapillomas. Fig. 12 and 13 show low and high power views of such a papilloma found 39 days after grafting MCA-treated skin to control hosts (Group B). The pictures show a denuded keratin pearl in the wake of a lymphocytic infiltration in the dermis of the papilloma.

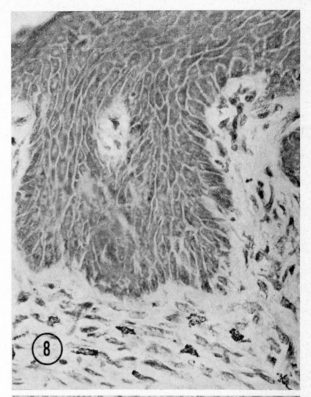

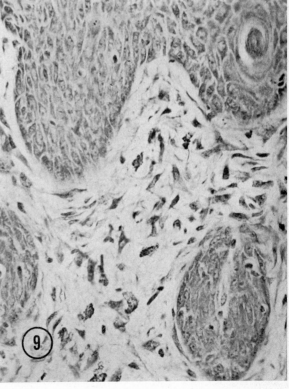

FIG. 8, 9. High power views of the stroma beneath papillomas similar to Fig. 3 developing in X-irradiated (Group C) or ALS-treated (Group D) hosts, respectively (21 days after grafting). Toluidine blue. × 350.

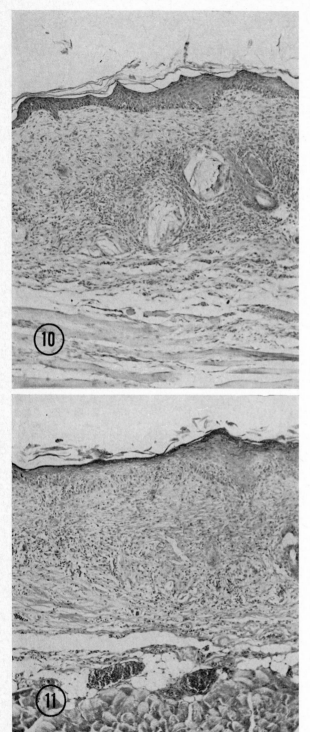

A high power view of the clump of epithelium indicated by the arrows in Fig. 12 and 13 is shown in Fig. 14. Large hyperplastic cells with prominent nucleoli present are seen in the center of the clump. Cells in the periphery where lymphocytes may be seen appear irregular and pyknotic. This pattern is interpreted as indicating immunologic destruction of the epithelium since it has not been observed in immunologically depressed hosts and is routinely seen in papillomas undergoing regression. An epithelial clump found in the dermis beneath a microscopic lesion similar to the one shown in Fig. 6 is shown in Fig. 15 for comparison. The pictures show the similarity in structure of the epithelial cells and the presence of mononuclear cells in the periphery. This type of appearance reinforces the impression of active immunologic destruction of micropapillomas in immunologically competent hosts.

The composition of the inflammatory infiltrate around such epithelial clumps includes both mononuclear cells and mast cells in immunologically competent hosts. Fig. 16 shows a portion of a microscopic papilloma in a MER-stimulated host as it appears with a toluidine blue stain. Lightly granulated mast cells are found to the right and below the clump, along with a mixed population of inflammatory cells. The picture shows the irregular outline of the clump and the pyknotic appearance of the epithelial cells; these cells should be compared with the more uniform hyperplastic cells within the epithelium to the left. The close association of mast cells with degenerating epithelial clumps is shown in Fig. 17. This is a high power view of Fig. 7, thought to represent the residua of a micro-

FIG. 10, 11. Focal inflammatory lesions showing lymphocyte exocytoses in MER-stimulated hosts (Group A) (39 days after grafting). Hematoxylin and eosin. × 90.

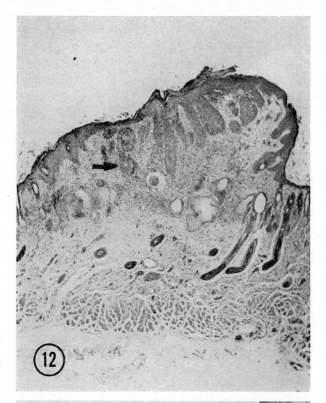

FIG. 12. Low power scan of submacroscopic papilloma undergoing lymphocytic infiltration shown 39 days after grafting to recipient in Group A. Hematoxylin and eosin. × 37.

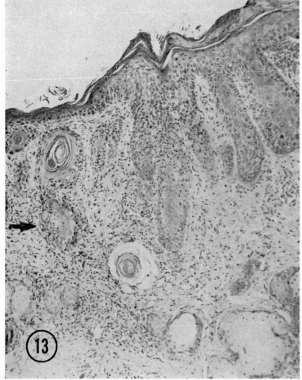

FIG. 13. Higher power view of a portion of the same lesion. Note presence of denuded keratin pearl and epithelial clump surrounded by lymphocytes. Hematoxylin and eosin. × 90.

59

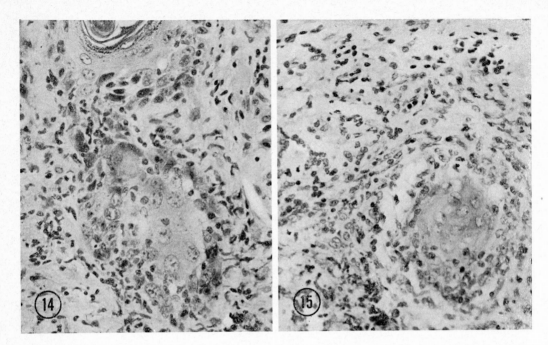

FIG. 14, 15.   Epithelial clumps in immunologically competent hosts (Groups B). Compare Fig. 14, which is a high power view of the clump shown in Fig. 13, with Fig. 15, which is a clump found in a focal inflammatory lesion. Note the dense mononuclear cell infiltrate in both lesions. Hematoxylin and eosin. × 310.

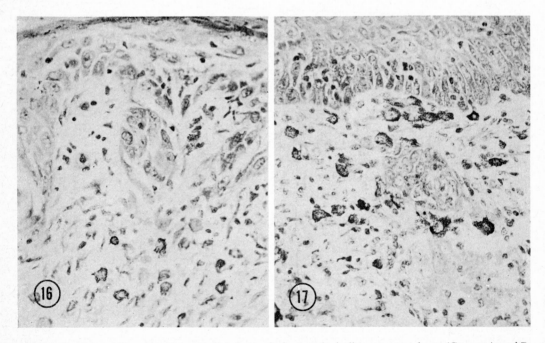

FIG. 16, 17.   Mast cell response to epithelial clumps in immunologically competent hosts (Groups A and B, respectively). Note the irregular outline of the clumps and the presence of pyknotic cells. Toluidine blue. × 310.

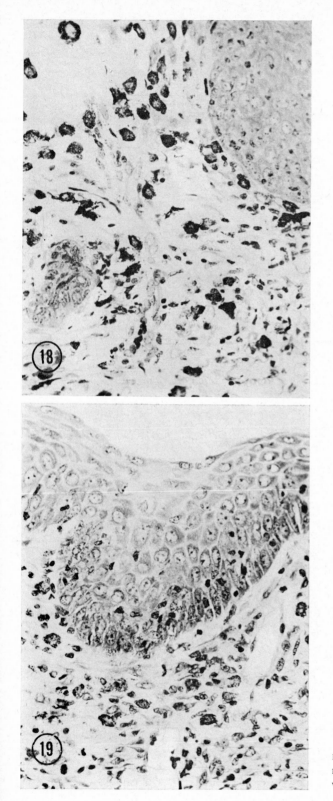

FIG. 18, 19.   Mast cell response in papilloma regression sites (Group B). Compare with Fig. 16 and 17. Toluidine blue. × 350.

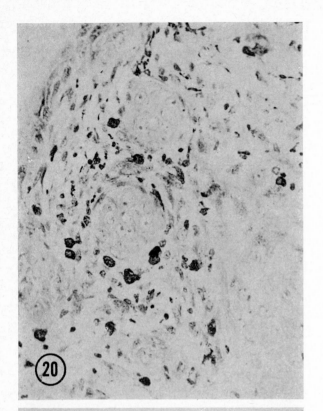

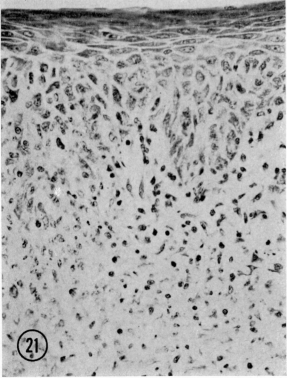

FIG. 20. Mast cell response to epithelial clumps in immunologically depressed hosts (Group C). Note the regular outline of the clumps and the good condition of the epithelial cells within them. Compare with Fig. 16 and 17. Toluidine blue. × 350.

FIG. 21. Mononuclear cell response in a malignant lesion recorded 39 days after grafting MCA-treated skin to a recipient in Group A. Note the complete absence of mast cells. Toluidine blue. × 350.

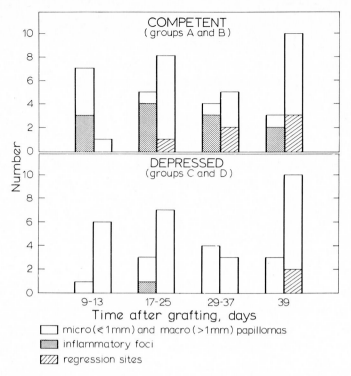

FIG. 22. Microscopic (left column) and macroscopic (right column) lesions in grafts transplanted to immunologically competent and depressed hosts.

scopic papilloma. The presence of mononuclear cells in the epithelium of this lesion is noted.

Fig. 18 and 19 show the mast cell and inflammatory response accompanying the regression of macroscopic papillomas in immunologically competent hosts. There is a halo of what appear to be degranulated mast cells around an epithelial clump in Fig. 18.

Mast cells also occur in close proximity to the hyperplastic epithelium of micropapillomas in immunologically depressed hosts. Fig. 20 shows an area beneath such a papilloma in an X-irradiated host. There is a definite uniformity of the cells within the two epithelial clumps, and a healthy regularity of their outlines. A few mononuclear cells are present to the left of the clumps. The characteristic plumpness of the mast cells here is in

contrast to those seen previously in immunologically competent hosts.

Several of the lesions seen soon after grafting appeared to be malignant. In contrast to the papillomas described above, these lesions completely lacked a mast cell response, although mononuclear responses were common. Shown in Fig. 21 is one such lesion; the basement membrane present to the right of the figure is lost in the left, and the cells exhibit marked atypia; there is a striking loss of polarity. Monocytes permeate the lesion but mast cells are absent.

Quantitation of lesions. Fig. 22 shows the frequency of occurrence of the major types of lesions recorded during the histological study. The lesions are divided into three categories: 1) intact microscopic and macroscopic papillomas (similar to Fig. 2 and 12 respectively);

63

2) inflammatory foci (similar to Fig. 6); 3) regression sites (similar to Fig. 10)*

The data are presented in two columns which represent microscopic (left) and macroscopic (right) lesions. Focal inflammatory lesions are scored in the "microscopic" column. For ease of comparison, the data from Groups A and B, and from Groups C and D were pooled to give profiles of papilloma development in "competent" and "depressed" hosts, respectively. Each pair of columns shown for a given interval represents the total number of lesions seen in serial sections examined from 13 to 17 grafts.

In the first interval (nine to 13 days), there were more microscopic lesions (micropapillomas and inflammatory foci) in competent hosts (total of seven) than in depressed hosts (total of one). Conversely, there were more macroscopic papillomas in depressed hosts than there were in competent hosts (total of six papillomas vs. one, respectively). It is noteworthy that both microscopic and macroscopic papillomas showed more inflammation in competent hosts than in depressed hosts at this time.

At each of the successive intervals (17 to 25; 29 to 37; and 39 days) there were approximately the same number of lesions in the microscopic columns of both groups. However, in competent hosts, most of these lesions were inflammatory foci (stippled) rather than intact microscopic papillomas (white).

The total number of microscopic and macroscopic papillomas recorded in competent hosts was 25 out of a total of 62 grafts (0.40 papillomas per graft) compared to 34 papillomas in the 56 grafts made to depressed hosts (0.61 papillomas per graft). This difference in papilloma incidence is highly significant ($t = 2.50$, $P < 0.01$) and is in keeping with previously reported results (5). The de-

ficit of papillomas in competent hosts can be accounted for by considering the numbers of microscopic inflammatory foci observed in both groups. When inflammatory foci are included in the tabulation of papilloma group totals, there are actually comparable numbers of lesions in the competent and depressed groups (37 and 35 respectively). This observation is consistent with the possibility that in competent hosts a portion of the incipient papillomas were destroyed at a microscopic level and were later scored as "inflammatory foci."

Taken together with the previous histological observations (5, 6), these data strongly suggest that the inflammatory foci reported here actually represent the residua of immunologically destroyed tumors predicted by the theory of immunological surveillance. This study thus reinforces the immunological interpretations given by various investigators to explain the results of studies showing longer papilloma latencies (2, 4, 5) or lower papilloma incidences (3, 5) in immunologically competent, relative to depressed, hosts.

DISCUSSION

The paucity of previous reports of microscopic foci or nodules (cf. 13) can now be explained. Microscopic foci of papilloma regression probably undergo a relatively rapid restitution. Both in the rabbit (14) and in the mouse (6), the debris accompanying macroscopic papilloma regression (mostly dermal keratin) is cleared within several days of the observed dissolution of a lesion. As Rous has previously emphasized (13, 14), papilloma regression (in the rabbit) leads to a complete restoration of a normal appearing epithelium within a few weeks of the initial event.

The apparent success of the search for microscopic foci in this study may be attributed in part to the opportunity afforded by the graft-promotion test system to confine observations to a strictly limited period during

---

* Regression sites were scored only where macroscopic papillomas had been previously recorded.

papilloma development. In addition, the presence of keratin debris from epithelial pearls undergoing destruction provided a suitable marker for detecting regression sites at both the microscopic and macroscopic level.

Observations of similar inflammatory foci in mice resistant to skin carcinogenesis such as those of Cramer and Simpson (15) and Okamoto (16), may be seen in retrospect as probable reports of immunologic surveillance. Both of these studies stressed the importance of mast cells in the generation of "host resistance" to carcinogenesis. The current findings also suggest a role for mast cells in the destruction of microscopic skin tumors. Mast cell degranulation may accompany papilloma regression on both a macroscopic (5) and microscopic level. Although such degranulation may be due to a variety of nonspecific causes, degranulation is also commonly caused by a specific local immune reaction (17). The absence of mast cells in malignant skin tumors (see Fig. 21) is consistent with the observation that successful immunological surveillance occurs almost exclusively at the premalignant level in this system (12). These facts, coupled with the recent demonstration that mast cell proliferation follows antigenic stimulation (18), suggest that mast cells may indeed form part of the total immunologic surveillance system against cancer.

This study has demonstrated the likely occurrence of the type of microscopic events originally predicted by Burnet (1), by using the system of isograft-promotion of MCA-treated skin. Whether or not it will be possible to demonstrate immunological surveillance against strictly autochthonous tumors remains to be determined.

Supported by a grant from the Anna Fuller Fund and in part by NIH Research Grant CA-05388 from the National Cancer Institute of the United States.

REFERENCES

1. BURNET, F. M. Immunologic recognition of self. *Science* **133**: 307, 1961.
2. MILLER, J. F. A. P., GRANT, G. A. and ROE, F. J. C. Effect of thymectomy on the induction of skin tumours by 3,4 benzopyrene. *Nature (Lond.)* **199**: 920, 1963.
3. GRANT, G., ROE, F. J. C. and PIKE, M. C. Effect of neonatal thymectomy on the induction of papillomata and carcinomata by 3,4 benzopyrene in mice. *Nature (Lond.)* **210**: 603, 1966.
4. JOHNSON, S. Effect of thymectomy on the induction of skin tumors by dibenzanthracene and of breast tumors by dimethylbenzanthracene in mice of the 1F strain. *Brit. J. Cancer* **22**: 755, 1969.
5. LAPPÉ, M. A. Evidence for the antigenicity of papillomas induced by 3-methylcholanthrene. *J. nat. Cancer Inst.* **40**: 823, 1968.
6. LAPPÉ, M. A. The role of immunologic surveillance during skin carcinogenesis in the mouse. Ph.D. thesis, University of Pennsylvania, 1968.
7. BURNET, F. M. Immunological factors in the process of carcinogenesis. *Brit. med. Bull.* **20**: 154, 1964.
8. BURNET, F. M. Immunological aspects of malignant disease. *Lancet* **i**: 1171, 1967.
9. THOENES, G. H. A simplified method for skin grafting. *Proc. Soc. exp. Biol. (N.Y.)* **132**: 68, 1969.
10. LEVEY, R. H. and MEDAWAR, P. B. Nature and mode of action of antilymphocytic serum. *Proc. nat. Acad. Sci. (Wash.)* **56**: 1130, 1966.
11. PEARSE, A. G. E. "Histochemistry: theoretical and applied," 2nd edn. London, J. and A. Churchill Ltd., 1960.
12. LAPPÉ, M. A. and PREHN, R. T. Immunologic surveillance at the macroscopic level: Nonselective elimination of premalignant skin papillomas. *Cancer Res.* **29**: 2374, 1969.
13. ROUS, P. The challenge to man of the neoplastic cell. *Science* **157**: 24, 1967.
14. ROUS, P. and KIDD, J. G. Conditional neoplasms and neoplastic states. A study of the tar tumor of the rabbit. *J. exp. Med.* **73**: 365, 1941.
15. CRAMER, W. and SIMPSON, W. L. Mast cells in experimental skin carcinogenesis. *Cancer Res.* **4**: 601, 1944.
16. OKAMOTO, Y. Stromal response in relation to invading forms of tumors. A histochemical and histopathological study. *Gann* **57**: 563, 1966.
17. CARTER, P. B., HIGGINBOTHAN, R. D. and DOUGHERTY, T. F. The local response of tissue mast cells to antigen in sensitized mice. *J. Immunol.* **79**: 259, 1957.
18. MILLER, J. J. and COLE, L. J. Proliferation of mast cells after antigenic stimulation in adult rats. *Nature (Lond.)* **217**: 263, 1968.

IMMUNOSUPPRESSIVE ACTIVITY OF THE ONCOGENIC PURINE DERIVATIVE 3-HYDROXYXANTHINE

M. N. TELLER and I. SMULLYAN

Division of Experimental Chemotherapy, Sloan-Kettering Institute for Cancer Research, New York, New York, USA

ABSTRACT

The immunosuppressive activity of the purine derivative 3-hydroxyxanthine was tested in rats, in which it is oncogenic. The reported immunosuppressants 3-methylcholanthrene, cortisone and cyclophosphamide, were included for comparisons and for positive controls. 3-hydroxyxanthine and 3-methylcholanthrene were only moderately active in depressing hemagglutinin antibody formation and homograft response. Cortisone, which was only moderately active in depressing antibody response, effectively reduced homograft response to permit growth of the mouse sarcoma 180 in rats. Cyclophosphamide, tested only for antibody suppression, was highly active. Cortisone increased tumor incidence and decreased tumor latency in rats treated with 3-hydroxyxanthine.

INTRODUCTION

The purine N-oxide derivative 3-hydroxyxanthine (1) was reported by Brown et al. (2), Sugiura and Brown (3) and Sugiura et al. (4) to be oncogenic in rats. Its ability to induce tumors at the subcutaneous site of injection and in the liver was confirmed by Teller et al. (5). Since immunodepressive activities have been shown for several chemical oncogens (6–13), the question of such activity for oncogenic purine N-oxides is relevant. This communication describes initial studies in which the effects of 3-hydroxyxanthine on both humoral and cellular immune responses in rats were measured. The moderate effect produced by this compound on immune reactivities led to an experiment to determine the effect of additional immune depression by cortisone on initiation and progression of neoplasms.

MATERIALS AND METHODS

Host. Young male CFN Wistar Rats (Carworth, New York, N.Y.) were used in tests for immune reactivity. Young male CD Sprague-Dawley rats were used for tumor induction (Charles River Breeding Laboratories, Wilmington, Del.).

Antibody titers. The hemagglutinin antibody test of Nathan et al. (14) was followed. Blood was collected from the hearts of ether-anesthetized rats 12 days after i.p. injection of the antigen, tanned sheep red blood cells. Titration of the blood serum was performed on each individual sample by serial twofold dilutions, and the titers were recorded as $\log_2$ of the reciprocal of the highest dilution showing microscopic hemagglutination. The time of administration of test compound is stated in relation to injection of antigen on day 0, and when given prior to day 0, is preceded by a minus sign. Where averages for two tests are given, the differences in titers were less than two tubes in the twofold dilution series.

Compounds. 3-hydroxyxanthine was prepared as a homogenized suspension in 0.5% carboxymethylcellulose in physiologic saline (CMC) so that the dose was administered in 0.5 ml of diluent. 3-methylcholanthrene (MC) was dissolved in sesame oil by heating in a water bath, and the dose was contained in 0.2 ml of oil. MC was administered two days before administration of antigen (12). Cyclophosphamide was injected immediately after it was dissolved in saline. Cortisone acetate was used as received (CORTONE® acetate, saline suspension). All compounds were injected s.c.

Homograft. The mouse tumor sarcoma 180 (S180) growing subcutaneously in the randomly bred Swiss mouse (Taconic Swiss Farms, Germantown, N.Y.) was used to measure homograft response in the rat. Although this is actually a heterograft, the response is usually spoken of as "homograft" reactivity. The tumor, removed from a mouse seven to nine days after implantation by trocar, was minced and prepared as a 50% suspension in saline. One-half ml of the tumor suspension was transplanted s.c. in the right flank of rats. The rats were killed seven days after tumor transplantation and the injection sites were examined grossly for tumor growth. Growth was classified as follows: a) negative, no growth; b) positive, type 1: solid, viable tumor tissue growing progressively; c) positive, type 2: mostly necrotic tumor tissue containing at least one area (usually a nodule) of viable tumor tissue.

Tumor induction. 3-hydroxyxanthine was injected s.c. in the interscapular area at a dose of 7 mg once a week for eight weeks. The rats were palpated for masses weekly until they died or were sacrificed at the termination of the experiment (18 months). Masses and grossly abnormal tissues were removed and examined microscopically after preparation and staining with hematoxylin and eosin.

Statistical evaluation. The significance of the differences between groups was determined according to Mainland and Murray (15).

RESULTS

Effects on hemagglutinin antibody. Young adult male CFN rats were treated at various intervals with single or multiple doses of 3-hydroxyxanthine to determine the effect on antibody formation. The oncogen MC, given as a single dose of 1 mg two days before injection of the sheep red blood cells, was included in the experiment because it is known to depress immune reactivity and to produce tumors at this dose. Cortisone and cyclophosphamide, also known immunosuppresants (16), were also included to provide additional positive controls for the hemagglutination test. Direct comparisons of the several results are not possible because it was not feasible to run all tests in parallel.

3-hydroxyxanthine depressed hemagglutinin antibody formation moderately when 7 mg were given on day 2, or with 1 mg given three times a week for two weeks (Table 1). Antibody titers were decreased moderately in those rats treated with 6 mg MC, a very high dose, but not in those treated with 1 mg. A similar titer was obtained with cortisone, but only when it was administered on days −4 and 3. However, cyclophosphamide almost completely suppressed antibody formation at the dose used (17).

Effects on homograft response. A suspension of minced S180 was implanted s.c. in young adult male CFN rats. At various intervals, groups of 10 rats were treated with 3-hydroxyxanthine or MC to determine their effects on homograft response. Cortisone-treated rats were also included as positive controls. In these experiments, all rats were sacrificed seven days after tumor transplantation. The results of two experiments are presented in Table 2.

The tumor developed in approximately the same numbers of rats following the different treatments in Experiment I. The numbers of tumors in any treated group did not differ significantly from those in the control groups, although there may have been a trend toward larger numbers in the treated animals. In

TABLE 1. *Effects of 3-hydroxyxanthine, MC, cortisone and cyclophosphamide on hemagglutinin antibody production in rats injected i.p. on day 0 with sheepred blood cells*

Compound	Dose (amount/injection)	Days administered[a]	No. of rats	Mean titer (log_2)	Remarks
3-hydroxyxanthine	7 mg	-4	5	8.3	
		-2	4	9.0	
		0	5	9.8	
		2	10	5.6	Average of 2 tests
	1 mg	-4, -2, 0, 3, 5, 7	5	5.6	
		-2, 0, 2, 5, 7, 9	4	7.3	
		0, 2, 4, 7, 9, 11	4	8.0	1 rat not responding was omitted
		2, 5, 7, 9	4	7.5	
MC	6 mg	-2	5	5.4	
		4	5	6.8	
	1 mg	-2	10	8.4	Average of 2 tests
Cortisone	20 mg	-1, 6	6	10.5	
		0, 7	5	9.0	
		-4, 3	5	4.4	
Cyclophosphamide	2.6 mg	-4 (hr), 1, 2, 3, 4	5	0.6	No titer in 3 rats
Sesame oil	0.2 ml	-2	10	9.1	Average of 2 tests
Saline	0.8 ml	-1, 6	5	12.0	
		0, 7	3	10.3	
CMC	0.5 ml	0, 2, 4, 7, 9, 11	5	9.2	
Untreated, unimmunized controls			5	0.4	No titer in 4 rats

[a] Precedence by a minus sign indicates time of administration prior to injection of antigen on day 0.

TABLE 2. *Effects of 3-hydroxyxanthine, 3-methylcholanthrene and cortisone on the growth of mouse tumor S180 in CFN rats*

Experiment	Treatment Compound	Dose (amount/injection)	Days administered[a]	Tumor growth[b] Type 1	Type 2	Total (%)
I	3-hydroxyxanthine	7 mg	-1	4	1	50
			0	2	3	50
		1 mg	0, 2, 5	2	0	20
	3-methylcholanthrene	1 mg	-2	2	2	40
	Cortisone	3 mg	0	4	0	40
	Sesame oil	0.2 ml	-2			
	CMC	0.5 ml	0, 2, 5	1	0	10
II	3-hydroxyxanthine	7 mg	0	1	7	80
		1 mg	0, 2, 4	1	4	50
	3-methylcholanthrene	1 mg	-2	2	0	20
	Cortisone	8 mg	0	10	0	100
		3 mg	0, 2, 4	6	3	90
	Sesame oil	0.2 ml	-2	0	2	20
	Saline	0.125 ml	0, 2, 4	0	0	0
	CMC	0.5 ml	0, 2, 4	0	2	20
	Untreated			2	1	30

[a] Precedence by a minus sign indicates time of administration prior to injection of antigen on day 0.
[b] Gross observation of tumor growth in 10 rats per group on day 7.

TABLE 3. *Effect of cortisone on tumor induction in male rats treated with 3-hydroxyxanthine*

Treatment	No. of rats	No. with tumors (cumulative) Month														% incidence
		5	6	7	8	9	10	11	12	13	14	15	16	17	18	
3-hydroxyxanthine[a]	20	0	2	3	6	6	7	—	—	—	7	8	—	8	9	45
3-hydroxyxanthine plus cortisone[b]	20	2	6	10	13	17	18	—	—	—	—	—	—	—	18	90
CMC plus cortisone	10	0	—	—	—	—	—	—	—	—	—	—	—	—	0	0

[a] 3-hydroxyqanthine in CMC was injected s.c. at a dose of 7 mg once weekly for eight weeks.
[b] Cortisone acetate in saline was administrated s.c. at a dose of 20 mg immediately after injection of 3-hydroxy xanthine.

Experiment II (Table 2), the results were essentially similar except for rats treated with cortisone. When 3 mg were administered on three alternate days, tumors grew in 90% of the hosts. When a single dose of 8 mg was given on the day of tumor implantation, neoplasms appeared in 100%. These results were significantly different from those for the controls ($P \leq 0.05$). In addition, the largest number of large, actively growing tumors (type 1) was in the cortisone-treated rats.

Effect on tumor induction. Experiments I and II indicate that, under the experimental conditions used, the immunosuppressive effects of 3-hydroxyxanthine were, at most, moderate. It was of interest, therefore, to determine the effects of additional immunodepression on tumor induction by this oncogen. For this purpose, 7 mg of 3-hydroxyxanthine were given once a week for eight weeks because this dose had previously been found to induce a 50% tumor incidence at the site of injection in 18 months (5). Cortisone was injected in a distal area shortly after each administration of 3-hydroxyxanthine.

Tumor incidence was 90% in rats treated with 3-hydroxyxanthine in combination with cortisone (Table 3). The 50% incidence point occurred at seven rather than at 18 months in the absence of cortisone, and 18/20 rats bore tumors by the 10th month. No tumors developed at the site of injection in the controls.

DISCUSSION

Few reports are available regarding the possible immunosuppressive activity of purine N-oxides. Brown et al. (18) reported no depression of hemagglutinin antibody in rats treated with 6-mercaptopurine 3-N-oxide, which has low oncogenic activity (3). Southam et al. (19) found that neither guanine 3-oxide nor 3-hydroxyxanthine, both potent oncogens (2–5) enhanced papilloma incidence in Swiss mice painted with MC.

The results reported here suggest that the immunosuppressive activity of 3-hydroxyxanthine is, at most, only moderate. Admittedly, this conclusion was reached with reservations because of the limited number of dose schedules and tests used. Administration of 3-hydroxyxanthine centered chronologically around injection of the antigen because of the report that 75% of the radioactivity of the labeled oncogen given s c. in the rat was accounted for in the urine by 6 hr and virtually all of it by 24 hr (20). The number, size of doses and time of administration of 3-hydroxyxanthine were those usually employed in tests for oncogenicity, i.e., 7 mg once a week or 1 mg 3 times weekly for a number of weeks. These schedules have been found to

69

provide high tumor incidences (5 and un-published results). The competence of the test system for hemagglutinin antibody was evidenced by the effectiveness of cyclophosphamide (Table 1). However, the lack of a greater immunosuppressive activity by cortisone (and MC) perhaps indicates the importance of the time the test agent is administered in relation to the antigen. It is of interest in this regard that Rubin (10) reported humoral antibody formation was not decreased by MC, whereas Stjernswärd (12), who used the spleen cell plaque-forming assay, noted decreased antibody-forming potential in mice treated with this substance.

Mouse tumor S180 was selected for measurements of homograft response because of previous experience with its growth characteristics in rats (21). The effect of 3-hydroxy-xanthine on the homograft response was only moderate, as revealed by the number of type 1 tumors seen at autopsy (Table 2). Cortisone, as expected, was effective, but few tumors developed in rats treated with 1 mg MC. In another, similar test with a small number of rats, a single dose of 6 mg MC resulted in tumor growths no different from those in the controls.

Cortisone very effectively increased tumor incidence of 3-hydroxyxanthine-treated rats from an expected maximum of about 50% at 18 months to 90% by 10 months, with a 50% incidence point at seven months. Whether 3-hydroxyxanthine and cortisone do, in fact, act in conjunction with respect to immunodepressive activity remains to be determined.

Reports that suppression of the immune responses potentiates chemical and viral tumor induction provide impressive evidence that host immunity does play a major role in neoplastic transformations and in the progression of neoplastic disease. Interest in the immunological parameter of oncogenesis was stimulated by the work of Miller et al. (22), among others, who reported the effect of thymectomy on tumor induction in mice; by the experiments of Davidsohn and Stern (23) describing a possible relationship between susceptibility to spontaneous tumors and general immunologic reactivity; by the investigations of Malmgren et al. (8), Davidsohn et al. (6), Rubin (10), Prehn (9) and Stjernswärd (11) on the immunosuppressive effects of chemical oncogens and of Peterson et al. (24) for viral oncogens; and by the studies of Teller et al. (25) regarding interrelationships between aging, immunity and cancer.

There are many facets that need to be explored more deeply, such as the chemical induction of tumors by quantities of agents not leading to measurable immunosuppressive effects, and determination of the degree of immunosuppression required for the initiation and progressive growth of neoplastic cells.

The foregoing, therefore, makes it imperative to study new oncogens from the viewpoint of immunosuppressive activity. In this way the possible relationship between oncogenicity and immunosuppressive activity might be elucidated.

We are indebted to Drs. C. C. Stock and G. B. Brown for helpful discussions, and to Dr. G. Stohr for gross and histological examinations. The technical assistance of E. Bruno is gratefully acknowledged. We are grateful, too, for generous supplies of the following: S180 tumor from Dr. G. S. Tarnowski and S. Banks; cyclophosphamide from the Cancer Chemotherapy National Service Center, National Cancer Institute; and cortisone (Cortone acetate) from Merck & Co., Inc.

Supported in part by National Cancer Institute Grant CA 08748 and by Grant DRG-1014 from the Damon Runyon Memorial Fund for Cancer Research, Inc.

REFERENCES

1. Wölcke, U. and Brown, G. B. Purine N-oxides. XXII. On the structures of 3-hydroxy-xanthine and guanine 3-oxide. J. org. Chem. 34: 978, 1969.
2. Brown, G. B., Sugiura, K. and Cresswell, R. C.

Purine N-oxides. XVI. Oncogenic derivatives of xanthine and guanine. *Cancer Res.* **25**: 986, 1965.

3. SUGIURA, K. and BROWN, G. B. Purine N-oxides. XIX. On the oncogenic N-oxide derivatives of guanine and xanthine and a nononcogenic isomer of xanthine N-oxide. *Cancer Res.* **27**: 925, 1967.

4. SUGIURA, K., TELLER, M. N., PARHAM, J. C. and BROWN, G. B. Purine N-oxides. XXXII. A comparison of the oncogenicities of 3-hydroxyxanthine, guanine 3-N-oxide and some related compounds. *Cancer Res.* **30**: 184, 1970.

5. TELLER, M. N., STOHR, G. and DIENST, H. Purine N-oxides XXXI. Studies on the oncogenicity of 3-hydroxyxanthine. *Cancer Res.* **30**: 179, 1970.

6. DAVIDSOHN, I., STERN, K. and SABET, L. Immune responses in mice and rats exposed to carcinogens. *Proc. Amer. Ass. Cancer Res.* **2**: 102, 1956.

7. LINDER, O. E. A. Survival of skin homografts in methylcholanthrene-treated mice and in mice with spontaneous mammary cancers. *Cancer Res.* **22**: 380, 1962.

8. MALMGREN, R. A., BENNISON, B. E. and McKINLEY, T. W. Reduced antibody titers in mice treated with carcinogenic and cancer chemotherapeutic agents. *Proc. Soc. exp. biol. (N.Y.)* **79**: 484, 1952.

9. PREHN, R. T. Function of depressed immunologic reactivity during carcinogenesis. *J. nat. Cancer Inst.* **31**: 791, 1963.

10. RUBIN, B. A. Carcinogen-induced tolerance to homotransplantation. *Progr. exp. Tumor Res. (Basel)* **5**: 217, 1964.

11. STJERNSWÄRD, J. Immunodepressive effect of 3-methylcholanthrene. Antibody formation at cellular level and reaction against weak antigenic homografts. *J. nat. Cancer Inst.* **35**: 885, 1965.

12. STJERNSWÄRD, J. Immunosuppression by carcinogens. *Antibiot. et Chemother. (Basel)* **15**: 213, 1969.

13. PARMIANI, G., COLNAGHI, M. I. and DELLA PORTA, G. Immunodepressive and leukemogenic effects of urethan in C3Hf and SWR mice. *Proc. Soc. exp. Biol. (N.Y.)* **130**: 828, 1969.

14. NATHAN, H. C., BIEBER, S., ELION, G. B. and HITCHINGS, G. H. Detection of agents which interfere with the immune response. *Proc. Soc. exp. Biol. (N.Y.)* **107**: 796, 1961.

15. MAINLAND, D. and MURRAY, I. M. Tables for use in fourfold contingency tests. *Science* **116**: 591, 1952.

16. MAKINODAN, T., ALBRIGHT, J. F., PERKINS, E. H. and NETTESHEIM, P. Suppression of immunologic responses. *Med. Clin. N. Amer.* **49**: 1569, 1965.

17. SANTOS, G. W. and OWENS, A. H., JR. A comparison of the effects of selected cytotoxic agents on the primary agglutinin response in rats injected with sheep erythrocytes. *Bull. Johns Hopk. Hosp.* **114**: 384, 1964.

18. BROWN, G. B., LEVIN, G., MURPHY, S., SELE, A., REILLY, H. C., TARNOWSKI, G. S., SCHMID, F. A., TELLER, M. N. and STOCK, C. C. Purine N-oxides. XV. The synthesis of 6-mercaptopurine 3-N-oxide. Its chemotherapeutic possibilities. *J. med. Chem.* **8**: 190, 1965.

19. SOUTHAM, C. M., TANAKA, S., ARATA, T., SIMKOVIC, D., MIURA, M. and PETRAPULOS, S. F. Enhancement of responses to chemical carcinogens by nononcogenic viruses and antimetabolites. *Progr. exp. Tumor Res. (Basel)* **11**: 194, 1969.

20. MYLES, A. and BROWN, G. B. Purine N-oxides. XXX. Biochemical studies of the oncogen 3-hydroxyxanthine. *J. biol. Chem.* **244**: 4072, 1969.

21. TELLER, M. N., WOLFF, R. and WAGSHUL, S. F. Host-tumor-drug relationships in experimental chemotherapy systems with allogeneic and xenogeneic host-tumor combinations. *Cancer Res.* **24**: 114, 1964.

22. MILLER, J.F.A.P., GRANT, G. A. and ROE, F.J.C. Effect of thymectomy on the induction of skin tumors. *Nature (Lond.)* **199**: 920, 1963.

23. DAVIDSOHN, I. and STERN, K. Heterohemoantibodies in inbred strains of mice. II. Immune agglutinins and hemolysins for sheep and chicken red cells. *J. Immunol.* **72**: 216, 1954.

24. PETERSON, R. D. A., HENDRICKSON, R. and GOOD, R. A. Reduced antibody forming capacity during the incubation period of Passage A leukemia in C3H mice. *Proc. Soc. exp. Biol. (N.Y.)* **114**: 517, 1963.

25. TELLER, M. N., STOHR, G., CURLETT, W., KUBISEK, M. L. and CURTIS, D. Aging and cancerigenesis. I. Immunity to skin and tumor grafts. *J. nat. Cancer Inst.* **33**: 649, 1964.

26. BERENBAUM, M. C. Effects of carcinogens on immune processes. *Brit. med. Bull.* **20**: 159, 1964.

BASIC PROTEINS AND SYNTHETIC POLYNUCLEOTIDES AS MODIFIERS OF IMMUNOGENICITY OF SYNGENEIC TUMOR CELLS

WERNER BRAUN, OTTO J. PLESCIA, JANA RASKOVA and DAVID WEBB

Institute of Microbiology, Rutgers University, State University of New Jersey,
New Brunswick, New Jersey, USA

ABSTRACT

Immunization of mice with chemically or virally-induced syngeneic tumor cells, complexed electrostatically to methylated bovine γ-globulin or conjugated covalently to bovine γ-globulin, produced a degree of protective immunity against subsequent challenge with isologous tumor cells. Also, in animals sensitized with 2,4-dinitrophenyl bovine serum albumin immunization with tumor cell 2,4-dinitrophenyl conjugates evoked some protective immunity against subsequent challenge. However, such protective responses were not obtained under conditions similar to those encountered in clinical cases, i.e. when animals were first sensitized to the tumor cell line under test, by implantation and subsequent excision of tumor tissue. Under such conditions, immunization following excision tended to decrease rather than increase resistance to challenge. In an effort to modify host responses in sensitized animals in the direction of protection, and presumably cell-mediated immunity, the effects of polyadenylic-polyuridylic acid (poly A:U), a known nontoxic stimulator of antibody formation and of cell-mediated immunity, were explored. Treatment of mice with poly A:U, after excision of syngeneic chemically-induced tumor cells or at the time of implantation of virus-induced syngeneic tumor cells, resulted in a lesser frequency of recurrence or a reduced rate of tumor growth, respectively. The effects of poly A:U, a poor interferon inducer, were as good as those obtainable with a good interferon inducer, namely toxic and pyrogenic polyinosinic-polycytidylic acid. This finding strengthens the belief that the antitumor effects of synthetic polynucleotides are attributable to a stimulation of classical immune responses, rather than to interferon effects.

INTRODUCTION

The presence of specific antigens in virus-induced or carcinogen-induced tumors is no longer in doubt (1–10), but the capacity of such antigens to evoke protective immune responses in autochthonous or syngeneic hosts is often limited. Among the factors presumably responsible for the inability of such antigens to evoke strong protective immunity are: a) a lack of sufficient "foreignness" of tumor cell antigens, and hence their immunological inactivity (5, 8, 10), b) a high degree of dependence of protective immunity on cell-mediated immunity, rather than on humoral antibody formation,* and present difficulties to attain selective stimulation of cell-mediated responses (5, 11–16), and c) a weakening of specific or general immunological responsiveness of the host, particularly in terms of cell-mediated immunity, in the course of tumor growth (6, 14–16).

In an attempt to circumvent the first cited factor, i.e. poor immunogenicity, we utilized an approach based on a simple procedure that we developed several years ago in attempts to convert ordinarily non-immunogenic oligomers and polymers of nucleic acids into potent immunogens (17, 18). We discovered that complexing of nucleic acids with foreign basic proteins, either methylated bovine serum albumin (MBSA) or methylated bovine γ-globulin (MBGG), endowed the ordinarily non-immunogenic molecules with a capacity to induce good antibody responses in rabbits. The formation of the immunogenic complexes was the result of electrostatic interactions between the basic methylated proteins and the acidic nucleic acids, and it turned out that the same phenomenon could be utilized to develop or potentiate the immunogenicity of certain other acidic, ordinarily non-immunogenic substances (18, 19). Thus antibodies specific for pneumococcal capsular polysaccharide (Type III), hyaluronic acid, and poly-L-glutamic acid were produced in rabbits with ease following the injection of such polymers as complexes with MBSA. Since then, MBSA has been used by many investigators as a "carrier" for converting non-immunogens into immunogens (18, 20). Subsequently, one of us (O.J.P.) discovered, in studies with

rabbit heart and kidney cells, that the same methodology permits the production of antibody responses to allogeneic cell-associated antigens, and that the same unusual responsiveness also can be evoked if an animal is first sensitized to a hapten [e.g. 2,4-dinitrophenyl (DNP) coupled to BSA] and then immunized with homologous cells to which the hapten (e.g., DNP) has been conjugated (19).

These findings prompted us to explore the applicability of such procedures to the immunization of mice with syngeneic tumor cells complexed to a protein carrier or conjugated to a hapten. As will be shown in this communication, such immunizations resulted in protection, provided that the host had not been exposed, prior to immunization, to the tumor cells from which the vaccine had been prepared. Since previously sensitized animals tended to show a decrease in protection following immunization compared to non-immunized animals, we subsequently focused our attention on procedures that might modify host responsiveness, specifically in the direction of cell-mediated immunity, and explored the effects of the synthetic double-stranded polynucleotide polyadenylic-polyuridylic acid (poly A:U), a known stimulator of antibody formation (21) and cell-mediated immunity (22), on host responses to syngeneic tumor cells. The initial results of these tests also will be reported here.

MATERIALS AND METHODS

Animals and tumor cell lines. C3H and C57Bl mice were used for the production of sarcomas by s.c. injections of methylcholanthrene (MC) or dibenzanthracene (DBZ) into 90-day-old female or male animals. Rauscher leukemia virus-induced ascites tumor cells (MCDV-12) in Balb/c mice served as a model for a tumor cell population known to be associated with a virus. The chemically-induced tumors were maintained by passage in syngeneic mice at intervals of about two weeks, the cells being injected s.c.; in addition, new chemically induced tumor lines were isolated approximately every six months. The

---

* It is likely that some protective immunity can be achieved by cytotoxic humoral antibodies early in tumor development, i.e. during periods when single tumor cells predominate, whereas cell-mediated immunity attains a predominant protective role as the disease progresses.

MCDV-12 cell line was also maintained by passage, injecting them i.p. into Balb/c mice at five-day intervals.

Challenge with living tumor cells. For challenge with chemically-induced tumor cell lines, tissue removed from the site of tumor growth was cut, teased, and then treated with 0.01% collagenase for 90 min at 37 C on a shaker. The suspension was then filtered through gauze, washed twice with saline, diluted in Eagle's medium, and counted. At the same time, samples were exposed to 1% trypan blue and the percentage of stained cells ascertained. Any preparation containing more than 20% stained cells was discarded. Dilutions of acceptable suspensions were titrated in syngeneic recipients; the cells were injected s.c. and weekly measurements were made of the size of the tumors as they developed at the site of injection. In general, approximately 3×10^5 cells produced "takes" in 100% of the animals. Most of the tests were carried out with MC-induced tumors in C3H or C57Bl mice. For challenge with virus-induced ascites tumor cells, diluted suspensions of peritoneal exudate cells from mice that had been previously injected i.p. with MCDV-12 cells were implanted intradermally into Balb/c hosts, usually at a dosage of 2×10^6 cells/mouse.

Preparation of vaccines and mode of immunization. Tumor cell homogenates or whole tumor cells, obtained by treatment of solid tumors with 0.01% collagenase as described above, were mixed with MBGG at room temperature for 60 min. For 1 ml of a 20% (wet cell volume) homogenate, 0.3 ml of a 1% MBGG solution was used. For 1 ml of a 10% suspension of cells, 0.3 ml of a 1% MBGG solution was also used. In later experiments cells were first frozen and thawed three times and then treated with MBGG. MBGG was prepared according to the procedure of Sueoka (23). The protein-complexed cell material (0.2 ml) was then injected i.m. in complete Freund's adjuvant, and at the same time 0.02 ml of pertussis vaccine (Eli Lilly vaccine, USP, V-1035) was injected i.p. This immunization procedure was repeated at weekly intervals for three weeks; then the animals were allowed to rest for two weeks and a fourth injection was given, followed by challenge one week later. A number of variations in routes of immunization and dosages, as well as omission of complete Freund's adjuvant or pertussis vaccine, were tested, but since they did not lead to any significant change in results they will not be detailed here.

Polynucleotide treatment. Poly A:U and poly-inosinic-polycytidylic acid (poly I:C) were obtained from Miles Laboratories and were injected i.p., in quantities of either 300 or 600 μg/mouse, on indicated days prior to, and following, implantation of tumor cell populations.

Implantation and excision of tumor cell populations. Pieces of tumor were implanted s.c. in the dorsal region with the aid of a trochar. At time of excision of the tumor mass, all the grossly detectable growth and surrounding tissue was excised.

Complement fixation test. Standard procedures, using 3 C_{H50} hemolytic units, were employed.

RESULTS

Immunization prior to challenge with syngeneic tumor cells. At the time of initiation of these studies, we had completed experiments that had shown that rabbits immunized with 1% phenol-extracted, DNA-rich materials from MC-induced mouse tumor cells (induced in C57Bl), complexed with MBSA, produced antibodies to the complexed cells just as they did when immunized with allogeneic heart or kidney cells complexed with MBSA. We therefore tested the response to the MBSA-complexed DNA-rich tumor cell fractions in mice, and failed to obtain responses in C3H, C57Bl, A/J and DBA animals. Calf thymus DNA complexed to MBSA, which in rabbits evokes antibody formation (24), also failed to produce detectable antibody responses in these mice. Since mice are notoriously poor responders to BSA, but respond to BGG, we explored the capacity of MBGG-complexed DNA-rich preparations to evoke responses. Since pertussis vaccine is a stimulator of responses to BGG in mice, we administered the MBGG-complexed material in complete Freund's adjuvant together with an i.p. administration of pertussis vaccine. This procedure resulted in a response in mice as measured by complement-fixation, and we therefore proceeded to test the effects of immunization of C57Bl mice with MBGG-complexed homogenates of tumor cells that had been obtained after MC treatment of C57Bl mice. The vaccine was administered in complete Freund's adjuvant with simultaneous administration of pertussis vaccine. The mice thus immunized showed a production of circulating antibodies to tumor cell homogenates as measured by complement-fixation, but these immune responses were not accompanied by significant protective effects, and in fact they tended to be associated with enhancement of tumor growth in animals subsequently challenged with syngeneic living tumor cells.

More encouraging results were obtained with whole tumor cells. In these tests, C57Bl males were vaccinated with syngeneic MC-induced tumor cells complexed with MBGG, or conjugated covalently with BGG through bisdiazotized benzidene (BDB), or conjugated covalently with DNP. All animals were immunized i.m. using complete Freund's adjuvant, as described above. Such immunization did not produce any detectable evidence of tumor growth at the site of injection, indicating that the various treatments had resulted in an inactivation of most or all of the cells.

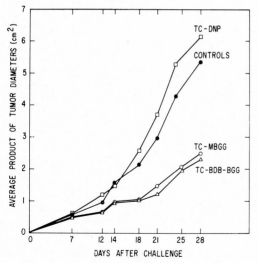

FIG. 1. Growth curves of tumors developing from isografts in C57Bl males immunized with 1) MC tumor cells BDB-BGG ($\triangle$); 2) MC tumor cells-DNP ($\blacksquare$); 3) MC tumor cells-MBGG (O). Non-immunized controls = ●.

The animals were challenged s.c., either with 1×10^6 or 3×10^5 collagenase-treated cells, one week after the last injection of vaccine. The results are presented in Fig. 1. It will be seen that differences in resistance became apparent only in some of the vaccinated groups challenged with 3×10^5 cells; challenge with 1×10^6 cells failed to reveal differences owing to the large inoculum. With the lower challenge dose, a slower rate of growth than in the non-vaccinated group was observed in the groups immunized with MBGG-complexed cells or with the BDB-BGG-conjugated tumor cells. In addition to these protective effects, evident from the large difference in the average size of the tumors, there were two animals in the MBGG group in which the growing tumors later regressed and disappeared.

Fig. 2 presents complement-fixation data for the experiment just described; the sera used were obtained from the animals just prior to challenge. A considerable variability in individual responses can be noted, but despite such variability there was clear evidence for the presence of complement-fixing antibodies (reacting with whole MC-C57Bl tumor cells) in all vaccinated groups. When these results are examined together with the protection data, a lack of correlation between complement-fixing antibodies and protection again becomes apparent. This is particularly true for the group vaccinated with MC-tumor cell-DNP. Mice in this group showed no immunity to challenge with viable tumor cells (cf. Fig. 1) but their sera contained complement-fixing antibody.

Since conjugation with DNP failed to elicit any protective effects, a modification of the immunization procedure was tested, utilizing a principle studied by Plescia in the case of other homologous antigens (9). The animals were first sensitized with DNP conjugated to BSA as a carrier. One week later, the sensitized animals were vaccinated with DNP-conjugated tumor cells, using the same immu-

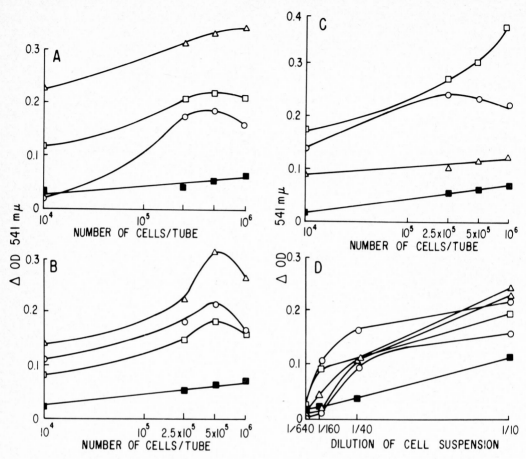

IG. 2. Analysis of mouse sera (C57Bl males) by complement-fixation The serum samples obtained from individual mice of a given immunization group were pooled into three groups, each pool containing the sera from five mice, except in group D (see below) which was divided into five subgroups of three each. The results for each pool are indicated by separate lines connecting the open symbols; results for the control sera (pre-immunization samples) are indicated by solid squares. A) Sera from animals immunized with MC-tumor cell-DNP; B) sera from animals immunized with MC-tumor cell-BDB-BGG; C) sera from animals immunized with MC-tumor cell-MBGG; D) sera from animals pretreated with BSA-DNP and then immunized with MC-tumor cell-DNP. Abscissa represents concentration of antigen, which was a suspension of tumor cells obtained from a solid tumor treated with collagenase, except for D in which mechanical disruption of tissue was employed. Ordinate represents a measure of complement-fixing antibody. A value of 0.350 represents complete fixation of complement added to test system.

nization schedule as described above. This procedure, sensitizing the mice to DNP prior to vaccinating them with tumor cell-DNP conjugate, was effective. They attained a degree of protection as measured in terms of the rate of growth of the tumor. The complement-fixation data for sera of these mice are shown in Fig. 2.

Similar results indicating that a degree of protection could be achieved when normal animals were immunized with MBGG-complexed or BGG-conjugated tumor cells were obtained in additional tests with other tumor cell lines that ordinarily produced no protective immunity, including virus-induced MCDV-12 tumor cells in Balb/c mice.

Immunization following sensitization to viable tumor tissue. An extension of the above described studies to tests in which the vaccine was prepared from one cell line and the challenge cells were derived from another line revealed that the achievable protection was specific for the cell line employed for immunization, and did not extend to independently derived tumor cell lines, including those induced by the same carcinogen in the same inbred strain of mice. In view of this confirmation of the antigenic individuality of independently derived tumor cell lines (25, 26), it became obvious that in the absence of common tumor antigens, the method of rendering tumor cells immunogenic by complexing with MBGG or by conjugation to carrier proteins could be of potential usefulness only in therapy rather than in prophylaxis. Accordingly we modified our test procedure to produce

conditions more like those encountered in clinical cases. Pieces of a given MC-induced tumor were implanted s.c. into syngeneic recipients and the resulting tumor growth was removed surgically seven to 10 days later. The animals were then divided into two groups, one of which received a vaccine prepared by freezing and thawing tumor cells which were then complexed with MBGG. The other group was not vaccinated and served as a control for efficacy of the vaccine. The vaccinated animals were immunized once a week for three weeks, and again two weeks after the third injection. One week after the last injection, all animals of this group and the control group that did not show recurrence of the original tumor growth were challenged with one of three graded doses of viable isologous tumor cells. Animals that had received neither the original tumor implant nor vaccine

TABLE 1. *Incidence of recurrence of excised tumors in vaccinated and nonvaccinated C57Bl female mice. Tumor cell line MC-14 (C57Bl)*

Group	% of animals showing recurrence of tumor at site of implantation on day				
	7	17	24	31	39 after excision
Tumor excised, nonvaccinated	22	35	44	48	48
Tumor excised, vaccinated	4	15	23	27	27

Average number of animals per group: 50

TABLE 2. *Incidence of tumor takes in C57Bl female mice after challenge with tumor cell line MC-14 (C57Bl)*

Group	Challenge dose	No. of animals/total no. showing takes on days				
		7	14	21	28	35 after challenge
Tumor excised, nonvaccinated	3×10^4	0/7	2/7	2/6	2/5	2/5
	1×10^5	2/6	2/5	2/5	2/5	2/5
	3×10^5	3/6	4/6	4/6	4/6	4/6
Tumor excised, vaccinated	3×10^4	1/6	2/6	2/4	2/4	2/4
	1×10^5	3/5	3/5	4/4	4/4	4/4
	3×10^5	5/5	5/5	5/5	5/5	5/5
No prior tumor, no vaccination (Controls)	3×10^4	8/10	9/10	10/10	10/10	10/10
	1×10^5	9/10	10/10	10/10	10/10	10/10
	3×10^5	9/9	9/9	9/9	9/9	9/9

served as controls for the viability of the challenge cells.

The results obtained in these experiments seemed to be dependent on the tumor cell line used. Three criteria were employed: 1) recurrence of the excised tumor at the site of implantation or metastasis or both, 2) percentage of take of the challenge and 3) rate of growth of the tumor resulting from challenge. An example of a positive effect in terms of criterion 1 is shown in Table 1. It should be noted, however, that in this experiment subsequent challenge did not reveal an increase in protection over that resulting from the initial tumor growth (Table 2); in fact, vaccinated animals showed a somewhat lower resistance than animals that had not been vaccinated following excision of the tumor

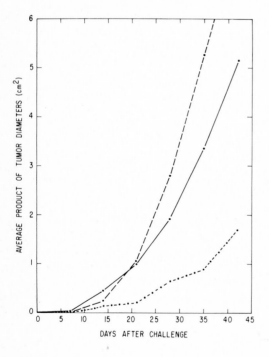

FIG. 3. Average rate of growth of tumors in C57Bl females following challenge with MC-14 (C57Bl) tumor cells (3×10^5/mouse). Three different groups of mice were used; untreated control group——; implant excised, immunized —·—; Implant excised, not immunized, – – –.

implant. However, their resistance, though diminished, was still appreciably greater than that of untreated animals. In terms of the average rate of growth of tumors in those animals showing positive takes (Fig. 3), it was observed that the growth rate was lower in animals of the excised, vaccinated group than in animals from the excised, nonvaccinated group. Animals of the excised, nonvaccinated group actually showed growth rates that were somewhat faster than the rate of growth of tumors in previously untreated controls. Similar results were obtained in tests with four other tumor cell lines derived from C3H and C57Bl mice.

Modification of host responses by polynucleotides. In view of the fact that vaccination following excision of a tumor implant tended to diminish host resistance conferred by the tumor implant against subsequent new challenge we searched for means of directing the response to tumor cell vaccines into a protective rather than an enhancing response. The most likely approach was to find ways of favoring the development of cell-mediated immunity rather than the formation of humoral antibody, which has long been suspected of being responsible for enhancement effects (26–32). Since we had evidence for the stimulatory effects of nontoxic, nonpyrogenic poly A:U on both antibody formation and cell-mediated immunity (21–22), we decided to test its influence on the frequency of recurrence of tumor growth in animals from which the tumor growth had been excised and also on the rate of growth of MCDV-12 ascites tumor cells in Balb/c mice.

For tests on the regrowth of excised tumor implants, we first had to determine the period of residence of the growing neoplastic tissue required for the attainment of partial and total protection against recurrence of tumor growth after removal of the primary focus. It was found, with tumor cell line MC-C57-15, that excision after three days provided little

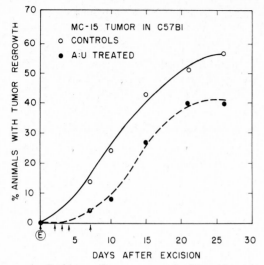

FIG. 4. Incidence of tumor regrowth (% positive animals) in C57Bl females following excision, E, of a MC-induced transplantable tumor. The tumor, implanted s.c. by trochar, was allowed to grow for four days prior to excision. Recurrence was judged by detection of measurable tumor growth. Poly A:U was injected i.v. (300 µg/mouse) on days indicated.

protection against recurrence; excision four or five days after implantation led to recurrence frequencies of 40 to 60%; and excision after seven days yielded a high degree of protection. Choosing the four-day period of growth prior to excision as a convenient parameter, animals were injected i.p. at the time of excision and on days thereafter, as shown in Fig. 4, with 300 µg poly A:U/mouse per day. As illustrated in Fig. 4, such treatment led to a reduction in the frequency of recurrence of tumor growth.

Poly A:U administration also suppressed the rate of growth of the MCDV-12 (Rauscher leukemia virus-induced) tumor cells in Balb/c mice. As illustrated in Fig. 5, maximum suppression occurred during the first week after implantation of the tumor cells, and i.p. injections of poly A:U one day before, on the day of implantation, and one day thereafter (–1, 0, +1) gave the best protection. Elimi-

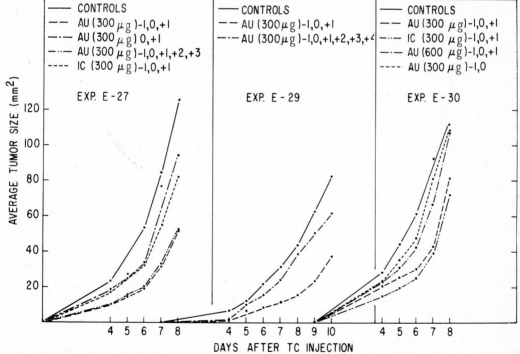

FIG. 5. Effect of poly A:U on growth of MCDV-12 ascites tumor cells in syngeneic Balb/c mice. Ascites cells (2 × 10⁶) were inoculated intradermally and the poly A:U was injected intravenously on the days and in the amounts indicated.

nation of the third injection $(+1)$ or the first injection (-1) reduced the effect. A prolonged series of injections (e.g., -1, 0, $+1$, $+2$, $+3$) did not improve the effects (Exp. E-27 in Fig. 5) or even reduced them (Exp. E-29 in Fig. 5). Doubling the amount of poly A:U given with each injection (i.e. 600 mμ instead of 300 mμ) reduced the effect instead of increasing it; this might be due to a stimulation of both the immune response and tumor cell multiplication by large amounts of polynucleotides. Nontoxic, nonpyrogenic poly A:U produced as good or even better effects than toxic and pyrogenic poly I:C (Fig. 5). Neither poly I:C nor poly A:U prevented death, presumably due to a generalized viremia, of the MCDV-12-infected Balb/c mice 10 to 12 days after the implantation of the tumor cells.

DISCUSSION

The foregoing results confirm prior observations on the potential immunogenicity of isogenic or autologous tumor cells (1–10), particularly when prevented from progressive growth by means such as excision (33), or under conditions of enhanced responsiveness of the host, or after modifications that result in a greater degree of foreignness of the neoplastic cell. Attempts to achieve the latter are no longer unique; a similar approach has been reported by Czajkowski et al. (34), Fahey et al. (35), and has also been considered by Attia and Weiss (30) as well as Cinader (36). However, an approach such as the one utilized by Czajkowski et al. depends on the chemical conjugation of foreign protein to components of the tumor cell membrane and thus might result in critical alterations in the structure of the tumor antigens. In contrast, basic proteins, which can complex with any acidic polymer, do so because of electrostatic interaction which does not lead to chemical denaturation of antigens of the tumor. In order to further avoid any undesirable auto-immune responses to normal antigens of tu-

mor cells, it would be desirable ultimately to utilize critical, purified tumor cell antigens, rather than the entire cell or its membrane, for the preparation of a vaccine evoking protective immune responses.

The utilization of synthetic polynucleotides for the stimulation of host resistance to syngeneic tumors is also no longer unique (37–40), but this approach was not prompted initially, as it was in our case, by attempts to increase cell-mediated immune responses, but rather by attempts to utilize the antiviral effects of certain synthetic polynucleotides (41–43). The actual results of the various successful tests of other workers indicated that the effects could not be due to interferon stimulation but must involve instead effects of these polynucleotides on other immune responses. This is now brought out more clearly by the present finding that poly A:U, an agent with poor capacity for interferon stimulation (22), is as effective as poly I:C, a potent interferon inducer (41–43), for the production of elevated tumor immunity. In view of the fact that poly I:C is pyrogenic and toxic whereas poly A:U is not pyrogenic and appears to be relatively free of toxic effects (44), it would appear highly desirable to utilize poly A:U rather than poly I:C in clinical studies. Finally, it should be noted that a modification of host responses to tumor antigens through the use of adjuvants has been observed in studies that preceded the area of utilization of polynucleotide in tumor studies (30).

It now remains to be determined whether a combination of the two approaches discussed here, i.e. the potentiation of the immunogenicity of syngeneic tumor cells and the stimulation of host-responses by polynucleotides, might result in good protective responses in animals that were previously sensitized to the tumor cell line from which the vaccine was prepared. In view of the fact that immunogenic tumor cell components can be prepared, it would appear that the only remaining block to individual immunotherapy remains our present inability to channel obtainable responses selectively or preferentially into protective cell-mediated immune responses. Once this block is removed, the way should be free for the clinical assessment of an approach that theoretically carries much promise, namely a combination of chemotherapy and immunotherapy utilizing potentiated antigens and host responses (22), or employing surgery plus such newer approaches to immunotherapy.

We are pleased to acknowledge the competent technical assistance of Miss Dolores Adams.

Supported by U.S.P.H.S. Grants AI-08493 and AM-8742, NSF Grants GB-8311 and B9-0301R, and ACS Grant T-501.

REFERENCES

1. PREHN, R. T. and MAIN, J. M. Immunity to methylcholanthrene-induced sarcomas. *J. nat. Cancer Inst.* **18**: 769, 1957.
2. KLEIN, G., SJÖGREN, H. O., KLEIN, E. and HELLSTRÖM, K. E. Demonstration of resistance against methylcholanthrene-induced sarcomas in the primary autochthonous host. *Cancer Res.* **20**: 1561, 1960.
3. HABEL, K. Resistance of polyoma virus immune animals to transplanted polyoma tumors. *Proc. Soc. exp. Biol. (N.Y.)* **106**: 722, 1961.
4. SJÖGREN, H. O., HELLSTRÖM, I. and KLEIN, G. Resistance of polyoma virus immunized mice to transplantation of established polyoma tumors. *Exp. Cell Res.* **23**: 204, 1961.
5. AMOS, D. B. and STETSON, C. Tumor immunity. *Ann. N.Y. Acad. Sci.* **101**: 1, 1962.
6. PREHN, R. T. Tumor specific immunity to non-viral tumors. *Canad. Cancer Conf.* **5**: 387, 1963.
7. SOUTHAM, C. M. Host defense mechanisms and human cancer. *Ann. Int. Pasteur* **107**: 585, 1964.
8. OLD, L. J. and BOYSE, E. A. Immunology of experimental tumors. *Ann. Rev. Med.* **15**: 167, 1964.
9. SJÖGREN, H. O. Transplantation methods as a tool for detection of tumor-specific antigens. *Progr. exp. Tumor Res. (Basel)* **6**: 289, 1965.
10. HADDOW, A. Immunology of the cancer cell: Tumor-specific antigens. *Brit. med. Bull.* **21**: 133, 1965.
11. KLEIN, E. and SJÖGREN, H. O. Humoral and cellular factors in homograft and isograft immunity against sarcoma cells. *Cancer Res.* **20**: 452, 1960.
12. OLD, L. J., BOYSE, E. A., CLARKE, D. A. and CARSWELL, E. A. Antigenic properties of chemically induced tumors. *Ann. N.Y. Acad. Sci.* **101**: 80, 1962.
13. ROSENAU, W. and MORTON, D. L. Tumor-specific inhibition of growth of methylcholanthrene-induced sarcomas *in vivo* and *in vitro* by sensitized isologous lymphoid cells. *J. nat. Cancer Inst.* **36**: 825, 1966.
14. MIKULSKA, Z. B., SMITH, C. and ALEXANDER, P. Evidence for an immunological reaction of the host directed against its own actively growing primary tumor. *J. nat. Cancer Inst.* **36**: 29, 1966.
15. HELLSTROÖ, I., HELLSTRÖM, K. E. and PIERCE, G. *In vitro* studies of immune reactions against autochthonous and syngeneic mouse tumors induced by methylcholanthrene and plastic discs. *Int. J. Cancer* **3**: 467, 1968.
16. BARSKI, G. and YOUN, J. K. Evolution of cell-mediated immunity in mice bearing an antigenic tumor. Influence of tumor growth and surgical removal. *J. nat. Cancer Inst.* **43**: 111, 1969.
17. PLESCIA, O. J. and BRAUN, W. Nucleic acids as antigens. *Advanc. Immunol.* **6**: 231, 1967.
18. PLESCIA, O. J. and BRAUN, W. "Nucleic acids in immunology." New York, Springer-Verlag, 1968.
19. PLESCIA, O. J. The role of the carrier in antibody formation. *Curr. Top. Microbiol. Immunol.* **50**: 78, 1969.
20. MAURER, P. H. and PINCHUCK, P. Immunogenicity of synthetic polymers of amino acids; role of carrier and genetic background, in: E. Mihich (Ed.), "Immunity, cancer and chemotherapy." New York, Academic Press, 1967, p. 319.
21. BRAUN, W., NAKANO, M., JAROSKOVA, L., YAJIMA, Y. and JIMENEZ, L. Stimulation of antibody-forming cells by oligonucleotides of known composition, in: Plescia, O. J. and Braun, W. (Eds.), "Nucleic acids in immunology." New York, Springer-Verlag, 1968.
22. BRAUN, W. New approaches to immunology as potential adjuncts to chemotherapy, in: "Progress in antimicrobial and anticancer chemotherapy." *Proc. 6th Int. Cong. of Chemotherapy.* Tokyo, University of Tokyo Press, 1970, v. 1, p. 17.
23. SUEOKA, N. and CHENG, T. Fractionation of nucleic acids with the methylated albumin column. *J. molec. Biol.* **4**: 161, 1962.
24. PLESCIA, O. J., BRAUN, W. and PALCZUK, N. C. Production of antibodies to denatured deoxyribonucleic acid (DNA). *Proc. nat. Acad. Sci.* **52**: 279, 1964.
25. KLEIN, G. Tumor antigens. *Ann. Rev. Microbiol.* **20**: 223, 1966.
26. HELLSTRÖM, K. E. and HELLSTRÖM, I. Immunological defenses against cancer. *Hosp. Pract.* **5**: 45, 1970.
27. FELDMAN, M. and GLOBERSON, A. Studies on the mechanism of immunological enhancement of tumor grafts. *J. nat. Cancer Inst.* **25**: 631, 1960.
28. KALISS, N. The elements of immunologic enhancement: a consideration of mechanisms. *Ann. N.Y. Acad. Sci.* **101**: 64, 1962.
29. WEISS, D. W., FAULKIN, L. J., JR. and DEOME, K. B. Acquisition of heightened resistance and susceptibility to spontaneous mouse mammary carcinomas in the original host. *Cancer Res.* **24**: 732, 1964.

30. Möller, G. and Möller, E. Studies *in vitro* and *in vivo* of the cytotoxic and enhancing effect of homoral isoantibodies. *Ann. N. Y. Acad. Sci.* **99**: 504, 1962.

31. Möller, G. Studies on the mechanism of immunological enhancement of tumor homografts. III. Interaction between humoral isoantibodies and immune lymphoid cells. *J. nat. Cancer Inst.* **30**: 1205, 1963.

32. Attia, M. A. M. and Weiss, D. W. Immunology of spontaneous mammary carcinomas in mice. V. Acquired tumor resistance and enhancement in Strain A mice infected with mammary tumor virus. *Cancer Res.* **26**: 1787, 1966.

33. Gershon, R. K., Carter, R. L. and Kondo, K. Immunologic defenses against metastases: impairment by excision of an allotransplanted lymphoma. *Science* **159**: 646, 1968.

34. Czajkowski, N. P., Rosenblatt, M., Cushing, F. R., Vazquez, J. and Wolf, P. L. Production of active immunity to malignant neoplastic tissue. Chemical coupling to an antigenic protein carrier. *Cancer (Philad.)* **19**: 739, 1966.

35. McEnany, M. T., Kelly, M. G. and Fahey, J. L. Effects of immunization with tumor cell-foreign protein conjugates on growth of syngeneic tumor grafts. *Proc. Amer. Ass. Cancer Res.* **9**: 46, 1968.

36. Cinader, B. Acquired tolerance, autoantibodies and cancer. *Canad. med. Ass. J.* **86**: 1161, 1962.

37. Levy, H. B., Law, L. W. and Rabson, A. S. Inhibition of tumor growth by polyinosinic-polycytidylic acid. *Proc. nat. Acad. Sci. (Wash.)* **62**: 357, 1969.

38. Larson, V. M., Clark, W. R. and Hilleman, M. R. Influence of synthetic (Poly I:C) and viral double-stranded ribonucleic acids on adenovirus 12 oncogenesis in hamsters. *Proc. Soc. exp. Biol. (N.Y.)* **131**: 1002, 1969.

39. Larson, V. M., Clark, W. R., Dagle, G. E. and Hilleman, M. R. Influence of synthetic double-stranded ribonucleic acid, poly I:C, on Friend leukemia virus. *Proc. Soc. exp. Biol. (N.Y.)* **132**: 602, 1969.

40. Youn, J. K., Barski, G. and Huppert, J. Inhibition de leucemigenese virale chez la souris par traitement avec polynucleotides synthetiques. *C.R. Acad. Sci. (Paris)* ser. D. **267**: 816, 1968.

41. Lampson, G. P., Tytell, A. A., Field, A. K., Nemes, M. M. and Hilleman, M. R. Inducers of interferon and host resistance, I. Double-stranded RNA from extracts of *Penicillium funiculosum*. *Proc. nat. Acad. Sci. (Wash.)* **58**: 782, 1967.

42. Field, A. K., Tytell, A. A., Lampson, G. P. and Hilleman, M. R. Inducers of interferon and host resistance. II. Multistranded synthetic polynucleotide complexes. *Proc. nat. Acad. Sci. (Wash.)* **58**: 1004, 1967.

43. Hilleman, M. R. Interferon induction and utilization. *J. cell Physiol.* **71**: 43, 1968.

44. Braun, W. Relationships between the effects of poly I. poly C and endotoxin. *Nature (Lond.)* **224**: 1024, 1969.

ERRATUM

On page 80, column 1, line 7: mμ should read μg.

STUDIES ON THE EFFECT OF
PHYTOHEMAGGLUTININ ON ASCITES TUMOR
IN MICE

E. ROBINSON and T. MEKORI

Department of Oncology, Rambam Government Hospital, Haifa, and Hebrew University–Hadassah
Medical School, Jerusalem, Israel

ABSTRACT

Mice were treated with phytohemagglutinin (PHA), BCG vaccine or typhoid vaccine before or after implantation of ascites tumor cells. In many of the treated animals, the tumor mass was significantly smaller than in the controls. Administration of the different substances elicited similar effects. PHA injection increased the peripheral leukocyte count both in normal and in tumor-bearing mice, and to a greater degree in the latter. PHA injected i.p. was more effective than i.v. administration in reducing tumor volume. Differential counts of peripheral blood and peritoneal cells showed that PHA increased the percentage of lymphocytes.

It is suggested that PHA acts both by stimulating the host defense mechanism and by destroying malignant cells directly.

Phytohemagglutinin (PHA), an extract of the kidney bean *Phaseolus vulgaris*, acts as a blastogenic agent in lymphocyte cultures and increases the peripheral leukocyte count *in vivo* (1). Recently it has been shown that PHA can retard the development of experimental tumors in mice and hamsters (2); a dose of 1 mg given to mice with ascites tumor was found to reduce tumor volumes significantly. These results led to the tentative use of PHA in cancer patients (3), in whom some temporary improvement was noted. The purpose of the present investigation was to study the effect on tumor growth of PHA given before, together with, or after tumor transplantation in mice with ascites tumor, and to examine the morphological changes in the tumor cells

after treatment. The effect of treatments with BCG and typhoid vaccine on tumor volumes, and of the three agents on the leukocytes of the tumor-bearing hosts, were also examined.

MATERIALS AND METHODS

Animals. The following animals were employed: Mice of the Swiss NIH inbred strain maintained at the Weizmann Institute of Science by brother and sister mating since 1959; Swiss albino mice from a closed isogenic colony bred at the Hebrew University since 1958; and Swiss Albino random-bred mice obtained from A. Lebenstein breeders Yoqneam, Israel. The animals weighed between 20 and 25 g at the time of experimentation, and were always employed in groups of 10 each.

Tumor. The Landschütz ascites tumor, obtained from the Department of Experimental Medicine and Cancer Research, Hebrew University–Hadassah Medical School, was used. This neoplasm has been passed for many years by weekly i.p. transfer of 0.2 ml ascites fluid containing approximately 10^6 viable cells. Unless indicated otherwise, challenge in the present experiments was also with 10^6 cells.

Phytohemagglutinin. Wellcome phytohemagglutinin was used (Wellcome Research Laboratories, England). The freeze-dried material, containing 50 mg/vial, was stored at 4 C. Before use, it was diluted with 5 ml of sterile water or sterile isotonic saline. An amount of 0.5 to 3 mg was injected i.v. into the tail vein or i.p. before, together with, or after the implantation of the ascites tumor cells.

Tumor cell volume. Seven or 14 days after ascites cell implantation, the mice were killed with ether. The peritoneal cavity was opened, irrigated with saline, and the ascites fluid collected into graduated tubes. The volume of packed cells was determined after centrifugation at 3,000 rpm for 10 min in an Ecco centrifuge, type 2.55, N-9053.

Incubation of ascites cells with PHA. Suspensions of ascites cells were incubated with PHA for 1 hr at 37 C immediately before the mixtures were injected.

Differential cell counts. Samples of venous blood were taken from the tail and blood smears prepared. The dry preparations were fixed with May-Grünwald fluid and stained with Giemsa stain for 10 min. For differential counts, 500 cells were counted. The same procedure was used for differential counts on preparations obtained from the sediments of the peritoneal fluid after centrifugation, except that the smears were stained for only 5 min.

BCG and typhoid vaccine treatment. In a number of experiments, animals were given living BCG, obtained from the Serum Institute, Copenhagen, or with living typhoid vaccine (*Salm. typhi*, 1×10^9 organisms, *Salm. paratyphi A* 5×10^8 organisms, *Salm. paratyphi B*, 5×10^8 organisms per ml, obtained from the Ministry of Health, Jerusalem). In each experiment, a similar number of untreated mice with tumor served as controls.

Statistical evaluation. The significance of the differences between the treated and the control groups was tested by the Scheffè method.

RESULTS

The effect of PHA on tumor development is shown in Tables 1 and 2. It is seen from the results of the experiments presented in Table 1

TABLE 1. Effect of PHA treatment on the development of ascites tumor[a]

Time of PHA administration in relation to tumor implantation	Dosage of PHA (mg)											
	0.5			1.0			2.0			3.0		
	Control	Treated	$P<$	Control	Treated	$P<$	Control	Treated	$P<$	Control	Treated	$P<$
120 hr before	—	—	—	1.61 (10)	2.61 (10)	0.001	1.61 (10)	2.82 (10)	0.001	1.61 (10)	1.81 (10)	0.001
72 hr before	1.95 (10)	1.71 (10)	0.05	1.89 (50)	0.66 (50)	0.01	1.85 (10)	1.90 (10)	NS	1.85 (10)	1.29 (10)	0.001
48 hr before	—	—	—	1.72 (10)	1.32 (10)	0.001	—	—	—	—	—	—
24 hr before	—	—	—	1.54 (10)	1.28 (10)	NS	—	—	—	—	—	—
0	1.96 (10)	1.66 (10)	0.01	2.13 (10)	1.39 (10)	0.001	—	—	—	—	—	—
48 hr after	1.96 (10)	1.09 (10)	0.001	—	—	—	—	—	—	—	—	—

[a] The numbers express the mean tumor volumes of packed cells (in ml) in the treated and control mice seven days after challenge with 10^8 cells. The figures in parentheses show the number of mice in each experiment.
The overall estimate of the standard deviations within each of the control and experimental cell volumes was 0.3591.   NS = Not significant

TABLE 2. *Effect of PHA in the development of ascites tumor. Relative tumor cell volumes[a]*

Time of PHA administration in relation to tumor implantation	Dosage (mg)	Route of administration	Treated	Non-treated
72 hr before	1	i.p.	29.5	41.3
72 hr before	1	i.v.	36.3	45.0
72 hr after	1	i.p.	37.5	29.8

[a] The numbers express tumor cell volumes (mean of 30 animals/group) as percentages of the total abdominal fluid volume, 14 days after challenge with 10^6 cells.

TABLE 3. *Differential counts of peritoneal cells of PHA-treated and control mice[a]*

Group	Large lymphocytes	Small lymphocytes	Tumor cells	Unclassified (most probably tumor cells)
Tumor only	26	6	423	45
1 mg PHA before tumor implantation	70	13	416	1
1 mg PHA after tumor implantation	29	0	471	0

[a] The numbers express the means of 20 values per group, taken on day 10 after tumor implantation. Five hundred cells were counted for each animal.

TABLE 4. *Effect of typhoid vaccine treatment on the development of ascites tumor*

No. of mice	Dose (ml)	Route of administration	Time of administration[a]	Tumor volume (ml) Control	Tumor volume (ml) Treated
20	1	s.c.	72 hr before	2.52	1.41
20	0.05	s.c.	24 and 96 hr after	1.1	0.55
20	0.05	s.c.	24 and 72 hr after	1.1	0.45

[a] In relation to tumor implantation.

TABLE 5. *The effect of BCG treatment on the development of ascites tumor*

No. of mice	Dose (ml)	Route of administration	Time of administration[a]	Tumor volume (ml) Control	Tumor volume (ml) Treated
20	0.1	i.v.	72 hr before	2.61	0.82
20	0.3	i.v.	72 hr before	2.61	1.1
20	0.2	i.v.	24 hr before	2.61	1.78
20	0.1	i.v.	at time of implantation	2.96	1.81
20	0.1	i.v.	24 hr after	2.30	0.82
20	0.1	i.p.	at time of implantation	2.30	0.57
20	0.5	i.p.	at time of implantation	2.96	2.38

[a] In relation to tumor implantation.

(challenge with 10^8 cells) that in the groups of mice in which PHA was injected before tumor transplantation, the greatest reduction in tumor cell volume was obtained when 1.0 mg was administered 72 hr prior to implantation. Tumor inhibition was also found when this quantity of PHA was given 48 or 24 hr before, or even on the day of the tumor transplantations, but when administration was 120 hr previously, there was a significant increase in tumor volume. Larger (2 to 3 mg) and smaller (0.5 mg) doses of PHA elicited a lesser effect, and with the larger quantities this was sometimes in the direction of increased tumor development. Administration of 0.5 mg PHA 48 hr after tumor transplantation also brought about a significant reduction in tumor volume.

Table 2 shows the results of another set of experiments employing 10^6 instead of 10^8 cells for challenge; the data represent mean tumor cell volumes as percentages of the whole abdominal fluid. The lowest percentage of tumor cells was found in the group of mice which received PHA i.p. 72 hr before tumor implantation. Administration of PHA 72 hr after implantation appeared to produce a slight increase in the relative tumor volume.

When 10^6 ascites tumor cells were first incubated with 1 mg PHA for 1 hr at 37 C and then injected into normal mice, the animals showed no indication of tumor development during a two-month observation period. In the corresponding control group injected with tumor cells only, all animals developed tumors within two weeks. Vital staining of the mixture before injection showed the death of 95% of the tumor cells.

The differential counts of peritoneal cells performed on PHA-treated and control animals on day 10 after ascites implantation is shown in Table 3. Administration of PHA before tumor transplantation increased the number of lymphocytes in the peritoneal cell population from 6.4 to 16.6%; administration

of the agent after tumor transplantation elicited no change.

The effects of typhoid vaccine and BCG administration on the tumor volumes are shown in Tables 4 and 5. Both agents reduced the tumor volumes significantly, and the differences between the treated and control groups were statistically significant.

In Fig. 1, the effect of injections of PHA and ascites tumor cells on the total number of blood leukocytes is seen. Implantation of

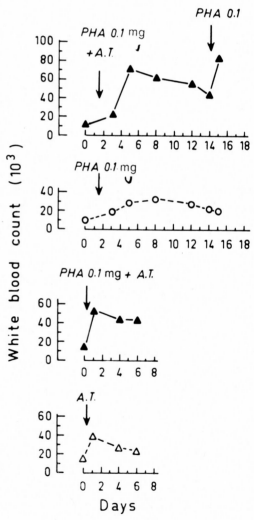

FIG. 1. The effect of ascites tumor (AT) and phytohemagglutinin on white blood count in mice.

the neoplastic cells increased the number of leukocytes. PHA elicited a similar but less marked effect, and exposure to both PHA and ascites cells caused a very pronounced increase in the total leukocyte counts. From Fig. 2 it is seen that increases in the dose of PHA raised the leukocyte counts correspondingly. The differential leukocyte counts of the peripheral blood of PHA-treated and untreated mice is shown in Table 6. Presence of the tumor cells reduced the percentage of lymphocytes, and PHA administration largely prevented the tumor-induced decrease in these cells.

DISCUSSION

Phytohemagglutinin causes small lymphocytes of the peripheral blood to enlarge, divide and synthesize RNA and protein *in vitro*. We have previously reported the impairment of certain functions of lymphocytes in cancer patients, but these lymphocytes still respond to PHA stimulation in culture (4). This prompted us to study the effect of PHA stimulation of hosts with malignant neoplasms. Mice with ascites tumor were chosen because

we had found them to show similar immunological impairment as did cancer patients with respect to foreign skin graft survival (5). The results presented here show that PHA, especially when administered prior to tumor implantation, inhibited the development of the neoplasm.

In contrast, Datta et al. did not find a protective effect of PHA against the growth of ascites tumor (6). The discrepancy between their finding and ours could have arisen from the use of different batches of PHA. Holm et al. (7) observed that unsensitized allogenic lymphocytes have a cytotoxic action on cultivated target cells after the addition of PHA. Möller (8) similarly noted cytotoxic effects on explanted tumor and normal embryonic cells subsequent to contact with normal allogenic lymphocytes in the presence of PHA, and it is possible that the *in vitro* and *in vivo* effects of PHA are based on similar mechanisms. The increase of lymphocytes and parallel reduction in tumor growth observed in the present experiments after PHA administration suggest that it may indeed be PHA "modi-

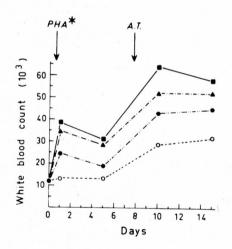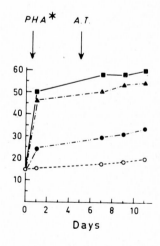

FIG. 2.   The effect of ascites tumor (AT) and various doses of phytohemagglutinin on white blood count in mice.

PHA 0.3 mg ■ ———— ■   PHA 0.1 mg ● —·—··●
PHA 0.2 mg ▲ —·—·—▲   No PHA, control ○ – – – ○

Table 6. *Effect of PHA and tumor cells on differential blood counts*[a]

Group	Lymphocytes (%)	Monocytes (%)	Segmented cells (%)	Stab cells (%)	Mitotic figures (%)
Control	65	4	31	0	0
Injected with tumor cells only	12	3	81	2	2
Injected with PHA only	55	3	39	2	1
Injected with 1 mg PHA and tumor cells[b]	42	6	49	0	2
Injected with tumor cells and PHA[c]	48	5	45	1	1

[a] The numbers express the means of 15 values taken on day seven after tumor implantation The PHA was administered 72 hr before the tumor cells.
[b] PHA given 72 hr prior to tumor challenge.
[c] PHA given 72 hr after tumor challenge.

fied" lymphocytes which are able to destroy the tumor target cells *in vivo*.

The administration of PHA to normal mice increased the total leukocyte count; the same phenomenon has also been observed in normal and irradiated rats. In the present study, it was seen that PHA injected into mice with ascites tumor increased their leukocyte counts to values above those found in untreated animals carrying the tumor or in normal mice given PHA. It is possible that this synergistic effect of PHA and tumor experience arises from a PHA-stimulated response to factor(s) liberated in the course of the host-tumor interaction.

PHA strongly retarded tumor development when given 72 hr before tumor transplantation. This is in accordance with the finding reported by Weiss et al. (10) who treated mice with a methanol-insoluble moiety of attenuated tubercle bacilli and found that this fraction increased the resistance of the animals to tumor implantation especially when it was administered some time before tumor challenge. On the other hand, when PHA was given 72 hr after tumor transplantation, tumor development in the treated groups was increased. It may be that PHA does not have the same effect in advanced malignancy as when given earlier. Further studies are being carried out in this connection.

No tumor growth accrued in animals given a mixture of tumor cells incubated with PHA *in vitro*, and it thus appears that PHA may also act directly on the target cells.

Supported in part by a grant from the Israel Cancer Association.

REFERENCES

1. Robinson, E. Phytohemagglutinin and marrow regeneration. *Lancet* i: 370, 1966.
2. Robinson, E. and Ashkenazi, A. Effect of phytohemagglutinin on ascites tumor and SV_{40} induced sarcoma of hamsters. *Israel J. med. Sci.* 3: 822, 1967.
3. Robinson, E. Treatment of mouse ascites tumor and human malignancies with phytohemagglutinin. *Harefuah* 81: 345, 1966 (in Hebrew).
4. Robinson, E. In vitro and in vivo studies of lymphocytes from cancer patients and normal donors, in: Yoffe, J. N. (Ed.), "The lymphocyte in immunology and haemopoiesis." London, Edward Arnold, 1966, p. 309.
5. Ben Hur, N., Biran, S. and Robinson, E. Comparison of the survival of homotransplanted skin grafts from normal mice and mice with ascites tumor. *Transplantation* 4: 205, 1966.
6. Datta, S. P., Cerin, M., Ghose, T. and Cerin, J. Effect of phytohemagglutinin on Ehrlich ascites carcinoma. *Brit. J. Cancer* 23: 616, 1969.
7. Holm, G., Perlman, P. and Werner, B. Phytohemagglutinin induced cytotoxic action of normal lymphoid cells on cells in tissue culture. *Nature (Lond.)* 203: 841, 1964.

8. Möller, E. Contact induced cytotoxicity by lymphoid cells containing foreign isoantigens. *Science* **147**: 873, 1965.

9. Delmonte, L., Liebelt, A. G. and Liebelt, R. A. Granulopoiesis and thrombopoiesis in mice bearing transplanted mammary cancer. *Cancer Res.* **26**: 149, 1966.

10. Weiss, W., Bonhag, R. S. and Leslie, P. Studies on the heterologous immunogenicity of a methanol insoluble fraction of attenuated tubercle bacilli. II. Protection against tumor isografts. *J. exp. Med.* **124**: 1039, 1966.

IMMUNOLOGICAL FACTORS IN NONSPECIFIC STIMULATION OF HOST RESISTANCE TO SYNGENEIC TUMORS

A Review

DIANE J. YASHPHE

Department of Immunology, Hebrew University–Hadassah Medical School, Jerusalem, Israel

The establishment of the germ theory of disease at the end of the 19th century laid the foundations for the development of a monistic view of disease and immunity: Specific agents cause characteristic and distinct pathological conditions, and may initiate states of specifically heightened resistance manifested only during a second exposure to that agent. To a great majority of investigators in the first half of this century, the suggestions that the host response may play a large role in the pathogenesis of microbial disease, or that the resistance to infections could be heterogeneous and induced nonspecifically seemed only somewhat short of heresy. It has only been very recently that attention has been paid to the true lability of host-parasite equilibria and to the large element of nonspecificity which is common to them.

Moreover, there developed an almost instinctive conceptual association between specificity and immunological mechanisms on the one hand, and nonspecificity and nonimmunological reactions on the other. That the mode of action of a nonspecifically elicited heightened resistance may nonetheless be based on specific immunological reactivity is, indeed, quite a new concept.

Nevertheless, there are early reports of experience with a microbial pathogen provoking increased refractoriness to another, unrelated one, and the observation has been recorded that such experience might lead as well to a better capacity to resist neoplastic cells. Thus, for example, it was noted that patients with active or quiescent tuberculosis seemed considerably more resistant to pneumonic plague (1), an observation which appears to have some experimental corroboration (2). Considerable attention was attracted by the claims of Holmgren, who reported postmortem confirmation of the efficacy of the tuberculin test as a tool for the differential diagnosis of neoplastic and non-neoplastic lesions of the gastrointestinal tract (3). There have, indeed, been numerous reports in the early decades of the century that survivors of acute tuberculosis are endowed with heightened resistance to cancer. This belief came under strong attack subsequently (4), but it may nonetheless be that infection with tubercle bacilli under some circumstances does elevate resistance to neoplasia.

At the turn of the century, a number of physicians suggested that bacterial infections might be effective in the therapy of malignant

90

TABLE 1. *Materials which have been found to nonspecifically stimulate the specific immune response or host resistance*

I. Microorganisms and sub-cellular fractions
  A. Mycobacteria
     Human and animal strains of mycobacteria, including BCG, MER, wax D
  B. Gram-negative bacilli
     Salmonella, Shigella, E. coli, Serratia, H. influenzae, B. pertussis, Brucella, endotoxin moieties
  C. Gram-positive cocci
     Staphylococci, Streptococci
  D. Gram-positive bacilli
     Corynebacterium parvum, Listeria
  E. Others
     Zymosan, lactic dehydrogenase virus

II. Nonbacterial materials
  A. Macromolecules
     Nucleic acids (DNA, RNA), synthetic polynucleotides
     DNA digests, antilymphocytic serum
  B. Small molecules
     1. Organic
        Vitamin A, fatty acids and lipids, epinephrine
     2. Inorganic
        Alum, bentonite, silica, beryllium

The materials listed are not distinct entities. Thus, wax D is responsible for the classical adjuvant properties of whole mycobacteria, but its role in the induction of resistance by MER and BCG is unknown; and the lipopolysaccharide portion of bacterial cell walls is at least one of the common active components of many other microorganisms.

diseases. Coley and Mantagne, for instance, based such impressions on clinical experience, and initiated the treatment of cancer patients with mixtures of bacterial toxins (5). It would appear from the vantage point today of an extensive literature on the nonspecific immunogenic potentials of bacterial endotoxins, mycobacterial moieties, and other microbial substances that these early attempts may have had a reasonable basis, although this basis was not necessarily recognized by their proponents.

It has only been in the last 15 years, however, that a variety of clinical observations, discoveries in basic immunology, recognition of the nature of bacterial resistance phenomena and advances in the understanding of neoplasia have converged to provide a suffi-

ciently cohesive picture to stimulate rational, inductive research in the area of nonspecific stimulation of host resistance to neoplastic variants. Most significantly, it has been shown beyond a doubt that most, if not all, tumors are immunogenic in autochthonous and syngeneic subjects, and that a variety of microbial and other entities can stimulate both the immunologic apparatus and tumor resistance.

Although many investigators are today focusing attention on specific immunotherapy by means of tumor-associated antigens, many others hold out greater hope for therapy based on the nonspecific activation of the organism's responsiveness to the tumor cells. However, only few investigators have as yet studied the effects of nonspecific immunological stimulators on resistance to tumors in the autochthonous host or in recipients of tumor isografts. These studies will be reviewed here, together with related observations on nonspecific stimulation of the immune response. They support the suggestion that this is indeed a useful approach to tumor immunotherapy.

NONSPECIFIC STIMULATORS* OF RESISTANCE
TO ISOGENIC AND AUTOCHTHONOUS TUMORS

A large number of different materials with a wide range of properties stimulate immunological reactivity nonspecifically (Table 1). Some of these also stimulate resistance to transplanted isogenic tumors or tumors in the primary host, and details of this work are summarized in Table 2.

Infection of experimental animals with living BCG has been used most commonly (6–14). When administered systemically, this

---

* A nonspecific stimulator here designates a material whose administration confers on the recipient the ability to respond, or respond more efficiently, to challenge with a non-cross reacting antigen, bacterium or tumor, as measured either by a heightened specific immune response or by increased resistance.

91

TABLE 2. *Nonspecific stimulation of tumor resistance*

Material	Reference	Dose	Route	Tumor or carcinogen	Host	Route of challenge	Time of treatment relative to challenge	Effect on tumor or host
BCG (living)	6	1 mg	i.v. i.p. s.c.	Ca755	C57F$_1$	s.c.	−17 days	Decreased tumor size, decreased mortality, regressions
	7	1 mg	i.v.	Mammary carcinoma	Balb/c	s.c.	−2 to −3 weeks	None
		1 mg	i.v.	Mammary carcinoma	C3H	s.c.	−2 to −3 weeks	None
		1 mg	i.v.	DBP fibrosarcoma	Balb/c	s.c.	−2 to −3 weeks	None
		1 mg	i.v.	Mammary carcinoma	(IXC3H)	s.c.	−7 days	Decreased tumor size, decreased mortality, regression
		1 mg	i.v.	DBP fibrosarcoma	Balb/c	s.c.	−7 days	
		1 mg	i.v.	DBP fibrosarcoma	(IXC3H)	s.c.	−8 days	
		1 mg	i.v.	MCA fibrosarcoma	Balb/c	s.c.	−7 days	
		1 mg	i.v.	Leukemia	AKR	Spontaneous	2 months old	Delay in appearance of leukemia
		1 mg	i.v.	Mammary carcinoma	(IXC3H)	Spontaneous	53 days old	Decreased tumor incidence
		1 mg	i.v.	MCA	Swiss	Induced	86 days post-MCA	Delay in appearance of MCA induced tumors, same final incidence
	8	1 mg	s.c.	Sr^{90}	CBA	Induced	Time of appearance of first tumor	Fewer tumors
	9	—	i.p. s.c.	Myeloid Leukemia	C57	s.c.	−17 weeks	Delayed death
	10, 11	1 mg	i.v.	E ♂ G2 leukemia	(DBAXC57)	i.p.	−15 days	Prolonged survival
	12	—	i.p.	Mammary carcinoma	C3H	Spontaneous	2 months and 5 months of age	Markedly decreased incidence tumors in breeding females
	13	1 mg	i.v.	L1210 leukemia	(DBAXC57)	s.c.	+1, 7 ×/30 days	Prolonged survival
	14	1 mg	s.c.	MCA-induced	CBA	s.c.	−3 days to −6 hr	Slightly enhanced growth
	15, 16	—	i.d.	Prolonged survival of patients with lymphoblastic leukemia after chemotherapy				
BCG (phenolized)	9	1 to 1.5 mg	i.p.	Uterine sarcoma	Balb/c	s.c.	−12 to −4 weeks	Decreased incidence of tumors
		0.5 to 1.5 mg	i.p.	MCA fibrosarcoma	Balb/c	s.c.	−3 weeks	Earlier appearance of tumors, decreased survival

Agent	Ref	Dose	Route	Tumor	Strain		Timing	Effect
MER	9	0.5 mg	i.p.	Uterine sarcoma	Balb/c	s.c.	-4 weeks	Decreased incidence of tumors
		0.25 mg	i.p.	Uterine sarcoma	Balb/c	s.c.	+1 and +7 days	Suggestion of delayed appearance
		0.5 mg	i.p.	Uterine sarcoma	Balb/c	s.c.	+7 and +14 days	Suggestion of delayed appearance
		0.25 mg	i.p.	Hepatoma (CCl_4)	C3H	s.c.	-2 weeks	Delay in appearance, prolonged survival
		0.5 mg	i.p.	Hepatoma (CCl_4)	C3H	s.c.	-4 weeks	Delay in appearance
		0.5 mg	i.p.	Mammary carcinoma	RIII	s.c.	-4 months	Delay in appearance
		0.3 mg	i.p.	Osteogenic sarcoma	C3Hf	s.c.	+2 and +7 days	Suggestion of delayed appearance
		0.5 to 1.0 mg	i.p.	MCA fibrosarcoma	Balb/c	s.c.	-3 weeks	Earlier appearance, decreased survival
	12	0.5 mg	i.p.	Fibrosarcoma	DBA/2	s.c.	-25 days	Earlier appearance, decreased survival
		2×0.4 mg	i.p.	Mammary carcinoma	RIII	Spontaneous	2 months and 5 months old	Lower incidence of spontaneous tumors in breeding females
	17	2.5 to 5 mg	i.p.	Mammary carcinoma	C3H	Spontaneous	Given to adults	Lower incidence of spontaneous tumors in breeding females
		0.5 mg	i.p.	Preneoplastic	C3H	Induced	After pituitary implants	Decreased incidence of preneoplastic nodules under hormonal stimulation
	18, 19	0.25 to 0.6 mg	i.p.	MCA-papillomas	Balb/c	Induced	15 days before graft of MCA-skin	Decreased incidence of papillomas on MCA-treated skin Decreased progression from papilloma to carcinoma
	Lappé, personal communication	—	i.p.	MCA-papillomas	Balb/c	Induced	15 days before graft of MCA-skin	Occasional increased incidence of papillomas in MCA-treated skin, and increased regression
C. parvum	20	0.5 mg	i.v.	Mammary carcinoma	A	s.c.	-2, +8 or +12 days	Delay in appearance of tumor, increased survival
		0.5 mg	i.v.	MCA-sarcoma	(CBAXA)F1	s.c.	-2 days	Delay in appearance, increased survival
	21	1 mg	i.p.	Leukemia	(CBAXAKR)	i.p.	-7 days	Prolonged survival time
	22	200 µg	i.d.	MCA-sarcoma	CBA	s.c.	18 days post-tumor (12 days post-cyclophosphomide)	30 to 70% regressions

Material	Reference	Dose	Route	Tumor or carcinogen	Host	Route of challenge	Time of treatment relative to challenge	Effect on tumor or host
B. pertussis	23	—	i.p.	YLI lymphoma	C57	s.c.	0	Earlier appearance of tumors
	24	—		Prolonged survival of patients with acute leukemia after chemotherapy				
Streptococci+ serratia	25	—	i.p.	Ca755	C57	s.c.	7 days after tumor reached 0.5 to 2.0 cm^2	None
			i.p.	Lymphosarcoma	C3H	s.c.		None
				Mammary carcinoma	C3H	Spontaneous		None
				MCA-induced	C3H	Induced		None
Bacterial toxins and infections	1, 26			Higher spontaneous regression rate in patients with variety of malignancies				
DNA digests	27	1 mg/week i.p.	i.p.	Mammary carcinoma	C3H	Spontaneous	8 months of age	Delay in appearance of tumor, longer survival in retired breeders
		1 mg/week i.p.	i.p.	C3H tumor	C3H	s.c.	-67 weeks	Decreased incidence
Polyadenylic-polyuridylic acid	28	300 µg	i.v.	MCA-induced	C57Bl	s.c.	5× in week following excision	Fewer regrowths
Polyinosinic-polycytidilic acid	29	100 µg 3×/week	i.p. i.v.	J96132 reticulum cell sarcoma	C57	s.c. or i.p.	+24 to 48 hr	Tumor regression increased survival time
				Lymphocytic lymphoma	SJL	s.c.	+24 to 48 hr	
				MT-1 (adenovirus)	Balb/c	s.c.	+24 to 48 hr	
				Fibrosarcoma	Balb/c	s.c.	+24 to 48 hr	
				L1210 leukemia	(C57BL/6 × DBA/2	i.p.	+24 to 48 hr	
	30	200 µg 5 to 7 doses	i.p.	DMBA-croton oil papillomas	Swiss	Induced	5 to 7 doses during -4 to +6 days with respect to DMBA	Little effect
		100 to 200 µg 3 × week	i.p.	DMBA-croton oil papillomas	Swiss	Induced	-4 days, 3×/week	Fewer tumors
		100 µg	i.p.	DMBA	Swiss	Induced	3 doses, 0 to 7 days following DMBA	Fewer tumors

DBP = 3, 4-9, 10 dibenzpyrene; DMBA = 7, 12-dimethylbenz(α)anthracene; MCA = 3-methylcholanthrene.

agent causes manifestations of toxicity and disease in laboratory animals, including appreciable weight loss (7). On the other hand, it has been used on a large scale and with considerable safety as an intradermal vaccine against tuberculosis in humans, and has recently been tried therapeutically in patients with malignant disease (15, 16). Phenolized BCG is better tolerated by animals, even in large quantities, but also suffers from the defect that it confers appreciable tuberculin sensitivity (31, 32). An active methanol-extraction residue (MER) of phenolized BCG (9, 12, 17–19, 33) was not toxic to mice or guinea pigs in effective quantities, and resulted only in weak tuberculin skin sensitivity (32). *Corynebacterium parvum* has recently been found to have tumor resistance-inducing properties in experimental animals (20–22), and *Bordetella pertussis* may prolong remissions of acute leukemia in man (24). Digests of DNA and synthetic polynucleotides increased resistance to tumors, but prolonged administration of polyinosinic-polycytidylic acid (poly I:C) was toxic to mice (27–30). A variety of bacterial toxins have been implicated in causing "spontaneous regressions" of human neoplasms (26). Endotoxins have been extensively studied as antitumor agents in allogeneic systems, but their toxicity would appear to preclude serious investigation of their beneficial properties in man, and they have not been tested widely in isogenic animal systems.

In laboratory studies, the effective dose for all these materials is similar: a single administration of 0.25 to 2 mg, or multiple doses totalling as high as 6 mg. Occasionally, a larger amount is less effective than a smaller one. The narrow dose range may reflect the slow degradation of bacterial cell walls. DNA digests and synthetic polynucleotides are probably degraded quite rapidly *in vivo*; they have been administered repeatedly in all successful experiments published.

The effective treatment-challenge interval varies; most materials are active only when administered before tumor challenge. In one series of experiments BCG proved efficacious when given one to two weeks (and in one case, 17 weeks) before tumor implantation, but resulted in better tumor growth when given within a few days of challenge (14). However, in another instance, multiple doses of BCG initiated after tumor implantation did succeed in slowing tumor growth (13).

MER was most effective against malignant tumors when the treatment-challenge interval was several weeks to months (9, 12, 17). *C. parvum* administered seven days before to 12 days after tumor challenge prolonged the survival time of the recipients (20, 21). BCG, MER and DNA digests decreased the incidence or delayed the appearance of spontaneous tumors in strains of mice carrying mammary tumor viruses when administered to breeding females before the appearance of tumors (7, 12, 13, 17, 27), and BCG was effective in delaying the development of methylcholanthrene (MCA)-and Sr^{90}-induced neoplasms (7, 8) when given at the time that tumors first started to appear. MER decreased the incidence of papillomas induced by MCA when given before the appearance of the lesions (18, 19). The growth of a variety of isogenic tumors was retarded when poly I:C was administered thrice weekly after tumor implantation (29). By comparison, mixtures of streptococci and serratia had no effect on tumor growth when administered after the tumors had grown to 0.5 to 2.0 cm^2 (25).

The importance of the treatment-challenge interval has not been studied in detail, but these results indicate that stimulation before tumor challenge, or before the appearance of spontaneous or induced tumors, is effective in increasing resistance, and may be more efficient than stimulation subsequent to tumor challenge. Only poly I:C markedly reduced tumor incidence when administered after tumor grafting (29). Treatment cannot be initiated prior to tumor appearance in a clinical situation, and a different approach must be taken from that of current laboratory models. In published clinical reports, two groups of physicians have combined chemotherapy and immunotherapy. Patients with acute leukemia were brought into remission with chemotherapy and then treated with BCG (15, 16) or *B. pertussis* (24) (nonspecific immunotherapy), or with killed tumor cells (15, 16) (specific immunotherapy). The treated patients stayed in remission longer than untreated ones, and the results, while not striking, seem promising.

Combination therapy has been studied in experimental systems with varying results. Pretreatment with BCG or methylhydrazine prolonged the survival of mice which had received grafts of a murine leukemia, but combining these treatments was less effective than chemotherapy alone (11). By comparison, cyclophosphamide given six days after the tumor implant potentiated the effect of *C. parvum* administered 12 days later; 70% of the implants of one tumor regressed, and 30% of another (22). This is a model worth pursuing: Decreasing the size of the tumor mass could decrease the size of antigenic challenge to one small enough to both stimulate the host's immune response and be susceptible to it.

This group of nonspecific stimulators has been shown to be effective against a wide variety of tumor types, in terms of the carcinogen, the tissue of origin, the strain of host, the nature of the host (primary or graft recipient), and whether preneoplastic or fully neoplastic cells are involved. Resistance has been induced to spontaneous tumors of unknown origin; to virus associated tumors [mammary carcinomas associated with the mammary tumor virus (MTV) in infected strains, and leukemias associated with murine leukemia viruses]; to tumors induced by chemical car-

cinogens such as MCA and 7, 12-dimethylbenz(α)anthracene (DMBA); and to tumors induced by physical agents (Sr^{90}). The tumors susceptible to resistance-stimulating materials have been of different tissue origins: leukemias, fibrosarcomas, osteosarcomas, mammary adenocarcinomas and papillomas. There is no strain specificity: many different strains of mice have served as isogenic or syngeneic tumor donors and hosts in these experiments.

Resistance to the same type of tumor can be increased whether it is studied in the primary host or in the secondary graft recipient. MER administered to RIII (MTV+) breeding females decreased the incidence of spontaneous tumors (12); administration of MER to RIII adults delayed the appearance of isografts of a mammary adenocarcinoma (9). BCG has been shown to be effective against both spontaneous (7) and grafted leukemias (10, 11, 13) in strains carrying murine leukemia viruses. Similarly, in the case of chemically induced tumors, BCG delayed the appearance of tumors induced by MCA in the primary host and stimulated resistance in recipients of grafts of MCA-induced neoplasms (7).

MER has been effective in two other experimental situations. Female mice of MTV+ strains undergoing continual hormonal stimulation develop hyperplastic alveolar nodules. These nodules rarely progress to mammary carcinomas, but they can be passaged indefinitely in the strain of origin, and are antigenic at least in those isogenic strains not carrying MTV (34). When MER was administered to mice during hormonal stimulation, fewer mice developed nodules, and the number of nodules arising per mouse was lower than in untreated animals (17). In another system, premalignant papillomas developed in skin painted with MCA and then grafted to isogenic recipients; in recipients treated with MER before grafting, papillomas appeared more slowly, with a lower incidence, and the proportion of those which regressed was higher (18, 19). There does not, therefore, seem to be any general limit on the type of tumor susceptible to increased nonspecific stimulation of host resistance. It would appear, of course, that tumors must be antigenic to be susceptible to such effects. Since antigenicity of experimental tumors has been well documented for both chemically induced (35) and virus-associated (36) tumors, it is assumed for the purpose of this discussion that such will be the case for all or at least most tumors.

IMMUNOLOGICAL FACTORS IN
ELEVATED HOST RESISTANCE TO NEOPLASIA

It should be made clear that there is not yet any direct evidence that materials such as MER, BCG, *B. pertussis* or others stimulate a specific immune response to tumors. The assumption that elevated host resistance is brought about by an elevated immune response is based on certain well-documented observations: 1) Tumors are immunogenic, and immunization of isogenic hosts protects against subsequent challenge with a graft of the same or of a cross-reacting tumor. 2) Some of these substances confer upon a host increased protection against autochthonous tumors and tumor isografts. 3) The same agents stimulate known immune responses as measured by both humoral and cellular reactivity to defined antigens.

Tumor resistance is more usually assayed by tumor growth in a host than by *in vitro* tests for the effector mechanism of host resistance which would measure the specificity of the response. For this reason, the effectiveness of nonspecific stimulators is still only an overall measurement of the ability of the host to defend itself against neoplastic cells. With increased refinement of *in vitro* methods for measuring cellular immune reactions, it should soon be possible to determine more precisely increased levels of antitumor activity in iso-

lated cell populations from isogenic hosts. In the meantime, studies on the mode of action of nonspecific stimulators are most often carried out by measuring specific antibody formation or a specific cellular immune response to other known antigens, and this information can then be applied indirectly to the analysis of tumor resistance. The importance of considering the effects of nonspecific stimulators on resistance to tumors and on defined immune responses in parallel will be clear when some factors influencing the host's immune response to neoplastic cells are examined.

Suppression of the immune response. Evidence has accumulated that suppression of the immune response may be a necessary precondition for tumor induction. A number of diverse materials are associated with both tumor induction and immunosuppression. Of a number of hydrocarbons tested, potent carcinogens such as MCA and DMBA were found to strongly inhibit the antibody response while noncarcinogens had no such effect (37, 38). Sr^{90} and X-irradiation (39, 40) induce tumor formation and suppress immunological responsiveness (41, 42). Antithymocyte serum (ATS) and antilymphocyte serum can depress antibody formation and cellular immunity (43–47) and can replace X-irradiation as the (immunodepressive) agent necessary for a high incidence of leukemia in C57BL mice (48). Administration of ATS also facilitates induction of other mouse tumors (49, 50). Mineral oil, a common component of many adjuvants, induces plasma cell tumors in BALB/c mice (51), and was found capable of depressing immunological responsiveness in that strain while not affecting oncogenesis-resistant C57BL animals (52). Some oncogenic viruses themselves appear to have the ability to suppress the immune response: This has been shown for Friend virus (53, 54), MTV (P. B. Blair et al. in preparation) and the murine leukemia virus (55), although a causal relationship between this property and their oncogenic potential has not been established.

In some cases, a nonspecific stimulator can both overcome the immunosuppression and increase resistance to tumors induced by the same agent. BCG was shown to elevate the antibody response to sheep red blood cells (SRBC) and to overcome the inhibition of the antibody response induced by MCA (56). BCG administered to mice close to the time that MCA-induced tumors begin to appear delayed tumor appearance (7). Sr^{90} induced tumors in mice after a long latent period, and the immune response to SRBC of mice exposed to Sr^{90} was depressed (41); animals infected with BCG at the time Sr^{90}-induced neoplasms appeared developed fewer tumors (8).

Other materials known to stimulate host resistance can overcome immunodepression. Endotoxin (57) and DNA digests (58) restored immunological competence in irradiated animals. MER offered some protection against the inhibition of antibody formation by ATS (59). It is noted that nonspecific stimulators of resistance have not yet been tested against tumors which arise due to these particular immunosuppressive agents, ATS and X-irradiation.

Poor immunological responsiveness also occurs naturally. The immune response of CBA mice was observed to increase with age and then decline (60), and resistance to tumor isografts paralleled this rise and fall (61). [The impairment of the immune response in old animals may be due to accumulation of virus. Older mice carrying MTV had a depressed response to allogeneic skin grafts and to SRBC as compared with isogenic mice free of the virus, and this depression coincided in time with the appearance of mammary adenocarcinomas (P. B. Blair et al., personal communication)]. Both endotoxin and synthetic polynucleotides proved effective in raising the immune response to SRBC of four-day-old mice and retired breeders above their normal

low levels (62–64). It would seem likely that other stimulators can also overcome agedependent immunosuppression, but they have not yet been tested on age-dependent susceptibility to tumors.

Immunological tolerance. Specific immunological tolerance to tumor antigens has been suggested as one important factor in the low level of host responsiveness to autochthonous tumors (65). The murine mammary tumor system illustrates this point well. It is difficult to immunize mice infected from birth with MTV against MTV-containing tumors. Isogenic mice not carrying the virus could be rendered resistant to tumor challenge by prior administration of MTV or of tissue containing MTV (34, 64–68). In the MTV (–) strains, C3Hf and BALB/c, immunity to MTV (+) tumors was cross-reactive, presumably directed to virus-associated antigens (66, 68). When MTV-containing tumors were shown to be immunogenic in virus-containing hosts, immunity was largely tumor specific and not usually cross-reactive (69, 70); that is, it appeared unrelated to the virus to which the host is tolerant. Cross-reactive immunity to virus-containing cancers could however, be elicited by MTV-infected tissue in A mice (71), suggesting that this strain is incompletely tolerant to MTV. MER stimulated resistance to the development of spontaneous MTV-associated tumors in hosts neonatally tolerant to the virus (RIII and C3H) (9, 17). Similarly, administration of living BCG to (IXC3H) F_1, an MTV (+) strain, lowered tumor incidence (7).

It is thus of interest that endotoxin, *B. pertussis*, *C. parvum*, and the lactic dehydrogenase virus (LDV), which stimulate antibody formation when administered with antigen, also can prevent the induction of specific immunological tolerance to specific protein antigens (72–85); that is, their administration with a dose of antigen which would normally lead to tolerance, enabled the recipient to respond normally to a second dose of the antigen. Some surface active agents have the same property (78, 85), and many of these stimulators have also been shown to activate macrophage lysosomal enzymes (86, 87). Dresser suggested that they may act by increasing the processing of soluble antigens by macrophages to a form necessary for the induction of antibody formation (78). It is not clear if this is the necessary or only mode of action of these materials in preventing tolerance or stimulating antibody formation, and it is even less clear if handling of antigen by macrophages is relevant to cellular immunity of the homograft type considered to be at work in tumor resistance. Nevertheless, the idea that nonspecific stimulators act by preventing specific immunological tolerance is a challenging one, and open to further experimentation.

Enhancement and resistance. Another factor controlling the fate of neoplastic cells in the host is the type of immune response mounted by the host. This consideration has already been well summarized by Kaliss and requires little elaboration here (88). Nonsolid tumors are susceptible *in vivo* to cytotoxic antibody, and they are also susceptible to sensitized lymphoid cells which may act synergistically with cytotoxic antibody. Solid tumors, on the other hand, appear to be susceptible largely to sensitized lymphoid cells, and their growth may be enhanced by specific antibody to the tumor (immunological enhancement). Under certain conditions, leukemias may also be enhanced by specific antibody (89).

Occasional experiments with nonspecific stimulators have resulted in increased tumor growth rather than resistance. This has been observed with BCG (14), MER (9, 18)* and

B. pertussis (23). Thus, the phenomenon of enhancement may be a major factor to be considered in immunotherapy.

The mechanism of antibody-mediated enhancement is not clear, but evidence from studies in allogeneic systems strongly suggests an impairment of the immune response to the tumor, rather than a change in the antigenicity of the tumor itself (90). Current studies attempt to distinguish among three possible foci of enhancing antibody activity: afferent, efferent, or central inhibition of the immune response (91). Most work on enhancement has been done with allogeneic tumors, but it can be induced in syngeneic systems as well. The Hellströms and co-workers have demonstrated an *in vitro* equivalent of enhancement with syngeneic tumors (92, 93); inhibition of tumor colony formation by sensitized lymphoid cells was reversed by antiserum from hosts with progressively growing cancers. Although this is a very elegant demonstration of the antagonism between cellular immunity and antibody formation to tumors, it is not yet clear whether the outcome of host-tumor interactions *in vivo* can be explained on this basis.

The type of immunoglobulin responsible for the enhancing activity is an important feature of the response. All evidence indicates that 7S rather than 19S immunoglobulin is responsible in allogeneic systems, and conflicting reports implicate either the γ-1 or γ-2 subclass (94–98). A central question is, accordingly, whether nonspecific stimulators might change the outcome of a tumor-host relationship by preferentially affecting one class of immunoglobulins or another. There is no evidence as yet that this is the case, although most nonspecific stimulators are known to elevate antibody levels during an immune response: Most of the materials listed in Table 1 have been shown to elevate levels of antibody or antibody-producing cells when given some time before or simultaneously with specific

---

* Enhancement and increased resistance may coexist. Thus, an MER-treated group of mice with a higher incidence of papillomas (18) eventually showed a higher incidence of regressions (Lappé, personal communication).

antigen. For example, in MER-treated mice, antibodies usually appeared earlier, higher levels were maintained longer, and both IgG and IgM antibodies were affected (99, 100). The ability to mount a better secondary response was observed in animals primed with antigen and *B. pertussis* or *C. parvum* (76, 77, 80). The affinity of antibodies often increased rapidly, indicating an earlier maturation of the immune response (80), and smaller doses of antigen were immunogenic (76). All of these results suggest a greatly increased level of efficiency of the antibody response.

Immunity to tumors appears to reside largely in populations of lymphoid cells. Other immune reactions of the cellular type include homograft immunity and delayed type hypersensitivity. The latter is, interestingly, a reaction long associated with mycobacteria, one of the most prominent nonspecific stimulators of tumor resistance. Delayed type hypersensitivity usually cannot be induced to soluble proteins unless administered with mycobacteria in Freund's adjuvant (101). Autoimmune diseases are usually induced experimentally with Freund's adjuvant, but can also be invoked with endotoxin (102) and *B. pertussis* (103). Many materials which stimulate resistance to isogenic tumors also stimulate homograft immunity as measured by resistance to allogeneic tumors: fewer tumors take, tumors are more rapidly rejected, or fewer recipients die when treated with nonspecific stimulators (6, 7, 104–109). In addition, BCG and MER can decrease the mean survival time of skin homografts (18, 110, 111).

One seeming exception to the association between agents which invoke cellular immunity and those which stimulate resistance to isogenic tumors is Freund's complete adjuvant. Immunization with tumor tissue or oncogenic virus in Freund's adjuvant can lead to enhancement of tumor growth (70, 112, 113). This may be due, however, to the administration of killed tissue rather than to the use of the adjuvant; immunization with dead tumor cells in allogeneic systems leads almost invariably to enhancement (90). Moreover, the slow release of antigen from the oil-in-water emulsion, rather than the content of mycobacteria, could be responsible for enhancement. It must also be considered that although enhancement and resistance are opposite manifestations of an immune response, minor changes in the experimental circumstances can tilt the equilibrium between them.

It is thus seen that many materials which stimulate tumor resistance can, under defined conditions, also affect either antibody formation or cellular immunity. The problem of primary importance is whether the immune response can be directed towards one of cellular immunity rather than antibody formation. Mechanisms of cellular immunity are not as easily studied as antibody formation, because the characteristics of the reactions are only now being defined on cellular and molecular levels. Thus studies on the mode of action of nonspecific stimulators in cellular immune responses have lagged behind similar studies in antibody formation. However, recent developments allow us to consider certain aspects of cellular immunity as part of the overall scheme of antibody formation, and suggest fruitful new approaches to mode of action studies (114).

Three cell types are currently held to be involved in antibody formation: 1) macrophages (115–117), which may be optional, to process or present the antigen to 2) thymus-processed antigen-sensitive cells, probably small lymphocytes, which then act synergistically with 3) nonthymus-processed small lymphocytes which differentiate to plasma cells and produce specific antibody (118–120). Different lines of evidence suggest that the thymus-processed cell is the effector cell in cellular immunity such as the homograft reaction, delayed sensitivity and some autoimmune diseases (114). This cell type may also carry immunological memory, and is identified by its susceptibility to antithymocytic serum (121, 122). By focusing on this distinction between the types of cells participating in the immune response, it may be possible to determine the effect of nonspecific stimulators on at least one parameter of cellular immunity.

OTHER ASPECTS OF HOST RESISTANCE

Nonspecific stimulation of host resistance to isogenic or autochthonous tumors can most profitably be discussed and explored within the framework of the immunological response. Evidence has been presented that materials which nonspecifically activate host resistance to tumors most likely also elevate the host's ability to mount a specific immune response to the tumor cells. There are, however, other factors which can be imagined to bear part, or perhaps even all, of the responsibility for the antitumor activities of such substances.

Many of the microorganisms and some of the nonbacterial materials listed in Table 1 both stimulate the reticuloendothelial system and induce interferon production (123–125). Both factors are beyond the scope of this review. However, since neither alone can account for all the effects of nonspecific stimulators of cancer resistance, their roles are seen, at most, as supplemental to the heightened specific immune response. Some agents may produce host resistance by modifying additional physiological processes: hormone levels, vascular permeability, release of pharmacological agents, inflammatory response, etc. Highly potent bacterial endotoxins, for example, provoke a Shwartzman reaction in spontaneous or transplanted allogeneic tumors, and this is often followed by complete regression of the neoplastic growth (126).

DISCUSSION

A number of materials have been observed to heighten nonspecifically host resistance to tumor isografts and to autochthonous tumors. Most of these materials are effective only when administered before tumor challenge, but some can be administered subsequent to tumor growth. Susceptible tumors include a wide spectrum with regard to oncogenic agent, tissue of origin and host strain. Future investigations of these materials should focus both on pertinent clinical models and on further understanding of their mode of action.

Clinical models should determine the optimal conditions for effectively stimulating resistance in tumor-bearing animals in conjunction with specific immunotherapy, chemotherapy, irradiation, surgery or all of these. Attempts should be made to decrease the tumor size (i.e., lower the antigen dose) with minimum damage to the normal immune apparatus, while raising the level of immunological reactivity with nonspecific stimulators. Although some nonspecific stimulators have been shown to overcome immunodepression, there is no evidence yet that this compensation is operative in all instances. These materials may only be effective when there is at least a minimum of immunologically reactive tissue available for stimulus. The use of nonspecific stimulators might sufficiently potentiate chemotherapy or irradiation to enable lower doses to be used, further sparing the immune response. It would be of importance in studies of this type to monitor immunological responsiveness of the host by immunization with an antigen unrelated to the tumor being studied, or by measuring the immune response to the tumor itself.

It is of equal importance to determine the conditions under which nonspecific stimulators will elevate host resistance rather than induce immunological enhancement. Such variables as the treatment-challenge interval, size of tumor challenge, immunogenicity of the tumor, tolerance to the tumor antigens, and immunization with living or dead tissues

101

should be tested. These results must lead, in turn, to a direct measurement of an increased immune response to specific tumor antigens *in vitro*. Here, one should be able to see if increased resistance is in fact due to an elevated immune response, and ask if increased immunological reactivity is due to an increased number of sensitized cells or to increased efficiency of a steady number.

Nonspecific stimulators have been shown to overcome the depression of the antibody response induced by some physical and chemical carcinogens. Studies on the mode of action of these materials also indicate that they can prevent the induction of tolerance to soluble antigens. Both of these effects on the immune response lend support to the concept that nonspecific stimulators of tumor resistance act by raising the level of effective immunological reactivity to tumor antigens. However, these observations provide little information on the exact function of these materials or the target cell or cells.

More direct experiments suggest that both macrophages and lymphocytes may be target cells. Lysosomal labilizers can prevent induction of tolerance to protein antigens *in vivo* (85); and these compounds can act on macrophages *in vitro* enabling the cells to process antigen into a more immunogenic form (86, 87). Single stranded synthetic polynucleotides enable populations of lymphoid cells to respond better to a primary antigenic stimulus *in vitro* (62). It has been suggested that synthetic polynucleotides, endotoxin and other membrane active agents mimic nonspecific activators, normally released from macrophages after antigenic stimulation, which alter stem cells to allow better antigenic stimulation of division and differentiation (62). Similarly, a soluble factor has been postulated to account for nonspecific bacterial resistance (127). A host with a high level of delayed-type hypersensitivity to one bacterium, may, upon secondary stimulation, release a soluble factor which activates macrophages and enables them to destroy more effectively non-cross-reacting organisms (127). Here, the nonspecific stimulator must be antigenic, and the host must be undergoing the corresponding immune response, although the effector cell is triggered and acts nonspecifically. It is not difficult to see a similarity between the nonspecific factors postulated to operate in the instances of stimulation by endotoxin and bacterial cross-resistance, except that in the former case the factors would be produced by macrophages and in the latter by specific lymphoid cells.

Clearly, each material, whether pure or crude, may have a variety of properties, one or more of which may determine its ability to elevate immunological responsiveness. It appears reasonable to assume that these materials trigger, or amplify, biochemical pathways and cellular differentiation which normally occur under specific antigenic stimulation. It is now of importance to determine the many steps of the immune response at which nonspecific stimulators can act, and the cells which they affect. Materials could then perhaps be selected or compounds designed which would act only on cell populations involved in a certain type of reaction—for example, stimulate cellular immunity to tumor antigens rather than antibody formation. Just as there are mediators of cellular immunity whose action, once elicited, is nonspecific (128), so there may be a variety of cellular functions which can be triggered by these nonspecific stimulators in place of antigen.

I am indebted to Professor David W. Weiss for his interest and advice during the preparation of this manuscript.

REFERENCES

1. Report of the International Plague Conference, Mukden, 1911.
2. GIRARD, G. and GRUMBACH, F. L'infection tuberculeuse de la souris entraîne sa résistance à l'infection pesteuse, expérimentale. *C.R. Soc. Biol. (Paris)* **152**: 280, 1958.

3 a. Holmgren, I. Fösök och iakttagelser över kancersjukas förhallande till tuberculin. *Hygiea (Stockh.)* **79**: 218, 1917.

b. Editorial. *Brit. med. J.* **2**: 297, 1917.

4. Cooper, F. G. The association of tuberculosis and carcinoma. *Amer. Rev. Tuberc.* **25**: 108, 1932.

5. Fowler, G. A. Enhancement of natural resistance to malignant melanoma with special reference to the beneficial effects of concurrent infections and bacterial toxin therapy. New York, New York Cancer Research Institute, 1969, monograph 9.

6. Old, L. J., Clarke, D. A. and Benacerraf, B. Effect of Bacillus Calmette-Gúerin (BCG) infection on transplanted tumors in the mouse. *Nature (Lond.)* **184**: 291, 1959.

7. Old, L. J., Benacerraf, B., Clarke, D. A., Carswell, E. A. and Stockert, E. The role of the reticuloendothelial system in the host reaction to neoplasia. *Cancer Res.* **121**: 1281, 1961.

8. Nilsson, A., Révész, L. and Stjernswärd, J. Suppression of strontium⁹⁰-induced development of bone tumors by infection with Bacillus Calmette-Gúerin (BCG). *Radiat. Res.* **26**: 378, 1965.

9. Weiss, D. W., Bonhag, R. S. and Leslie, P. Studies on the heterologous immunogenicity of a methanol-insoluble fraction of attenuated tubercle bacilli (BCG). II. Protection against tumor isografts. *J. exp. Med.* **124**: 1039, 1966.

10. Amiel, J. L. Immunothérapie active non spécifique par le B.C.G. de la leucémie virale E♂G2 chez des receveurs isogéniques. *Rev. franç. Étud. clin. biol.* **12**: 912, 1967.

11. Amiel, J. L. and Berardet, M. Essais de traitements de la leucémie E♂G2 associant chimiothérapie et immunothérapies actives non spécifique et spécifique. *Rev. franç. Étud. clin. biol.* **14**: 685, 1969.

12. Weiss, D. W. Immunology of spontaneous tumors, in: Lecam, L. and Neyman, J. (Eds.), "Proceedings of the Fifth Berkeley Symposium on Mathematical Statistics and Probability." Berkeley, University of California Press, 1967, p. 657.

13. Mathé, G. Immunothérapie active de la leucémie L1210 appliquée après la greffe tumorale. *Rev. franç. Étud. clin. biol.* **13**: 881, 1968.

14. Stjernswärd, J. Immune status of the primary host towards its own methylcholanthrene-induced sarcomas. *J. nat. Cancer Inst.* **40**: 13, 1968.

15. Mathé, G. Approaches to the immunological treatment of cancer in man. *Brit. med. J.* **4**: 7, 1969.

16. Mathé, G., Amiel, J. L., Schwarzenberg, L., Schneider, M., Cattan, A., Schlumberger, J. R., Hayat, M. and de Vassal, F. Active immunotherapy for acute lymphoblastic leukemia. *Lancet* **i**: 697, 1969.

17. Weiss, D. W., Lavrin, D. H., Dezfulian, M., Vaage, J. and Blair, P. B. Studies on the immunology of spontaneous mammary carcinomas of mice, in: Burdette, W. J. (Ed.), "Viruses inducing cancer." Salt Lake City, University of Utah Press, 1966, p. 138.

18. Lappé, M. A. Evidence for the antigenicity of papillomas induced by 3-methylcholanthrene. *J. nat. Cancer Inst.* **40**: 823, 1968.

19. Lappé, M. A. and Prehn, R. T. Immunologic surveillance at the macroscopic level: Nonselective elimination of pre-malignant skin papillomas. *Cancer Res.* **29**: 2374, 1969.

20. Woodruff, M. F. A. and Boak, J. L. Inhibitory effect of injection of *Corynebacterium parvum* on the growth of tumor transplants in isogenic hosts. *Brit. J. Cancer* **20**: 345, 1966.

21. Lamensans, A., Stiffel, C., Mollier, M. F., Laurent, M., Mouton, D. and Biozzi, G. Effect protecteur de *Corynebactérium parvum* contre la leucémie greffée AKR. Relations avec l'activité catalasique hépatique et la fonction phagocytaire du système réticuloendothélial. *Rev. franç. Étud. clin. biol.* **13**: 773, 1968.

22. Currie, G. A. and Bagshawe, K. D. Active immunotherapy with *Corynebacterium parvum* and chemotherapy in murine fibrosarcomas. *Brit. med. J.* **1**: 541, 1970.

23. Floersheim, G. L. Facilitation of tumor growth by *Bacillus pertussis*. *Nature (Lond.)* **216**: 1235, 1967.

24. Guyer, R. J. and Crowther, D. Active immunotherapy in treatment of acute leukemia. *Brit. med. J.* **4**: 406, 1969.

25. Havas, H. F. and Donnelly, A. J. Mixed bacterial toxins in the treatment of tumors. IV. Response of methylcholanthrene-induced, spontaneous, and transplanted tumors in mice. *Cancer Res.* **21**: 17, 1961.

26. Nauts, H. C. The apparently beneficial effects of bacterial infections on host resistance to cancer. New York, New York Cancer Research Institute, 1969, Monograph 8.

27. Braun, W., Lampen, J. O., Plescia, O. J. and Pugh, L. Effects of nucleic acid digests on spontaneous and implanted tumors of C3H mice, in: "Conceptual advances in immunology and oncology." New York, Hoeber Med. Div., Harper and Row, Inc., 1963, p. 450.

28. Braun, W. New approaches to immunology as potential adjuncts to chemotherapy, in: *Proceedings of the 6th International Congress of Chemotherapy, 1969*, (in press).

29. Levy, H. B., Law, L. W. and Rabson, A. S. Inhibition of tumor growth by polyinosinic-polycytidylic acid. *Proc. nat. Acad. Sci. (Wash.)* **62**: 357, 1969.

30. Gelboin, H. V. and Levy, H. B. Polyinosinic-polycytidylic acid inhibits chemically induced tumorigenesis in mouse skin. *Science* **167**: 205, 1970.

31. Weiss, D. W. and Wells, A. Q. Vaccination against tuberculosis with nonliving vaccines. II. Vaccination of guinea pigs with phenol-killed tubercle bacilli. *Amer. Rev. resp. Dis.* **81**: 518, 1960.

32. Weiss, D. W. and Wells, A. Q. Vaccination against tuberculosis with nonliving vaccines. III. Vaccination of guinea pigs with fractions of phenol-killed tubercle bacilli. *Amer. Rev. resp. Dis.* **82**: 339, 1960.

33. Weiss, D. W., Bonhag, R. S. and DeOme, K. B. Protective activity of fractions of tubercle

bacilli against isologous tumors in mice. *Nature* (*Lond.*) **190**: 889, 1961.

34. LAVRIN, D. H., BLAIR, P. B. and WEISS, D. W. Immunology of spontaneous mammary carcinomas in mice. III. Immunogenicity of C3H preneoplastic hyperplastic alveolar nodules in C3Hf hosts. *Cancer Res.* **26**: 293, 1966.

35. PREHN, R. T. Cancer antigens in tumors induced by chemicals. *Fed. Proc.* **24**: 1018, 1965.

36. OLD, L. J. and BOYSE, E. A. Antigens of tumors and leukemias induced by viruses. *Fed. Proc.* **24**: 1009, 1965.

37. STJERNSWÄRD, J. Immunodeppressive effect of 3-methylcholanthrene. Antibody formation at cellular level and reaction against weak antigenic homografts. *J. nat. Cancer Inst.* **35**:885, 1965.

38. STJERNSWÄRD, J. Further immunological studies of chemical carcinogenesis. *J. nat. Cancer Inst.* **38**: 515, 1967.

39. LIEBERMAN, M, HARAN-GHERA, N. and KAPLAN, H. S. Potentiation of virus leukaemogenesis in C57BL mice by X-irradiation or urethane. *Nature* (*Lond.*) **203**: 420, 1964.

40. HARAN-GHERA, N. The mechanism of radiation action in leukaemogenesis. The role of radiation in leukaemia development. *Brit. J. Cancer* **21**: 739, 1967.

41. STJERNSWÄRD, J. Immunosuppression by carcinogens. *Antibiot. et Chemother.* (*Basel*) **15**: 213, 1969.

42. TALIAFERRO, W. H. and TALIAFERRO, L. G. Effect of X-rays on hemolysin formation following various immunization and irradiation procedures. *J. infect. Dis.* **95**: 117, 1954.

43. WAKSMAN, B. H., ARBOUYS, S. and ARNASON, B. G. The use of specific "lymphocyte" antisera to inhibit hypersensitive reactions of the "delayed" type. *J. exp. Med.* **114**: 997, 1961.

44. WOODRUFF, M. F. A. and ANDERSON, N. A. Effect of lymphocyte depletion by thoracic duct fistula and administration of antilymphocytic serum on the survival of skin homografts in rats. *Nature* (*Lond.*) **200**: 702, 1963.

45. MONACO, A. P., WOOD, M. L., GRAY, J. G. and RUSSELL, P. S. Studies on heterologous antilymphocyte serum in mice. II. Effect on the immune response. *J. Immunol.* **96**: 229, 1966.

46. JAMES, K. Anti-lymphocytic antibody—a review. *Clin. exp. Immunol.* **2**: 615, 1967.

47. BARTH, R. F., SOUTHWORTH, J. and BURGER, G. M. Studies on heterologous antilymphocyte and antithymocyte sera. I. Serologic specificity and immunosuppressive activity of rabbit anti-mouse sera on the primary immune response. *J. Immunol.* **101**: 282, 1968.

48. HARAN-GHERA, N. and PELED, A. The mechanism of radiation action in leukemogenesis. IV. Immune impairment as a coleukemogenic factor. *Israel J. med. Sci.* **4**: 1181, 1968.

49. ALLISON, A. C., BERMAN, L. D. and LEVEY, R. H. Increased tumor induction by adenovirus type 12 in thymectomized mice and mice treated with antilymphocyte serum. *Nature* (*Lond.*) **215**: 185, 1967.

50. VREDEVOE, D. L. and HAYS, E. F. Effect of antilymphocytic and antithymocytic sera on the development of mouse lymphoma. *Cancer Res.* **29**: 1685, 1969.

51. POTTER, M. and BOYCE, C. R. Induction of plasma-cell neoplasms in strain BALB/c mice with mineral oil and mineral oil adjuvants. *Nature* (*Lond.*) **193**: 1086, 1962.

52. KRIPKE, M. L. and WEISS, D. W. Immunological parameters in the induction of murine plasma cell tumors by mineral oil, in: Severi, L. (Ed.), "Immunity and tolerance in oncogenesis" *Proc. IV. Quadrennial Int. Conf. on Cancer, Perugia, 1969* (in press).

53. CEGLOWSKI, W. S. and FRIEDMAN, H. Immunosuppression by leukemia viruses. I. Effect of Friend disease virus on cellular and humoral hemolysin responses of mice to a primary immunization with sheep erythrocytes. *J. Immunol.* **101**: 594, 1968.

54. WEDDERBURN, N. and SALAMAN, M. H. The immunodepressive effect of Friend virus. II. Reduction of splenic haemolysin-producing cells in primary and secondary responses. *Immunology* **15**: 439, 1968.

55. PELED, A. and HARAN-GHERA, N. Immunosuppressive effect of the radiation leukemia virus on cellular and humoral antibody formation. *Israel J. med. Sci.* **6**: 458, 1970.

56. STJERNSWÄRD, J. Effect of Bacillus Calmette Guérin and/or methylcholanthrene on the antibody-forming cells measured at the cellular level by a hemolytic plaque test. *Cancer Res.* **26**: 1591, 1966.

57. TALIAFERRO, W. H. and JAROSLAV, B. N. The restoration of hemolysin formation in X-rayed rabbits by nucleic acid derivatives and antagonists of nucleic acid synthesis. *J. infect. Dis.* **107**: 341, 1960.

58. FELDMAN, M., GLOBERSON, A. and NACHTIGAL, D. The reactivation of the immune response in immunologically suppressed animals, in: "Conceptual advances in immunology and oncology." New York, Hoeber Med. Div., Harper and Row Publishers, Inc., 1963, p. 427.

59. YASHPHE, D. J. and HARAN-GHERA, N. Modulation of the immune response by a methanol extraction residue of BCG: Studies on the mode of action. *Israel J. med. Sci.* **6**: 446, 1970.

60. WIGZELL, H. and STJERNSWÄRD, J. Age-dependent rise and fall of immunological reactivity in the CBA mouse. *J. nat. Cancer Inst.* **37**: 513, 1966.

61. STJERNSWÄRD, J. Age-dependent tumor-host barrier and effect of carcinogen-induced immunodepression on rejection of isografted methylcholanthrene-induced sarcoma cells. *J. nat. Cancer Inst.* **37**: 505, 1966.

62. BRAUN, W., YAJIMA, Y., JIMENEZ, L. and WINCHURCH, R. Activation, stimulation and the occasional non-specificity of antibody formation, in: Sterzl, J. (Ed.), "Developmental aspects of antibody formation and structure." New York, Academic Press, 1970.

63. HECHTEL, M., DISHON, T. and BRAUN, W. Influence of oligodeoxyribonucleotides on the immune response of newborn AKR mice. *Proc. Soc. exp. Biol.* (*N.Y.*) **119**: 991, 1965.

64. WINCHURCH, R. and BRAUN, W. Antibody for-

mation: Premature initiation by endotoxin or synthetic polynucleotides in newborn mice. *Nature* (*Lond.*) **223**: 843, 1969.

65. CINADER, B. Perspectives and prospects of immunotherapy. Autoantibodies and acquired immunological tolerance. *Canad. Cancer Conf.* **5**: 279, 1963.

66. DEZFULIAN, M., ZEE, T., DEOME, K. B., BLAIR, P. B. and WEISS, D. W. Role of the mammary tumor virus in the immunogenicity of spontaneous mammary carcinomas of BALB/c mice and in the responsiveness of the host. *Cancer Res.* **28**: 1759, 1968.

67. MORTON, D. L. Acquired immunological tolerance and carcinogenesis by the mammary tumor virus. I. Influence of neonatal infection with the mammary tumor virus on the growth of spontaneous mammary adenocarcinoma. *J. nat. Cancer Inst.* **42**: 311, 1969.

68. MORTON, D. L., GOLDMAN, L. and WOOD, D. A. Acquired immunological tolerance and carcinogenesis by the mammary tumor virus. II. Immune responses influencing growth of spontaneous mammary adenocarcinomas. *J. nat. Cancer Inst.* **42**: 321, 1969.

69. VAAGE, J. Nonvirus-associated antigens in virus-induced mouse mammary tumors. *Cancer Res.* **28**: 2477, 1968.

70. MORTON, D. L., MILLER, G. F. and WOOD, D. A. Demonstration of tumor-specific immunity against antigens unrelated to the mammary tumor virus in spontaneous mammary adenocarcinomas. *J. nat. Cancer Inst.* **42**: 289, 1969.

71. ATTIA, M. A. M. and WEISS, D. W. Immunology of spontaneous mammary carcinomas in mice. V. Acquired tumor resistance and enhancement in strain A mice infected with mammary tumor virus. *Cancer Res.* **26**: 1787, 1966.

72. BRAUN, W. and NAKANO, M. Influence of oligodeoxyribonucleotides on early events in antibody formation. *Proc. Soc. exp. Biol.* (*N.Y.*) **119**: 701, 1965.

73. FRANZL, R. E. and MCMASTER, P. D. The primary immune response in mice. I. The enhancement and suppression of hemolysin production by a bacterial endotoxin. *J. exp. Med.* **127**: 1087, 1968.

74. MERRIT, K. and JOHNSON, A. G. Studies on the adjuvant action of bacterial endotoxins on antibody formation. V. The influence of endotoxin and 5-fluoro-2-deoxyuridine on the primary antibody response of the Balb mouse to a purified protein antigen. *J. Immunol.* **91**: 266, 1963.

75. MERRIT, K. and JOHNSON, A. G. Studies on the adjuvant action of bacterial endotoxins on antibody formation. VI. Enhancement of antibody formation by nucleic acids. *J. Immunol.* **94**: 416, 1965.

76. FINGER, H., EMMERLING, P. and OFFENHAMMER, A. Increased primary immune response and priming in mice to subimmunogenic doses of sheep erythrocytes by *Bordetella pertussis*. *Experientia* (*Basel*) **25**: 866, 1969.

77. FINGER, H., EMMERLING, P. and BRÜSS, E. The influence of *Bordetella pertussis* on the preparation of mouse spleens for the secondary immune response. *Canad. J. Microbiol.* **15**: 814, 1969.

78. DRESSER, D. W. An assay for adjuvanticity. *Clin. exp. Immunol.* **3**: 877, 1968.

79. NEVEU, T., BRANELLEC, A. and BIOZZI, G. Propriétés adjuvantes de *Corynebacterium parvum* sur la production d'anticorps et sur l'induction de l'hypersnesibilité retardée envers les proteines conjuguées. *Ann. Inst. Pasteur* **106**: 771, 1964.

80. PINCKARD, R. N., WEIR, D. M. and MCBRIDE, W. H. Factors influencing the immune response. II. Effects of the physical state of the antigen and of lymphoreticular cell proliferation on the response to intraperitoneal injections of bovine serum albumin in rabbits. *Clin. exp. Immunol.* **2**: 343, 1967.

81. NOTKINS, A. L., MERGENHAGEN, S. E., RIZZO, A. A., SCHEELE, C. and WALDMANN, T. A. Elevated γ-globulin and increased antibody production in mice infected with lactic dehydrogenase virus. *J. exp. Med.* **123**: 347, 1966.

82. BROOKE, M. S. Conversion of immunological paralysis to immunity by endotoxin. *Nature* (*Lond.*) **206**: 635, 1965.

83. PINCKARD, R. N., WEIR, D. M. and MCBRIDE, W. H. Factors influencing the immune response. III. The blocking effect of *Corynebacterium parvum* upon the induction of acquired immunological unresponsiveness to bovine serum albumin in the adult rabbit. *Clin. exp. Immunol.* **3**: 413, 1968.

84. MERGENHAGEN, S. E., NOTKINS, A. L. and DOUGHERTY, S. F. Adjuvanticity of lactic dehydrogenase virus: Influence of virus infection on the establishment of immunologic tolerance to a protein antigen in adult mice. *J. Immunol.* **99**: 576, 1967.

85. DRESSER, D. W. Effectiveness of lipid and lipidophilic substances as adjuvants. *Nature* (*Lond.*) **191**: 1169, 1961.

86. UNANUE, E. R., ASKONAS, B. A. and ALLISON-A. C. A role of macrophages in the stimula, lation of immune responses by adjuvants. *J. Immunol.* **103**: 71, 1969.

87. SPITZNAGEL, J. K. and ALLISON, A. C. Mode of action of adjuvants: Retinol and other lysosome-labilizing agents as adjuvants. *J. Immunol.* **104**: 119, 1970.

88. KALISS, N. The transplanted tumor as a research tool in cancer immunology. *Cancer Res.* **21**: 1203, 1961.

89. BOYSE, E. A., OLD, L. J. and STOCKERT, E. Immunological enhancement of a leukemia. *Nature* (*Lond.*) **194**: 1142, 1962.

90. KALISS, N. The elements of immunologic enhancement: A consideration of mechanisms. *Ann. N.Y. Acad. Sci.* **101**: 64, 1962.

91. TAKASUGI, M. and HILDEMANN, W. H. Regulation of immunity toward allogeneic tumors in mice. II. Effect of antiserum and antiserum fractions on cellular and humoral responses. *J. nat. Cancer Inst.* **43**: 857, 1969.

92. HELLSTRÖM, I., HELLSTRÖM, K. E., EVANS, C. A., HEPPNER, G. H., PIERCE, G. E. and YANG, J. P. S. Serum-mediated protection of neoplastic cells from inhibition by lymphocytes immune to their tumor-specific antigens. *Proc. nat. Acad. Sci.* (*Wash.*) **62**: 362, 1969.

93. HEPPNER, G. H. Studies on serum-mediated inhibition of cellular immunity to spontaneous mouse mammary tumors. *Int. J. Cancer* **4**: 608, 1969.

94. IRVIN, G. L., III., EUSTACE, J. C. and FAHEY, J. L. Enhancement activity of mouse immunoglobulin classes. *J. Immunol.* **99**: 1085, 1967.

95. TOKUDA, S. and MCENTEE, P. F. Immunologic enhancement of sarcoma I by mouse γ-globulin fractions. *Transplantation* **5**: 606, 1967.

96. CHARD, T. Immunological enhancement by mouse isoantibodies: The importance of complement fixation. *Immunology* **14**: 583, 1968.

97. VOISIN, G. A., KINSKY, R., JANSEN, F. and BERNARD, C. Biological properties of antibody classes in transplantation immune sera. *Transplantation* **8**: 618, 1969.

98. TAKASUGI, M. and HILDEMANN, W. H. Regulation of immunity toward allogeneic tumors in mice. I. Effect of antiserum fractions on tumor growth. *J. nat. Cancer Inst.* **43**: 843, 1969.

99. YASHPHE, D. J., STEINKULLER, C. B. and WEISS D. W. Modulation of immunological responsiveness by pretreatment with a methanol-insoluble fraction of killed tubercle bacilli. *Israel J. med. Sci.* **5**: 259, 1969.

100. YASHPHE, D. J. and WEISS, D. W. Modulation of the immune response by a methanol-insoluble fraction of attenuated tubercle bacilli. Primary and secondary responses to sheep red blood cells and T$_2$phage. *Clin. exp. Immunol.* **7**: 269, 1970.

101. WHITE, R. G., BERNSTOCK, L., JOHNS, R. G. S. and LEDERER, E. The influence of components of *M. tuberculosis* and other mycobacteria upon antibody production to ovalbumin. *Immunology* **1**: 54, 1958.

102. DAVIES, A. M., GERY, I., ROSENMANN, E. and LAUFER, A. Endotoxin as adjuvant in autoimmunity to cardiac tissue. *Proc. Soc. exp. Biol. (N.Y.)* **114**: 520, 1963.

103. KALDEN, J. R., WILLIAMSON, W. G. and IRVINE, W. J. The effect of *Bordetella pertussis* vaccine on the development of experimental thyroiditis in rats immunized by the intralymph node route or into a hind footpad. *Clin. exp. Immunol.* **5**: 549, 1969.

104. BRADNER, W. T., CLARKE, D. A. and STOCK, C. C. Stimulation of host defense against experimental cancer. I. Zymosan and sarcoma 180 in mice. *Cancer Res.* **18**: 347, 1958.

105. HAVAS, H. F., GROESBECK, M. E. and DONNELLY, A. J. Mixed bacterial toxins in the treatment of tumors. I. Methods of preparation and effects on normal and sarcoma 37-bearing mice. *Cancer Res.* **18**: 141, 1958.

106. BIOZZI, C., STIFFEL, C., HALPERN, B. N. and MOUTON, D. Effet de l'inoculation du bacille de Calmette-Guérin sur le développement de la tumeur ascitique d'Erlich chez la souris. *C.R. Soc. Biol. (Paris)* **153**: 987, 1959.

107. MALKIEL, S. and HARGIS, B. J. Influence of *B. pertussis* on host survival following S-180 implantation. *Cancer Res.* **21**: 1461, 1961.

108. OLD, L. J., CLARKE, D. A., BENACERRAF, B. and STOCKERT, E. Effect of prior splenectomy on the growth of Sarcoma 180 in normal and bacillus Calmette-Guérin infected mice. *Experientia (Basel)* **18**: 335, 1962.

109. HALPERN, B. N., BIOZZI, C., STIFFEL, C. and MOUTON, D. Inhibition of tumor growth by administration of killed *Corynebacterium parvum*. *Nature (Lond.)* **212**: 853, 1966.

110. BALNER, H., OLD, L. J. and CLARKE, D. A. Accelerated rejection of male skin isografts by female C57BL mice infected with *Bacillus Calmette-Guérin* (BCG). *Proc. Soc. exp. Biol. (N.Y.)* **109**: 58, 1962.

111. VITALE, B. and ALEGRETTI, N. Influence of Bacillus Calmette-Guérin infection on the intensity of homograft reaction in rats. *Nature (Lond.)* **199**: 507, 1963.

112. BENTVELZEN, P., VAN DER GUGTEN, A., HILGERS, J. and DAAMS, J. H. Breakthrough in tolerance to eggborne mammary tumor viruses in mice, in: Severi, L. (Ed.), "Immunity and tolerance in oncogenesis." *Proc. IV Quadrennial Int. Conf. on Cancer, Perugia, 1969* (in press).

113. TER-GRIGOROV, V. S. and IRLIN, I. S. The stimulating effect of complete Freund's adjuvant on tumor induction by polyoma virus in mice and by Rous sarcoma virus in rats. *Int. J. Cancer* **3**: 760, 1968.

114. ROITT, I. M., GREAVES, M. F., TORRIGIANI, G., BROSTOFF, J. and PLAYFAIR, J. H. L. The cellular basis of immunological responses. *Lancet* **ii**: 367, 1969.

115. GALLILY, R. and FELDMAN, M. The role of macrophages in the induction of antibody in X-irradiated animals. *Immunology* **12**: 197, 1967.

116. UNANUE, E. R. and ASKONAS, B. A. The immune response of mice to antigen in macrophages. *Immunology* **15**: 287, 1968.

117. MITCHISON, N. A. The immunogenic capacity of antigen taken up by peritoneal exudate cells. *Immunology* **16**: 1, 1969.

118. CLAMAN, H. N., CHAPERON, E. A. and TRIPLETT, R. F. Thymus-marrow cell combinations. Synergism in antibody production. *Proc. Soc. exp. Biol. (N.Y.)* **121**: 236, 1966.

119. MILLER, J. F. A. P. and MITCHELL, G. F. Cell to cell interaction in the immune response. I. Hemolysin-forming cells in neonatally thymectomized mice reconstituted with thymus or thoracic duct lymphocytes. *J. exp. Med.* **128**: 801, 1968.

120. DAVIES, A. J. S. The thymus and the cellular basis of immunity. *Transplant. Rev.* **1**: 43, 1969.

121. MARTIN, W. J. and MILLER, J. F. A. P. Cell to cell interaction in the immune response. IV. Site of action of antilymphocyte globulin. *J. exp. Med.* **128**: 855, 1968.

122. LEUCHARS, E., WALLIS, V. J. and DAVIES, A. J. S. Mode of action of antilymphocyte serum. *Nature (Lond.)* **219**: 1325, 1968.

123. STINEBRING, W. R. and YOUNGNER, J. S. Patterns of interferon appearance in mice injected with bacteria or bacterial endotoxin. *Nature (Lond.)* **204**: 712, 1964.

124. FIELD, A. K., TYTELL, A. A., LAMPSON, G. P. and HILLEMAN, M. R. Inducers of interferon and host resistance. II. Multistranded syn-

thetic polynucleotide complexes. *Proc. nat. Acad. Sci.* (*Wash.*) **58**: 1004, 1967.

125. LAMPSON, G. P., TYTELL, A. A., FIELD, A. L., NEMES, M. R. and HILLEMAN, M. R. Inducers of interferon and host resistance. I. Double-stranded RNA from extracts of *Penicillium funiculosum*. *Proc. nat. Acad. Sci.* (*Wash.*) **58**: 782, 1967.

126. DURAN-REYNALS, F. Reaction of spontaneous mouse carcinomas to blood-carried bacterial toxins. *Proc. Soc. exp. Biol.* (*N.Y.*) **32**: 1517, 1935.

127. MACKANESS, G. B. The influence of immunologically committed lymphoid cells on macrophage activity *in vivo*. *J. exp. Med.* **129**: 973, 1969.

128. LAWRENCE, H. S. and LANDY, M. "Mediators of cellular immunity." New York, Academic Press, 1969.

TUMOR ANTIGENS AND THE NATURE
OF THE IMMUNE RESPONSE
TO NEOPLASTIC CELLS

IMMUNOLOGICAL STUDIES ON A HUMAN TUMOR

Dilemmas of the Experimentalist

GEORGE KLEIN

Institute for Tumor Biology, Karolinska Institutet, Stockholm, Sweden

RECENT ADVANCES IN EXPERIMENTAL TUMOR IMMUNOLOGY

Experimental tumor immunology has developed at an unexpected rate during the last decade. Following the demonstration that chemically induced mouse sarcomas can induce rejection reactions in genetically compatible (syngeneic) hosts (1, 2) and even in the original, primary host (3) and the even more puzzling finding that both DNA (4, 5) and RNA (6, 7) virus induced tumors are susceptible to rejection reactions induced in the syngeneic host by homologous virus or tumor inoculation, new information has accumulated rapidly in many different laboratories. Isograft or autograft reactions of varying intensity have been demonstrated against a large number of chemically and virally induced tumors in different species and some spontaneous tumors as well (for reviews see 8–14). It seems fair to say that at least weak responses have been shown to exist in all systems that have been thoroughly investigated, unless tolerance was shown to prevail; so far, this has only been found with tumors induced by some vertically transmitted, non-cytopathogenic RNA viruses (15–17).

Another important concept that has emerged from the experimental studies is the idea of immune surveillance, i.e. the continuous elimination of neoplastic cell clones *in statu nascendi*, by a process involving immune recognition. It was surmised (18) that this could be the biological basis of the homograft reaction. One important feature of the tumor specific rejection reactions is their relativity, i.e. their inability to deal with more than a relatively small number of tumor cells. Although the ceiling level is different for different systems, it is as a rule promptly overwhelmed by excessive cell numbers.

It is often emphasized that the relative nature of tumor specific rejection responses has some important practical consequences in relation to immunotherapy. Radiotherapy and chemotherapy act by single-hit kinetics and the same dose of therapy is required for each tenfold decrease of the tumor cell population, no matter whether the population is large or small. This imposes severe limitations on the attempts to eradicate the whole population, since the risks of toxicity and other side effects will increase for each logarithmic unit of population decrease. An immune rejection that can act against a ceiling of, say, 10^5 cells will have no practical significance for a population of 10^9 but it will achieve decisive importance when the population size has been brought down to 10^5 by other forms of therapy. The high specificity of the immune rejection, its ubiquitous action in the organism (except certain "sheltered" sites) and its non-toxic nature are other important aspects. The major significance of potential immunotherapeutic approaches lies, in other words, in the protection against recurrence and metastases, in combination with other forms of therapy. This would also be in line with the basic surveillance function of the rejection mechanism.

From the biological point of view, it makes sense that a surveillance mechanism, operating in the normal organism, should protect against small numbers of neoplastic cells, localized as incipient clonal foci, or scattered throughout the body, depending on the habits of the cell, rather than against large tumors. The development of frank neoplasia would then signal a breakdown of the system, e.g. by immunosuppression or, what is probably more important, by old age (19, 20). This may be one reason why most tumors occur in older people. In young patients, tumor development may reflect an overwhelming carcinogenic noxa, perhaps a potent oncogenic virus, operating on a favorable genetic background, or transmitted vertically, and setting surveillance specifically out of function by inducing tolerance.

What is the evidence for the existence of a surveillance mechanism? Most compelling is the demonstration (21–30) that neonatal thymectomy or treatment with antilymphocytic serum increases the incidence of chemically and virally induced tumors. The effects were particularly striking with tumors induced by the oncogenic DNA viruses, such as polyoma or SV_{40}. With chemically induced tumors, the results were less clear cut, although there is no doubt about their reality (e.g. 22, 30). One may recall in this context that certain chemical carcinogens, and aromatic hydrocarbons in particular, have a prolonged immunosuppressive effect (31, 32). This may contribute to their oncogenic effect, particularly in adult, immunocompetent animals, in contrast to some of the oncogenic viruses that require immunologically immature or hyporeactive hosts. The immunosuppressive component of chemical carcinogenesis may explain why the effects of neonatal thymectomy are no more dramatic in increasing tumor incidence: this will depend on the differential that can be obtained between the immunosuppressive action of the chemical carcinogen and the further abolition of the residual rejection potential by thymectomy.

There are two important exceptions from the tumor-amplifying effect of neonatal thymectomy. One is represented by the systems where immunological tolerance against tumor specific antigens plays a major role, such as in the genesis of mammary carcinoma in mice that received the mammary tumor agent (MTV) neonatally (15). Surveillance does not seem to function in this situation or is so inefficient that neonatal thymectomy has nothing to add and there is no significant increase in tumor incidence (28). The other exception can be exemplified by the virus-induced murine lymphomas that originate from thymus-dependent lymphoid tissues, e.g. the lymphomas induced by the Gross or the Moloney virus. Here, neonatal thymectomy prevents the development of lymphoma more or less completely (33–35), due to the fact that the differentiation of the neoplastic target cell cannot occur in the absence of the thymus. Obviously, it would be meaningless to look for evidence of surveillance by neonatal thymectomy in this situation, since the purpose of the experiment is counteracted at the outset. It is therefore of great interest that recent experiments of Allison and Law (27) have shown that the incidence of lymphomas and reticulum cell sarcomas can be increased by antilymphocyte serum in immunocompetent leukemia virus recipients. This is another important demonstration of immune surveillance and it also shows how one can distinguish between systems where neonatal thymectomy fails to increase tumor incidence due to tolerance (in these cases, ALS should not do it either) and the systems where the thymus dependence of the neoplastic target cell itself is responsible.

In this context, it is of interest that recent evidence points towards an increased incidence of tumors in patients receiving immunosuppressive therapy after kidney grafting. So far, the tumors that have appeared in frequencies above the expected level were mainly neoplasms of the lymphoreticular system (36). It is possible that the immunosuppressive treatment has acted by the inhibition of the surveillance function—and this would be the first indication of the existence of this function in man. In view of the fact that the tumors arise in the target tissue of the immunosuppressive action, it cannot be excluded, however, that a more direct oncogenic mechanism is involved. The classical demonstration by Haddow of growth inhibition as an early step in carcinogenic action may be recalled (37).

SEARCH FOR TUMOR SPECIFIC ANTIGENS IN BURKITT'S LYMPHOMA (BL)

A few years ago, we asked ourselves the question whether the main facts of experimental tumor immunology, as briefly recapitulated in the previous discussion, might open the way for similar studies on human tumors, and we began searching for a system that could be expected to give at least some meaningful answers. It was obvious that the choice of tumor was quite critical. BL was selected for the following three reasons: a) A viral etiology has been postulated, on reasonable grounds (38). A tumor of viral origin can be expected to carry distinctive antigens common for all tumors induced by the same virus, rather than antigens that differ for each individual tumor. b) Clinical observations (39–41) strongly suggested that host defense reactions may play an important role in this disease and

decisively influence that outcome of chemotherapy. c) Lymphoma cells lend themselves readily to the preparation of free cell suspensions; all tests designed for the study of cell surface antigens require suspensions that contain a high percentage of intact viable cells.

The first question we asked appeared quite straightforward: Was it possible to obtain evidence, by testing the reactivity of living BL cells with patients' sera, and in comparison with appropriate controls, that would indicate the existence of characteristic cell membrane associated antigens, in analogy with the virally induced murine leukemias and, if so, could this information help to elucidate the etiology of the disease, as well as the possible role of host defense reactions that may influence its clinical course? To approach this problem, we chose the technique that was most sensitive in the experimental leukemia studies (42, 43), i.e. membrane immunofluorescence with viable target cells (44). The findings, summarized briefly in the following sections, essentially confirmed the expectations, but they have also led to many unexpected observations and raised new dilemmas. Some of them may serve to exemplify the problems encountered during the transition from the experimental to the human situation.

STUDIES ON BL BIOPSY CELLS

During the first phase of this work, fresh BL biopsy cells were exposed to the sera of BL patients and various other donors, and we searched for attached immunoglobulins by the indirect membrane fluorescence technique (45–47). The sera of BL patients reacted more frequently than African control sera from donors with other neoplastic or non-neoplastic diseases. The possibility that the reactivity of the BL sera was due to isoantibodies became unlikely when it was found that autochthonous serum-cell combinations gave positive reactions in five of six cases where this could be tested. It turned out, furthermore, that the

113

most regularly positive sera have been derived from patients whose tumors have gone to total regression after chemotherapy. For this reason, the autochthonous target cell was frequently unavailable as far as the highly positive serum donors were concerned. To exclude isoantibodies, such sera were tested in parallel series against lymphoma cells and normal bone marrow cells derived from the same allogeneic BL donor. Lymphoma cells, but not bone marrow cells, reacted regularly in such tests, thus increasing the probability that the reactivity of the BL serum-cell combinations could not be simply due to the presence of isoantibodies. This was further reinforced by the finding that lymphoid cells of normal donors and of donors with different types of leukemias and other lymphoreticular diseases also failed to react.

While this was encouraging, further studies on the specificity of the reaction were hampered by the great variability of the biopsy preparations. One major source of the difficulty was the variable degree of immunoglobulin coating on the surface of the biopsy cells. This coating was detected by direct membrane immunofluorescence with conjugated anti-immunoglobulin reagents. It could be of two basically different kinds: IgM or IgG, or both, showing not only a difference in class specificity but also a difference in behavior in relation to the course of the disease (48, 49). In cases where the cell surface reacted with anti-IgM conjugates, reactivity was usually expressed on 100% or nearly 100% of the cells. When such cells were converted into established lines *in vitro*, it was found that their "IgM-ring" was maintained during long-term propagation. The membrane-IgM reactive lines did not secrete IgM into the medium (R. van Furth et al., personal communication). Preliminary characterization of the reactive substance in membrane fractionation experiments (50) indicates, at least as far as one cell of this type is concerned,

that 7S-size IgM subunits with μ- and κ-chain specificities are integrated into the cell membrane. Conceivably, this is the neoplastic variety of a normal lymphoid cell that incorporates molecules of this type into its plasma membrane as part of its normal differentiation. Lymphoid cells of this type have been postulated to play an important role in immunological memory or delayed hypersensitivity, or both (51). The lymphoma cells may represent the neoplastic variant in the same way as myeloma cells project normal immunoglobulin secreting plasma cells into a magnified, neoplastic image. The phenomenon is not exclusive for BL; a Swedish case of chronic lymphatic leukemia has been found with the same cellular characteristics (52).

Whatever the nature of the cell that carries membrane-associated immunoglobulins, it is important to note in relation to the present discussion that this property has always behaved as a cell marker when repeated biopsies were taken from the same patient. If it was present on the cells of a given tumor, it was maintained unchanged in the course of repeated biopsies; if it was absent, it remained absent. It was also maintained following successful heterografting of a membrane-IgM positive BL cell to the rat (53).

The IgG coat behaved quite differently. It was rarely present on untreated BL biopsy cells, but it tended to appear if the tumor persisted in spite of treatment. It accumulated following a recurrence that was presumably due to the selection of a tetraploid, probably immunoresistant, BL cell variant (49, 54). "Self-enhancement," i.e. the accumulation of "blocking" antibodies that prevent the access of immune lymphoid cells (13) is an obvious possibility.

Whether these considerations are realistic or not, the changing pattern of IgG coating with time and its failure to persist on derived *in vitro* lines (48, 55), indicates that it is due to coating from the outside, unlike the membrane associated IgM, that appears to represent a special type of production from within the cell.

The presence of performed immunoglobulin on the cell surface may interfere with the indirect membrane immunofluorescence reaction and, when present in subliminal degree, it probably explains some of the variability encountered when biopsy cells are used as targets. In order to avoid this variability, we started looking for more standardized target cells and turned to established culture lines.

EXPERIMENTS WITH ESTABLISHED

TISSUE CULTURE LINES

A number of BL-derived lymphoblastoid cell lines growing in stationary suspension cultures were tested against BL sera that reacted regularly with BL biopsy cells and were free of demonstrable isoantibodies (56). The pattern which appeared was strange but interesting. Four BL-derived lines gave positive membrane immunofluorescence reactions in the indirect test, after exposure to the reference serum "Mutua" (derived from a BL patient in long-term regression), whereas three BL-derived lines were negative. Eight control lines derived from various leukemias and, in one case, from a normal donor, were negative as well. At first, we could not understand this pattern. A clue was obtained, however, when these results were compared with the reactivity of the same cell lines in the Henle test (57) known to detect Epstein-Barr virus (EBV) (probably nucleocapsid) antigens. In carrier cultures, these antigens are present in a small frequency of the cells, as a rule. These cells show degenerative features and, when simultaneous immunofluorescence and electron microscopy is performed (58), turn out to be loaded with herpes-type EBV (59) particles. The first comparison of the membrane and EBV test revealed (60) that the four membrane positive lines contained EBV-antigens in more than 1% of the cells whereas the

membrane-negative lines were either EBV-negative or contained a very small frequency of positive cells (less than 1%).

This suggested that the membrane antigen detected by this reference serum may be determined by the genome of the EBV. More conclusive evidence was obtained in a prospective study (60). Fourteen new lines were established from biopsies received from Nairobi, and the frequency of EBV-positive and of membrane reactive cells was determined in parallel, on coded specimens, at two different laboratories. The same relationship was found as in the preliminary retrospective study: only the lines that carried a relatively high "EBV-load" showed a positive membrane antigen reactivity. In the reactive lines, the frequency of membrane positive cells was approximately ten times higher than the frequency of EBV-positive cells. The biopsies from which the lines were derived were membrane positive, but EBV-negative, as a rule. EBV reactivity appeared during the first week in culture. This suggests that the production of the viral nucleocapsid antigen is suppressed in the tumor cell *in vivo*. The suppressive factor could be antibody, but there are many other possibilities. Another curious observation was that repeated establishment of parallel lines from the same patient, derived from successive biopsies, led to lines with fairly similar EBV levels, whereas lines derived from different patients were quite different (61). This suggests that the viral "load" per cell, or the "activatability" of the virus, or both, are characteristic for the individual tumor. Since the membrane-associated IgM marker, mentioned above, and another study with glucose-6-phosphate dehydrogenase-isozyme markers (62) strongly indicate that the BL process has a clonal origin, this may reflect the virus-cell relationship that characterizes a particular clone.

The postulate that the membrane antigen is determined by the EBV was directly confirmed when it was found that it can be induced to appear in EBV-negative lines by infection with EBV concentrates (63) or by the admixture of heavily irradiated EBV-carrying cells (64).

Although the relationship between EBV and the membrane antigen was clarified by these studies, this applies only to the EBV-carrier cultures *in vitro*, and it must be kept in mind that similarly compelling evidence is lacking as to the connection between the membrane antigens detected on the biopsy cells and the virus, although there are strong indications that the biopsy cells probably express the same membrane antigen as the carrier cultures (65).

The antigenic components entering the EBV-determined membrane and the intracellular nucleocapsid complex differ with regard to immunological specificity. By absorbing sera that reacted with the membrane and the intracellular EBV complex as well with large numbers of intact, viable membrane antigen positive cells, it was possible to remove the membrane reactive antibodies, with only a minor reduction in the anti-EBV titer (66). Moreover, some sera could be found with antibodies against the membrane antigen, or the EBV antigen, but not both. Although such "discordant" sera were a minority, their existence is in line with the immunological distinctness of the two antigen types.

Further analysis of the two antigen systems revealed (67) that both the membrane and the intracellular antigens must be regarded as antigen complexes, with several distinct subcomponents. Sera that contain antibodies against several subcomponents of the intracellular EBV complex also tend to carry, as a rule, several antibody components against various parts of the membrane antigen complex, but the relationship is not absolute, and many combinations can be found. Patients with large, persisting tumors frequently had a larger number of serum antibody compo-

nents against both antigen complexes than sera from healthy, EBV-positive individuals, or convalescent sera from donors after infectious mononucleosis, or sera from BL patients whose tumors have gone to long-term regression following chemotherapy.

The nature of the membrane antigen, in terms of virus-cell relationships and in relation to the virus cycle, is an interesting problem that remains to be clarified. The ability of different sera to neutralize an artificial EBV infection of EBV-negative culture lines (such as Raji or 6410) was related to the titer of membrane reactive antibody, and not to the anti-EBV titer (68). This was particularly apparent when a series of sera were tested that were discordant with regard to their anti-EBV and membrane reactivity. In another series of tests, the sera of rabbits immunized with EBV concentrates were able to block the membrane antigen reaction specifically (69); this indicated that the membrane antigen was present in the immunizing material, either as a constituent or as a contaminant of the viral particles.

It has been shown that herpes simplex virus (HSV) is capable of inducing new membrane antigens in the cells it infects (70, 71). In viral mutants with different envelope characteristics, the membrane changes they induce are also different and in a way that closely parallels their envelope properties (72). It has been concluded that the appearance of viral envelope material is responsible for the changes in the cell membrane. Presumably, the virus changes the cellular membrane in order to facilitate the process of its own envelopment. In view of the parallel between EBV neutralization and membrane reactive antibody levels, it is conceivable that the EBV-associated membrane antigen represents viral envelope material as well. This is of interest because, for HSV, a relationship has been demonstrated between the changed "social behavior" of infected cells and their membrane modifications after exposure to different mutants of HSV (72). The understanding of the role which EBV-induced membrane changes may play in cell behavior may elucidate the relationship between this agent and the neoplastic diseases with which it is most regularly associated.

DISEASE-RELATED SEROLOGICAL PATTERNS

This topic can be discussed at two levels: a) the relationship between EBV-associated serological reactivity and clinical and pathological diagnosis, and b) changes in EBV-related serological patterns during the clinical course of EBV-associated diseases.

a) It can be stated first that the serological anti-EBV reactivity, as determined by the Henle test (57), is extremely widespread in all human populations. If the level of significant reactivity is set at a 1:10 serum dilution, as customary (73), the large majority of adult populations is EBV-positive. It may be questioned whether the 10 to 15% negatives (with titers < 10) are real or spurious. Specific antibodies may occur at titers below 10 and may be missed, due to the various test artefacts that arise at high serum concentrations (73). On the other hand, whereas some of the < 10 "negatives" may hide specific reactivity, at least part of them must be real negatives in the biological sense. A prospective study (74) has shown that EBV-positive young adults are protected from infectious mononucleosis, whereas a significant proportion of the "EBV-negatives" (i.e. < 10) developed the disease and became EBV-positive, in the course of a two- to four-year observation period.

The causal relationship between EBV and at least one form of infectious mononucleosis (75) is most clearly established by this prospective study. If this is accepted, it immediately leads to the question of whether EBV plays any etiological role in other diseases, and particularly the neoplastic diseases with which it is most regularly associated.

The serological patterns that are now known can be evaluated in different ways. In the Henle type anti-EBV test, BL and nasopharyngeal carcinoma (NPC) are distinguished by outstandingly high anti-EBV titers, so far unparalleled among other lymphoproliferative diseases and other carcinomas of the head and neck region (75–78). The geometric mean anti-EBV titer of BL patients was eight times higher than in various control groups. There were no significant differences between control sera collected from areas with a high or a low incidence of BL. With the exception of a few, moribund cases, low (< 1:80) anti-EBV titers were very rare among BL patients and there are no histologically confirmed cases with negative (< 1:10) titers. Occasionally, long-term regression cases tended to show falling titers after some years, but this was by no means the rule.

The serological behavior of BL and NPC sera is also exceptional in the precipitin test developed by Old et al. (79, 80), performed against a soluble antigen extracted from the EBV-carrying P3J lines. NPC sera from Africa and the USA were positive in 85 to 87% of the cases, and 59% of the African BL sera gave positive precipitin reactions. Other neoplasias, including lymphoproliferative diseases and carcinomas of different kinds, gave a much lower incidence of positives, with the exception of chronic lymphatic leukemia and lymphosarcoma that came close to the reactivity of the BL sera. Two distinct precipitin lines (B and P) could be identified regularly, but there was no obvious disease related difference between the two.

The antibodies against the EBV-associated membrane antigens can be most easily evaluated by the blocking of the direct membrane fluorescence reaction, obtained with specific reference conjugates (81, 82). When the Mutua conjugate was used, already referred to in the previous paragraph, only very exceptional normal sera showed any significant blocking at all and most of them were negative. Head and neck tumor sera, other than BL and NPC were negative in the majority of instances, but occasional highly positive sera have been encountered. The difference between the regularly high-reactive African or Chinese NPC sera and the predominantly low-reactive Indian hypopharyngeal and oropharyngeal carcinoma sera was particularly remarkable (77). Most BL and NPC sera with histologically confirmed diagnosis (and this means, for the NPC, the poorly differentiated or anaplastic type) gave significant and, in most cases, high to complete blocking reactions.

In a "tripartite" study, the anti-EBV (Henle)-test, the blocking of direct membrane fluorescence, and the precipitin reaction have been compared with 151 coded sera (83). There was a clear over-representation of BL and NPC sera within the "triple-high" reactivity group, and they were virtually absent from the "triple-low" group. The opposite was true for the two main groups of control sera, derived from healthy relatives of BL patients and from donors with head and neck tumors other than BL and NPC.

One interesting question concerns the relationship between geographical localization and serological reactivity. NPC are more easy to evaluate in this respect, since they represent a clear pathological entity and are not readily confused with other conditions. The EBV-associated serological reactivity of African, Swedish, French, Chinese and American cases was uniformly high and appeared to be characteristic for the anaplastic or poorly differentiated types (76, 77, 80).

The evaluation of BL outside Africa presents a more difficult problem, because the pathological picture alone does not permit a sharp distinction against other lymphomas. The combined clinical and pathological picture has readily recognizable features in the high-endemic areas but they are less charac-

teristic in other regions, and the classification becomes more arbitrary. If one nevertheless examines the data on the serological behavior of "Burkitt-like" lymphomas outside Africa, it appears that the results are partly in line with the African BL (83, 84), and partly differ from the African cases, i.e. have no distinctively high EBV-associated reactivity defined as high anti-EBV titer or high membrane blocking index, or both, and thus resemble ordinary lymphosarcomas rather than "true" BL. This picture cannot be interpreted meaningfully at present since serology cannot serve as the basis for classification if the problem is to decide whether non-African cases have an African-Burkitt-like serology or not; the argument becomes circular. Speculatively at least, one may nevertheless consider the possibility that the non-African Burkitt-like cases are heterogeneous. Some of them would be "true Burkitts," i.e. have the same etiology as the African cases, whereas others would be different and comparable to "ordinary" lymphosarcomas. Whether this classification can be based on the EBV-associated serological reactions depends on the question whether the relationship of the EBV to Burkitt's disease is of an essential or of an accidental nature.

b) Another approach to the study of disease-related EBV patterns is to follow the antibody titers against the various EBV-associated antigens horizontally, during the course of "EBV-associated" diseases, such as BL and NPC. For comparison, one may choose EBV-positive individuals with more or less related neoplastic diseases that are not regularly associated with high anti-EBV titers. Studies of this type are now becoming feasible; some preliminary information is already available. At an early stage, the indirect membrane test, performed with BL biopsy cell targets indicated (45, 46) that the most highly reactive sera are found in patients whose tumors have gone to long-term regression. Later, when the more specific and sensitive blocking of direct membrane fluorescence replaced the indirect test as the main method to detect antibodies against the EBV-associated membrane antigen complex on established culture lines, it turned out (82, 83, 85) that nearly all histologically confirmed African BL sera have a high blocking activity, i.e. show a complete or nearly complete cross reactivity with the reference conjugate. The few exceptions have come from moribund patients. This monotonously uniform blocking activity, obtained with the undiluted sera, hides large quantitative differences, however. When compared by serial titration against the same reference coniugate, the blocking titer of various BL patients' sera (taking a blocking index of 0.5 as the endpoint) could vary between 1:1 and 1:600 (85). In the individual patient, the titers may change considerably in the course of the disease, but, as a rule, they remain within the same order of magnitude: most changes are restricted to relatively few dilution steps up or down and the patients can therefore be classified into groups of low, medium and high reactivity.

Our preliminary findings indicate that the blocking titer differences between patients, as well as the horizontal changes, are influenced by a number of factors. In the course of rapid and extensive tumor growth, antibody levels probably fall due to adsorption to tumor cell membranes. When the patient receives chemotherapy and the tumor regresses, there is often an increase in titer. At first sight, this may seem paradoxical, in view of the immunosuppressive effect of chemotherapy. It is known, however, that chemical immunosuppression inhibits new primary antibody responses against antigens administered after the drug, but is much less efficient against immune reactions established before treatment.

An increase in blocking antibody titers was particularly apparent in BL and NPC patients who received local radiotherapy (86), including cases where therapy did not lead to complete tumor regression. In view of the fact that X-irradiated tumor cells are relatively good immunogens in experimental systems (3), this is of considerable interest. It may also be relevant that in EBV-carrier cultures with a relatively low membrane antigen reactivity, X-rays induce the appearance of the membrane antigen on a large fraction of the cells (87).

In BL patients with recurring tumors that continue to grow in spite of chemotherapy, blocking antibody levels that have fallen to low levels at or around the time of recurrence rise again (e.g. 49). Subsequently, the lymphoma cells become coated with IgG, as a rule, if the tumor persists. It is conceivable that such cells represent immunoresistant variants, similar to what has been found in experimental systems (88). This is supported, indirectly at least, by the history of two patients whose tumors recurred after several years of total regression and contained a high frequency of near-tetraploid cells (54), in contrast to more than 20 other BL biopsies examined (G. Manolov, personal communication) with a shorter clinical history, that were all in the near-diploid range. Tetraploid cells can frequently outgrow host responses that efficiently reject diploid cells of the same lineage (89).

The immunoglobulin coat acquired by the tumors that persist in spite of therapy may be the equivalent of enhancing antibody or of blocking antibody in Hellström's sense (13). This is not necessarily an alternative to the possibility that membrane-reactive antibodies may have a growth inhibitory action, but rather another facet of the same complex picture. An antibody that has cytotoxic or growth inhibitory properties against immunosensitive cells may exert an enhancing effect (i.e. protect the target cell against the cell mediated immune response) when it interacts with an immunoresistant cell without killing it. In addition, different antibodies no doubt differ; some can be cytotoxic and others enhancing towards the same target cell. In the course of chemotherapy that falls short of a total tumor kill, and the subsequent regrowth of the residual tumor with more antigen release and antibody binding, the immunosensitivity of the tumor cell population and the killing vs. enhancing power of the antibody population must obviously change in a complex way. This would require a multicomponential experimental analysis, that is not yet within reach.

In addition to the changes in membrane reactive antibody levels brought about by the tumor itself (i.e. changes due to absorption, antigen release, effect of tumor growth on the immune response, etc.), the antibody titer may change for other, tumor-unrelated reasons, and this may, in turn, influence tumor growth. This possibility has been brought into focus by the history of a BL patient (49) who was in total tumor regression for a period of four and one-half years and subsequently developed widespread abdominal metastases. Her membrane reactive antibody level, determined by the blocking test, fell markedly more than six months prior to recurrence, at a time when there was no reason to suspect the presence of any metastases. When the abdominal recurrence became manifest half a year later, the membrane reactive antibody level was still low, and the tumor cells were not yet coated with IgG. In the course of the subsequent two months, the serum antibody level increased again and the lymphoma cells became IgG-coated. This sequence of events decreases the probability that the fall of the antibody level that preceeded recurrence by six months was due to absorption to an as yet cryptic tumor: In that case, a period of slow tumor growth would have followed during the subsequent six-month period, and the secondary increase in antibody level, as well as the coating of the lymphoma cells with immunoglobulins would be expected to have occurred in the interim, appearing already at the time of

clinical recurrence. Indirect as this reasoning is, it has nevertheless raised the question whether a fall in antibody levels may be sometimes the cause, rather than merely the consequence, of tumor recurrence, and whether it could act by facilitating the outgrowth of "dormant" neoplastic cells.

One considerable gap in the information on the kinetics of recurrence is the lack of procedures that would permit the quantitative assessment of cell mediated immunity. This is probably the largest single unknown factor in the BL picture. Speculatively, one may recall the curious fact (90, 91) that the jaw tumors occur with the highest frequency at five and six years of age, testicular and ovarian tumors around the time of puberty, long bone tumors in adolescence, and one of the vary rare documented cases in an adult is a bilateral breast tumor in a lactating woman that went to spontaneous regression when the patient stopped nursing. This suggests that cell proliferation in or around the tissue of primary localization may contribute to the outgrowth of the tumor, perhaps by interfering with cell mediated immune surveillance, or, alternatively by imposing a growth stimulating effect on premalignant cell clones. Analogous events may trigger recurrence in long-term regression patients, and it is particularly interesting that recurrence occurs frequently at sites far removed from the primary site.

There is also some preliminary evidence indicating that the antibodies against the soluble EBV-associated antigens detected by immunoprecipitation show a different disease related pattern, appearing at the time of progressive tumor growth and frequently absent in patients whose tumors are in complete regression (49, 83). Although there are numerous exceptions to this, a relationship of this type appeared clearly when the horizontal history of the patient already mentioned above was followed during long-term regression and subsequent recurrence (49). This may also explain why high anti-EBV titered NPC sera are more frequently precipitin-positive than BL sera with comparably high titers: in NPC, the serum material is mainly derived from patients with residual or progressively growing tumors, while a collection of BL sera includes progressor and regressor sera as well.

The tumor-related presence of precipitating antibodies is reminiscent of some DNA-virus induced experimental tumor systems, and particularly the case of antibodies against "T-antigens." In polyoma, SV_{40} and adenovirus induced tumors, it is the "tumored hamster," i.e. the host of nonvirus producing, T-antigen positive tumors that tends to develop antibodies against T-antigens. The antibody levels usually fall when the tumor is removed or rejected and eventually disappear. T-antigens are intracellular, like the soluble antigens in the present system. They appear temporarily, as "early" components of the viral cycle, and they are regularly present in transformed cells. It is not known, however, whether they can be released from growing tumor cells by some kind of a secretory process or whether they represent necrotic tissue products.

Another type of intracellular, EBV-determined antigen that appears to show a similar relationship to tumor status is the "early antigen" (EA) that appears during an acute productive or abortive infection, after the exposure of EBV-negative blastoid cell lines to living EBV-concentrates (92). Antibodies against EA are most regularly present in the sera of tumor-bearing BL and NPC patients, and tend to be absent or only rarely present in EBV-positive sera from BL patients in long-term regression or from normal donors. In contrast to anti-EA, "ordinary" anti-EBV antibodies as detected by the original Henle test (57) and directed, in all probability, against nucleocapsid antigens, show little change with the stage of the disease. It might be speculated that the relatively constant anti-EBV levels are maintained by periodical virus produc-tion, perhaps in analogy with the "activation" of HSV.

Further clarification of the relationship between the dynamics of antibody formation against different EBV-determined antigens and the clinical course of the "high-EBV-associated diseases," such as BL and NPC, may be helpful in elucidating important virus-tumor-host relationships, particularly if compared to EBV-positive sera from patients with other tumors that are not characterized by a regularly high EBV-association.

IMPLICATIONS AND DILEMMAS

Four main dilemmas arise from this pattern of findings; they are interrelated, but all have their specific aspects. They can be briefly stated as follows:

a) *The etiological dilemma.* Can the occurrence of distinctive, tumor associated antigens give any clues about the etiology of the disease?

b) *The problem of neoplastic behavior.* Are the changes in the composition of the cell membrane, or other cellular organelles, as reflected by the appearance of new antigenic specificities, fundamentally involved in the neoplastic behavior of the cell, or, in other words, does the unresponsiveness of the cell to growth control depend on the change in composition or structure that is revealed by the immunological tests?

c) *The therapeutic problem.* Can any of the immunological reactions now identified serve to measure the patient's reactivity to its own tumor, in connection with various therapeutic procedures, including attempts at immuno-therapy?

d) *The prevention problem.* Are there any prevention approaches in sight?

Concerning the etiological dilemma, it is a useful point of departure that all virally induced experimental tumors share the same antigen, as long as they are induced by the same virus, at least as far as the transplanta-

121

tion-type, membrane-associated antigens are concerned. The reverse, the assumption of a common viral etiology on the basis of common antigens found in tumors of unknown origin is not necessarily justified, however. It has been shown (93–98) that virally induced new antigens can be made to appear by superinfecting normal cells or tumors of unrelated etiology with oncogenic and even with some nononcogenic viruses. The only difference between this secondary "antigenic conversion" and the primary event that occurs in direct relation to tumor induction is the lesser stability of the former, particularly in immune hosts (14), as well as a more irregular association between antigen and tumor, depending on the accidental nature of superinfection.

As discussed above, high anti-EBV titers and high antibody levels against EBV-associated membrane antigens and soluble antigens are regularly associated with at least two neoplastic diseases: BL and NPC. For NPC, it is clear that this serological pattern is independent of geographic or ethnic origin. A similar situation may exist for BL, but the lack of reliable criteria by which the identity of the disease can be established outside the endemic areas and distinguished from ordinary lymphomas makes a similar evaluation of the non-African cases more difficult.

It is important to stress that the main difference between BL and NPC and other normal or neoplastic serum donor categories investigated is not EBV-positivity, nor the occurrence of high titered reactions in occasional donors, since such donors may be found in most other categories as well, but the regular and consistent association of high titered reactions according to all three tests. Looking at it from this perspective, BL and NPC are unique. One may question, however, whether this perspective can be justified or, more specifically, what it implies.

As a starting point, we may take the convincing demonstration that EBV is causally related to at least one form of infectious mononucleosis (74, 75). This form afflicts EBV-seronegative adolescents, as a rule, is frequently positive for heterophile antibodies, and is regularly accompanied by seroconversion to anti-EBV positivity. As indicated by a prospective study (74), anti-EBV individuals are apparently protected from this disease.

The serological screening of many different human populations also showed (63, 73) that there is another, "early" seroconversion to anti-EBV positivity, culminating round four years of age, and particularly frequent in low socioeconomic groups. This early infection does not lead to infectious mononucleosis or any other disease identity so far recognized.

Viewed against this background, the relationship of EBV infections to BL and NPC may be considered in terms of the following alternatives:

a) The virus that causes infectious mononucleosis is also responsible for these two tumors; if this is true, intrinsic or extrensic cofactors have to be postulated to explain the malignant conversion (the "cofactor hypothesis");

b) Different virus subtypes are responsible for the different clinical entities (the "multiple virus hypothesis"); or

c) The virus is a relatively harmless inhabitant of lymphoid tissues, although it may cause temporary proliferation (mononucleosis) under certain conditions. When lymphoid tissues proliferate for other reasons, e.g. in malignancies due to other, unrelated causes, the virus travels along as a passenger, with increased antigen production and high-titered antibody formation as a result. This "passenger hypothesis" is the logical analogue of the "antigenic conversion" of established tumors by etiologically unrelated viruses, discussed above. In view of the high regularity of association, a requirement for a particular trophic relationship between EBV and the target (lymphoid) tissue may be added in the present case.

The passenger hypothesis cannot be excluded at present, but it appears less likely in view of the fact that lymphoproliferative diseases other than BL and anaplastic carcinomas other than NPC do not show a regular high-titered EBV-association. This statement includes malignancies occurring in the same or closely adjacent anatomical areas, such as reticulum cell sarcoma, Hodgkin's disease (at least the granulomatous form), lymphosarcoma, etc., and carcinomas that arise in or close to the tissues of the Waldeyer ring, such as the hypopharynx, oropharynx, the tonsil, base of the tongue, soft palate, etc. Carcinoma of the maxilla is a possible exception, but larger groups remain to be investigated. Although this reasoning does not exclude the passenger hypothesis, some assumptions have to be made to maintain it, e.g. by postulating a specific trophic relationship between the virus and the kind of lymphocyte that gives rise to BL and is particularly abundant in NPC, that would not apply to the lymphoid cells that proliferate in the various other malignancies, used as controls. No valid objection can be raised against such a hypothesis, but it appears rather far fetched in view of the fact that EBV-carrying blastoid cell lines can be regularly isolated from EBV positive individuals, including donors with lymphoreticular malignancies of the "control" type, i.e. diseases that do not show a consistently high EBV-positive serology.

The possibility that EBV acts together with some cofactor in causing neoplastic disease or, to phrase the same thesis differently, it acts by increasing the likelihood of neoplastic transformation brought about by other factors, has been recently proposed by Burkitt (99) as far as the etiology of BL is concerned. In order to fit the geographic distribution of the disease with a ubiquitous virus, Burkitt proposed that an insect-transmitted cofactor is responsible for the malignant manifestation and specified it as chronic holoendemic malaria. This was based on the absence of BL from certain areas where malaria control has been enforced for some time and its presence in adjacent regions where malaria control was not regularly practised.

It may be agreed that interactions between viruses and other agents, capable of stimulating the proliferation of a target tissue may lead to malignant transformation in experimental systems where neither the virus nor the other agent is oncogenic per se (100). Since chronic malaria exerts a strong proliferative stimulus on the reticuloendothelial system, Burkitt's modified theory is reasonable, although an objection may be raised that the same picture would result from the transmission of any etiological factor or cofactor mediated by the appropriate insect, and this includes other viruses. Recently, some preliminary evidence has been obtained concerning the frequency of the sickling trait in BL patients (R. H. Morrow and M. C. Pike, personal communication), however, that seems to indicate, albeit indirectly, that malaria may play a role in the causation of the disease.

The third possibility, the multiple virus hypothesis, implies the existence of closely related but biologically different EBV-viruses with differences in their oncogenic power and their target tissue preference. In light of the information derived from experimental oncogenic viruses, this is a realistic alternative as well. As far as leukemia viruses of the RNA type are concerned, it will be recalled that prior to the discovery of the interference test for avian leukosis virus classification (101), it was not possible to distinguish by morphological or immunological means between the viruses that were responsible for the different lympho- and myeloproliferative diseases or for fowl sarcoma. It is now known that the avian leukosis-sarcoma virus group has many closely related members; some induce solid tumors with highly distinctive properties, others are responsible for myeloid or erythromyeloid leukemia, or lymphomatosis, and still others cause no recognizable disease at all. A closely similar development can be noticed in the murine leukosis-sarcoma field. The Friend, Moloney, Rauscher, Gross, Kaplan, Rich, Graffi, Mazurenko, etc. agents are similar antigenically and indistinguishable by ultrastructure, but they induce distinct and characteristic clinical and pathological disease entities, specific for the viral agent (102). In the DNA field, a possibly relevant example is the series of HSV mutants, studied by Roizmann and his colleagues (72). Although this is not known to be an oncogenic system, it is important that different viral mutants induce different membrane changes in infected cells and, concomitantly, the cells are altered in their "social behavior" in ways that are characteristic for the virus mutant. Although a lytic virus obviously cannot transform its targets, the cellular changes are nevertheless concerned with intercellular relationships. Conceivably, other, nonlytic viruses of the same family might induce membrane changes compatible with cellular viability and reproductive integrity, and a social behavior changed in the direction of disobedience to growth regulation—or, in other words, neoplasia. It may be recalled in this connection that the agents of at least two neoplastic diseases, Marek's neurolymphomatosis in the chicken (103) and Lucké's carcinoma in the frog (104) were recently identified as herpes type viruses. A simian lymphoma is probably also due to a herpes type virus (F. Rauscher, personal communication).

The immunological tests so far performed on EBV-associated antigens, including those referred to in the previous sections, are not necessarily competent to reveal finer differences between closely related but biologically different agents with cross-reactive or overlapping antigenic components. A preliminary study of the membrane antigens carried on EBV-positive lymphoblastoid cell lines derived from BL and NPC did not show any difference in the reactivity patterns (105), but this may simply reflect the insufficient discriminating ability of the test.

Further studies are needed to distinguish between these possibilities. In order to narrow down the passenger hypothesis, more extensive tests are desirable on tumor categories where occasional sera gave high EBV-associated reactivity but only limited samples have been tested. Representative groups should include 20 to 30 sera at least and they should be tested preferably for antibodies to membrane, capsid and soluble antigens as well. More refined analytical methods are needed for the attempts to dissect different virus variants. The recent developments in the herpes simplex field suggest that biochemical studies on viral envelopes and altered cell membranes may be particularly rewarding. Nucleic acid hybridization may help to distinguish different variants as well and can also elucidate the function of the viral genome in different cells.

As far as the sero-epidemiology of EBV-infections is concerned, it has to be emphasized that there were no significant differences between low and high BL-endemic areas with regard to the distribution of anti-EBV titers in relation to age (73); a comparison of titers in normal populations is therefore unlikely to elucidate the possible role of this virus in BL. A prospective sero-epidemiological study may be more rewarding. It may be relevant in this connection that BL is essentially a childhood disease, with a peak incidence between four and seven years. This fact, together with the clinical and serological evidence indicating a relatively high antigenicity in the autochthonous host would speak for a short latency period during the oncogenic process: In experimental systems, highly antigenic tumors arise with short latency periods, as a rule; or, to put it in other words, highly antigenic tumors cannot escape rejection unless they grow out rapidly after their inception (8, 10, 106).

If this reasoning is essentially correct and the latency period of BL is relatively short, a prospective sero-epidemiological study may be decisive. In the populations of risk within the high endemic areas, like in other populations, there is a relatively small minority of EBV-negative children and another, even smaller minority with high anti-EBV titers. The majority consists of low-titered positives (73). The question is whether BL develops in one of the two minority groups or at random and irrespective of anti-EBV titer. Provided that a sufficiently large number of sera could be collected and stored under appropriate identification, tests may become feasible on predisease sera from individuals who develop BL within a few years' time. The objection may be raised that the sensitivity threshold of the anti-EBV test may be too high (1:10) and a fraction of anti-EBV positive sera may be classified as false negatives. Since more concentrated sera cannot be tested safely due to the nonspecific artefacts that tend to appear, this is probably true. It is also clear, however, that at least a substantial part of the "anti-EBV negative" donors, as defined by the 1:10 threshold, must be negative in the biological sense, since the prospective study on infectious mononucleosis has clearly shown (74) that the disease develops only in this group, and not in persons classified as anti-EBV positive according to the same criteria.

Concerning the relationship between EBV and NPC, the same types of hypotheses can be discussed as for BL. The multiple virus hypothesis would imply an NPC-specific EBV-variant. The cofactor hypothesis would lead to a consideration of both genetic and environmental factors, in light of the information on the incidence of the disease in migrant high-risk populations (107). A prospective serological study of this question would be very difficult at the present time, since NPC, unlike BL, occurs over an extremely wide age range.

The possible significance of the cell membrane changes reflected by the appearance of new antigens for the understanding of neoplastic cell behavior cannot be assessed at present, but it may be pertinent to point out that cell membrane changes are among the most seriously considered parameters of neoplastic behavior at present. They are almost invariably found when comparable normal and transformed cells are studied in parallel. They may concern changes in behavior, such as contact inhibition (108), or altered expression of phytoagglutinin receptors (109, 110) that may reflect a change in the synthesis of certain glycolipids (111), and they are perhaps linked to the appearance of new surface antigens (112). Membrane antigen changes have been demonstrated in all experimental tumors that have been thoroughly studied (8–14), and although the details concerning antigenic strength and patterns of cross reactivity vary from system to system, they must reflect some remodelling of the membrane structure. Growth regulating mechanisms, including both the forces that act via long range, humoral arms and the short range, contactual signals as well, must transmit their message to the target cell via receptors on the outer membrane. Nonlytic virus-cell interactions may result in the incorporation of virally determined (or virally derepressed) components into the membrane that render the appropriate receptors insensitive to regulation and, if this is compatible with continued cell growth and division, this may trigger neoplastic development. Since infection with potentially oncogenic viruses and the concomitant surface antigenic changes are not limited to the oncogenic target tissue but can occur in other cells as well that remain normal (i.e.

subject to regulation), a tissue or cell type specificity must be added to explain transformation. Since different tissues must obey different types of growth regulation, this is not surprising. Also, virally determined antigens may be retained while *in vivo* tumorigenic properties decrease or are lost from cell hybrid lines (113) or from the "revertant" forms that may arise from transformed cultures *in vitro* (114–116). Further studies on such systems will be most interesting, not only for the understanding of neoplastic behavior and the possible role of membrane changes in it, but also for the understanding of normal growth responsiveness at the cell level.

Meanwhile, the question whether EBV associated membrane antigens are essential for the neoplastic behavior of BL and NPC cells is not clear. As far as NPC is concerned, such membrane antigens have been demonstrated on derived lymphoblastoid cell lines (105) but it is not known whether they are present on the surface of the carcinoma cells. Established culture lines of BL cells carry EBV, as a rule, although at very different levels (60, 61). The membrane antigen can only be demonstrated in lines with a relatively high "EBV-load" (60) and is subject to environmental fluctuations (117). There is at least one BL line (Raji) which contains no demonstrable EBV antigen or virus particles (118). Very recently, however, it was found (H. zur Hausen, personal communication) that the Raji line contains DNA that will hybridize specifically with EBV DNA. Since the Raji line can be superinfected with EBV (90), the absence of virus production is presumably not due to repressors. If it carries genetic information derived from EBV, it is probably a defective viral genome, lacking the cistrons that specify the membrane, capsid and early protein antigens. If there would be any assurance that the Raji represents a neoplastic cell, this would imply that the membrane antigen is not required for neoplastic behavior. Since this question can-

not be tested directly with a human cell, however, a conclusive answer is not available. Further studies on the presence of viral DNA and virus specific messenger-RNA in BL derived lines, in comparison with EBV carrying blastoid cell lines of other origin may prove very informative. In this connection, it is interesting that infectious mononucleosis derived lines are reportedly more prone to loose their EBV than BL derived lines (119). Thus, whereas EBV is clearly helpful in inducing lymphoblastoid transformation and facilitates the establishment of stationary suspension cultures (120–122), there is no doubt that blastoid cell lines can exist without EBV.

Turning now to the therapeutic problems, it seems clearly established that the host immune response plays an important part in BL. This is indicated by the documented occurrence of spontaneous regression (91), by the substantial fraction of long-term survivors, sometimes after only mild chemotherapy (39–41, 90), by the reactivity of the autochthonous host against its own tumor cells, indicated by the presence of humoral antibodies reacting with the surface of viable cells (45, 46), by the positive C'1-a fixation test (123), and by the transformation of host lymphocytes when confronted with mitomycin treated autochthonous lymphoma cells in the mixed lymphocyte-target cell interaction test (124). In addition, the progressive accumulation of an IgG coating on the cell surface of tumors that persist in spite of therapy (48, 49) together with the tetraploid (immunoresistant?) constitution of tumors that have recurred after long-term regression (54) suggests that the dynamics of immunoselection may also apply to this human system, as they do for experimental tumors (89). Immunoresistance may be as important as drug resistance, if not more so, in frustrating therapy.

The host response to an autochthonous tumor is no less complex than other immune responses against viable cells. Different effector components interact in ways so that rejection, or its opposite, enhancement, will dominate the eventual outcome. Humoral antibodies are cytotoxic in some situations, whereas in others they lack demonstrable growth inhibitory effects but nevertheless manage to attach and thereby prevent the access of host lymphoid cells (10, 125). Recent evidence indicates that such "blocking antibody" may play an important role in counteracting the cell mediated host response in experimental (126) and human (127) tumors as well.

The main therapeutic dilemma is what the proper stimuli are, specific or nonspecific, and how they are best administered to the immune system, in order to achieve the objective, rejection, and avoid its opposite, enhancement. The rationale of introducing immune stimuli at a time when the tumor load confronting the host is minimal, i.e. after regression has been induced by chemotherapy, is obvious (128, 129), but the optimal form of stimulus and the best mode and timing of its administration is not. No *a priori* guidance can be given from experimental studies, because the same mode of administration, dosage, vehicle, etc. of the same preparation may favor rejection in one system and enhancement in another, and the differences depending on host species, tumor type and individual characteristics of the tumor line are immense. Ideally, it would be desirable to develop methods that allow the quantitative assessment of cell bound immunity and the synergistic or antagonistic action of humoral antibodies in relation to it in each untreated patient, and follow it subsequently during treatment. While this should be feasible, at least in principle, its practical application is still in the future. Meanwhile, an empirical approach, based on as much rational reasoning as the experimental models will allow, may yield important information, as the work of Mathé and his group clearly indicates (129).

Obviously, the prevention approach will have to await the further clarification of the relationship between serum conversion and tumor development, preferably from a prospective study. A discussion of this beyond the general statement that the ultimate goal of an immunological approach must be prevention rather than therapy appears premature at the present time.

Much of the work reported here has been carried out in collaboration with Drs. Peter Clifford, W. Henle, G. Henle, J. Yata, J. Stjernswärd, E. Klein, T. Tachibana, K. Nishioka, G. Goldstein, G. Pearson and L. Gergely as reported in the technical publications listed.

Supported by Grant CA-04747 and Contract NIH-69-2005 from the National Institutes of Health, Bethesda, Md., USA, and by grants from the Swedish Cancer Society and Magnus Bergvall's Foundation.

REFERENCES

1. FOLEY, E. J. Antigenic properties of methylcholanthrene-induced tumors in mice of the strain of origin. *Cancer Res.* **13**: 835, 1953.
2. PREHN, R. T. and MAIN, J. M. Immunity to methylcholanthrene-induced sarcomas. *J. nat. Cancer Inst.* **18**: 769, 1957.
3. KLEIN, G., SJÖGREN, H. O., KLEIN, E. and HELLSTRÖM, K. E. Demonstration of resistance against methylcholanthrene-induced sarcomas in the primary autochthonous host. *Cancer Res.* **20**: 1561, 1960.
4. SJÖGREN, H. O., HELLSTRÖM, I. and KLEIN, G. Transplantation of polyoma virus-induced tumors in mice. *Cancer Res.* **21**: 329, 1961.
5. HABEL, K. Resistance of polyoma virus immune animals to transplanted polyoma tumors. *Proc. Soc. exp. Biol. (N.Y.)* **106**: 722, 1961.
6. KLEIN, G., SJÖGREN, H. O. and KLEIN, E. Demonstration of host resistance against isotransplantation of lymphomas induced by the Gross agent. *Cancer Res.* **22**: 955, 1962.
7. SJÖGREN, H. O. and JONSON, N. Resistance against isotransplantation of mouse tumors induced by Rous sarcoma virus. *Exp. Cell Res.* **32**: 618, 1963.
8. KLEIN, G. Experimental studies in tumor immunology. *Fed. Proc.* **28**: 1739, 1969.
9. KLEIN, G. Tumor antigens. *Ann. Rev. Microbiol.* **20**: 223, 1966.
10. OLD, L. J. and BOYSE, E. A. Immunology of experimental tumors. *Ann. Rev. Med.* **15**: 167, 1964.
11. PASTERNAK, G. I. Antigens induced by the mouse leukemia viruses. *Advanc. Cancer Res.* **12**: 1, 1969.
12. DEICHMANN, G. I. Immunological aspects of carcinogenesis by deoxyribonucleic acid tumor viruses. *Advanc. Cancer Res.* **12**: 101, 1969.
13. HELLSTRÖM, K. E. and HELLSTRÖM, I. Cellular immunity against tumor antigens. *Advanc. Cancer Res.* **12**: 167, 1969.

127

14. SJÖGREN, H. O. Transplantation methods as a tool for detection of tumor specific antigens. *Progr. exp. Tumor Res.* (*Basel*) **6**: 289, 1965.
15. WEISS, D. W., LAVRIN, D. H., DEZFULIAN, M., VAAGE, J. and BLAIR, P. B. Studies on the immunology of spontaneous mammary carcinomas of mice, in: Burdette, W. J. (Ed.) "Viruses inducing cancer, implications for therapy." Salt Lake City, Univ. of Utah Press, 1966, p. 138.
16. AXELRAD, A. A. Changes in resistance to the proliferation of isotransplanted Gross virus-induced lymphoma cells, as measured with a spleen colony assay. *Nature* (*Lond.*) **199**: 80, 1963.
17. KLEIN, E. and KLEIN, G. Antibody response and leukemia development in mice inoculated neonatally with the Moloney virus. *Cancer Res.* **25**: 851, 1965.
18. BURNET, M. F. Somatic mutation and chronic disease. *Brit. med. J.* **1**: 338, 1965.
19. STJERNSWÄRD, J. Age-dependent tumor-host barrier and effect of carcinogen-induced immuno-depression on rejection of isografted methylcholanthrene-induced sarcoma cell. *J. nat. Cancer Inst.* **37**: 505, 1966.
20. CELADA, F. The immunologic defence in relation to age, in: Engel, A. and Larson, T. (Eds.), "Cancer and aging." Stockholm, Thule International Symposium, 1968, p. 97.
21. DEFENDI, V., ROOSA, R. A. and KOPROWSKI, H. Effect of thymectomy at birth on response to tissue, cells, and virus antigens, in: Good, R. A. and Gabrielsen, A. E. (Eds.), "The thymus in immunobiology." New York, Harper and Row, 1964, p. 504.
22. GRANT, G. A. and MILLER, J. F. A. P. Effect of neonatal thymectomy on the induction of sarcomata in C57BL mice. *Nature* (*Lond.*) **205**: 1124, 1965.
23. KIRSCHSTEIN, R. L., RABSON, A. S. and PETERS, E. A. Oncogenic activity of adenovirus 12 in thymectomized BALB/c and C3H/HeN mice. *Proc. Soc. exp. Biol.* (*N.Y.*) **117**: 198, 1964.
24. MILLER, J. F. A. P., GRANT, G. A. and ROE, F. J. C. Effect of thymectomy on the induction of skin tumors by 3, 4-benzopyrene. *Nature* (*Lond.*) **199**: 920, 1963.
25. MILLER, J. F. A. P., TING, R. C. and LAW, L. W. Influence of thymectomy on tumor induction by polyoma virus in C57BL mice. *Proc. Soc. exp. Biol.* (*N.Y.*) **116**: 323, 1964.
26. NOMOTO, K. and TAKEYA, K. Immunologic properties of methylcholanthrene-induced sarcomas of neonatally thymectomized mice. *J. nat. Cancer Inst.* **42**: 445, 1969.
27. ALLISON, A. C. and LAW, L. W. Effects of antilymphocyte serum on virus oncogenesis. *Proc. Soc. exp. Biol.* (*N.Y.*) **127**: 207, 1968.
28. LAW, L. W. Studies of thymic function with emphasis on the role of the thymus in oncogenesis. *Cancer Res.* **26**: 551, 1966.
29. LAW, L. W. Immunologic factors in susceptibility and resistance to tumor induction by viruses, in: Engel, A. and Larson, T. (Eds.), "Cancer and aging." Stockholm, Thule International Symposium 1968, p. 111.
30. JOHNSON, S. The effect of thymectomy and of the dose of 3-methylcholanthrene on the induction and antigenic properties of sarcomas in C57BL mice. *Brit. J. Cancer* **22**: 93, 1968.
31. STJERNSWÄRD, J. Immunodepressive effect of 3-methylcholanthrene. Antibody formation at the cellular level and reaction against weak antigenic homografts. *J. nat. Cancer Inst.* **35**: 885, 1965.
32. LINDER, O. E. A. Survival of skin homografts in methylcholanthrene-treated mice and in mice with spontaneous mammary cancers. *Cancer Res.* **22**: 380, 1962.
33. FURTH, J. Prolongation of life with prevention of leukemia by thymectomy in mice. *J. Geron.* **1**: 46, 1964.
34. LAW, L. W. Recent advances in experimental leukemia research. *Cancer Res.* **14**: 695, 1954.
35. KAPLAN, H. S. On the etiology and pathogenesis of the leukemias: a review. *Cancer Res.* **14**: 535, 1954.
36. PENN, I., BRETTSCHNEIDER, L. and STARZL, T. E. Malignant lymphomas in transplantation patients. *Transplant. Proc.* **1**: 106, 1969.
37. HADDOW, A. Chemical carcinogens and their modes of action. *Brit. med. Bull.* **14**: 79, 1958.
38. BURKITT, D. A lymphoma syndrome in tropical Africa. *Int. Rev. exp. Pathol.* **2**: 69, 1963.
39. CLIFFORD, P. Further studies in the treatment of Burkitt's lymphoma. *E. Afr. med. J.* **43**: 179, 1966.
40. BURKITT, D. Chemotherapy of jaw tumors, in: Burchenal, J. H. (Ed.), "Treatment of Burkitt's tumor." UICC Monograph Series, Heidelberg, Springer Verlag, 1967, v. 8. p. 94.
41. NGU, V. A. The African lymphoma (Burkitt tumors): Survivals exceeding two years. *Brit. J. Cancer* **19**: 101, 1965.
42. KLEIN, E. and KLEIN, G. Antigenic properties of lymphomas induced by the Moloney agent. *J. nat. Cancer Inst.* **32**: 547, 1964.
43. KLEIN, G., KLEIN, E. and HAUGHTON, G. Variation of antigenic characteristics between different mouse lymphomas induced by the Moloney virus. *J. nat. Cancer Inst.* **36**: 607, 1966.
44. MÖLLER, G. Demonstration of mouse isoantigens at the cellular level by the fluorescent antibody technique. *J. exp. Med.* **114**: 415, 1961.
45. KLEIN, G., CLIFFORD, P., KLEIN, E. and STJERNSWÄRD, J. Search for tumor specific immune reactions in Burkitt lymphoma patients by the membrane immunofluorescence reaction. *Proc. nat. Acad. Sci.* (*Wash.*). **55**: 1628, 1966.
46. KLEIN, G., CLIFFORD, P., KLEIN, E. and STJERNSWÄRD, J. Search for tumor specific immune reactions in Burkitt lymphoma patients by the membrane immunofluorescence reaction, in: Burchenal, J. H. (Ed.), "Treatment of Burkitt's tumor." UICC Monograph Series, Springer Verlag, 1967, v. 8, p. 209.
47. KLEIN, E., CLIFFORD, P., KLEIN, G. and HAMBERGER, C. A. Further studies on the membrane immunofluorescence reaction of Burkitt lymphoma cells. *Int. J. Cancer* **2**: 27, 1967.
48. KLEIN, E., KLEIN, G., NADKARNI, J. J., NADKARNI, J. S., WIGZELL, H. and CLIFFORD, P. Surface IgM-kappa specificity on a Burkitt

lymphoma cell *in vivo* and in derived culture lines. *Cancer Res.* **28**: 1300, 1968.

49. KLEIN, G., CLIFFORD, P., HENLE, G., HENLE, W., OLD, L. J. and GEERING, L. EBV-associated serological patterns in a Burkitt lymphoma patient during regression and recurrence. *Int. J. Cancer* **4**: 416, 1969.

50. ESKELAND, T. and KLEIN, E. Surface IgM on lymphoid cells. *Exp. Cell Res.* (in press).

51. SINGHAL, S. K. and WIGZELL, H. Cognition and recognition of antigen by cell associated receptors. *Progr. Allergy* **15**, 1970 (in press).

52. JOHANSSON, B. and KLEIN, E. Cell surface localized IgM-kappa immunoglobulin reactivity in a case of chronic lymphocytic leukaemia. *Clin. exp. Immunol.* **6**: 421, 1970.

53. LEVIN, A. G., FRIBERG, S. and KLEIN, E. Xeno-transplantation of a Burkitt lymphoma culture line with surface immunoglobulin specificity. *Nature (Lond.)* **222**: 997, 1969.

54. CLIFFORD, P., GRIPENBERG, N., KLEIN, E., FENYÖ, E. M. and MANOLOV, G. Treatment of Burkitt's lymphoma. *Lancet* **ii**: 517, 1968.

55. NADKARNI, J. S., NADKARNI, J. J., CLIFFORD, P., MANOLOV, G., FENYÖ, E. M. and KLEIN, E. Characteristics of new cell lines derived from Burkitt lymphomas. *Cancer (Philad.)* **23**: 64, 1969.

56. KLEIN, G., CLIFFORD, P., KLEIN, E., SMITH, R. T., MINOWADA, J., KOURILSKY, F. M. and BURCHENAL, J. H. Membrane immunofluorescence reactions of Burkitt lymphoma cells from biopsy specimens and tissue cultures. *J. nat. Cancer Inst.* **39**: 1027, 1967.

57. HENLE, G. and HENLE, W. Immunofluorescence in cells derived from Burkitt's lymphoma. *J. Bact.* **91**: 1248, 1966.

58. HENLE, G. and HENLE, W. Immunofluorescence, interference, and complement fixation technics in the detection of herpes-type virus in Burkitt tumor cell lines. *Cancer Res.* **27**: 2442, 1967.

59. EPSTEIN, M. A. and BARR, Y. M. Cultivation in vitro of human lymphoblasts from Burkitt's malignant lymphoma. *Lancet* **i**: 252, 1964.

60. KLEIN, G., PEARSON, G., NADKARNI, J. S., NADKARNI, J. J., KLEIN, E., HENLE, G., HENLE, W. and CLIFFORD, P. Relation between Epstein-Barr viral and cell membrane immunofluorescence of Burkitt tumor cells. I. Dependence of cell membrane immunofluorescence on presence of EB virus. *J. exp. Med.* **128**: 1011, 1968.

61. NADKARNI, J. S., NADKARNI, J. J., KLEIN, G., HENLE, W., HENLE, G. and CLIFFORD, P. EB viral antigens in Burkitt tumor biopsies and early cultures. *Int. J. Cancer* (in press).

62. FIALKOW, P. J., KLEIN, G., GARTLER, S. M. and CLIFFORD, P. Clonal origin for individual Burkitt tumors. *Lancet* **ii**: 384, 1970.

63. HENLE, W. and HENLE, G. *Proc. Int. Symp. Comp. Leukemia Res.*, Cherry Hill, 1969. Basel, S. Karger, (in press).

64. KLEIN, G., KLEIN, E. and CLIFFORD, P. Search for host defense in Burkitt lymphoma: Membrane immunofluorescence tests on biopsies and tissue culture lines. *Cancer Res.* **27**: 2510, 1967.

65. SMITH, R. T., KLEIN, G., KLEIN, E. and CLIFFORD, P. Studies of the membrane phenomenon in cultured and biopsy cell lines from the Burkitt lymphoma, in: Dausset, J., Hamburger J., and Mathé, G. "Advances in Transplantation."Copenhagen, Munksgaard, 1967, vol. 779, p. 484.

66. PEARSON, G., KLEIN, G., HENLE, G., HENLE, W. and CLIFFORD, P. Relation between Epstein-Barr viral and cell membrane immunofluorescence in Burkitt tumor cells. IV. Differentiation between antibodies responsible for membrane and viral immunofluorescence. *J. exp. Med.* **129**: 707, 1969.

67. SVEDMYR, A., DEMISSIE, A., KLEIN, G. and CLIFFORD, P. Antibody patterns in different human sera against intracellular and membrane-antigens and neutralization of EBV infectivity. *J. nat. Cancer Inst.* **44**: 595, 1970.

68. PEARSON, G., DEWEY, S., KLEIN, G., HENLE, G. and HENLE, W. Correlation between antibodies to Epstein-Barr virus (EBV)—induced membrane antigens and neutralization of EBV infectivity. *J. nat. Cancer Inst.* (in press).

69. BREMBERG, S., KLEIN, G. and EPSTEIN, A. Direct membrane fluorescence reaction of EBV-carrying human lymphoblastoid cells: Blocking tests with xenogeneic antisera. *Int. J. Cancer* **4**: 761, 1969.

70. ROIZMAN, B. and ROONE, P. R., Jr. Studies of the determinant antigens of viable cells. I. A method, and its application in tissue culture studies, for enumeration of killed cells, based on the failure of virus multiplication following injury by cytotoxic antibody and complement. *J. Immunol.* **87**: 714, 1961.

71. ROIZMAN, B. and SPRING, S. B. Alteration in immunologic specificity of cells infected with cytolytic viruses, in: Trentin, J. J. (Ed.), *Proc. Conf. Cross Reacting Antigens and Neo-antigens.* Baltimore, Williams & Wilkins Co., 1967, p. 85.

72. ROIZMAN, B. Herpes-viruses, membranes, and the social behaviour of infected cells. *Proc. Int. Symp. on Applied and Medical Virology. Fort Lauderdale, Florida.* Dec. 1969.

73. HENLE, G., HENLE, W., CLIFFORD, P., DIEHL, V., KAFUKO, G. W., KIRYA, B. G., KLEIN, G., MOOROW, R. H., MUNUBE, G. M. R., PIKE, P., TUKEI, P. M. and ZIEGLER, J. L. Antibodies to Epstein-Barr virus in Burkitt's lymphoma and control groups. *J. nat. Cancer Inst.* **43**: 1147, 1969.

74. NIEDERMAN, J. C., EVANS, A. S., SUBRAHMANYAN, L. and McCOLLUM, R. W. Prevalence, incidence and persistence of EB virus antibody in young adults. *New Engl. J. Med.* **282**: 361, 1970.

75. HENLE, G., HENLE, W. and DIEHL, V. Relation of Burkitt's tumor-associated herpes-type virus to infectious mononucleosis. *Proc. nat. Acad. Sci. (Wash.)* **59**: 94, 1968.

76. HENLE, W., HENLE, G., BURTIN, P., CACHIN, Y., CLIFFORD, P., DE SCHRYVER, A., DE THÉ, G., DIEHL, V., HO, H. C. and KLEIN, G. Antibodies to Epstein-Barr virus in nasopharyngeal carcinoma, other head and neck neoplasms, and control groups. *J. nat. Cancer Inst.* **44**: 225, 1970.

77. DE SCHRYVER, A., FRIBERG, S., JR., KLEIN, G., HENLE, W., HENLE, G., DE THÉ, G., CLIFFORD,

P. and Ho, H. C. Epstein-Barr virus-associated antibody patterns in carcinoma of the post-nasal space. *Clin. exp. Immunol.* **5**: 443, 1969.

78. JOHANSSON, B., KLEIN, G., HENLE, G. and HENLE, W. Epstein-Barr virus (EBV)-associated antibody patterns in malignant lymphoma and leukemia. I. Hodgkin's disease. *Int. J. Cancer* **6**: 450, 1970.

79. OLD, L. J., BOYSE, E. A., OETTGEN, H. F., DE HARVEN, E., GEERING, G., WILLIAMSON, B. and CLIFFORD, P. Precipitating antibody in human serum to an antigen present in cultured Burkitt's lymphoma cells. *Proc. Nat. Acad. Sci. (Wash.)* **56**: 1699, 1966.

80. OLD, L. J., BOYSE, E. A., GEERING, G. and OETTGEN, H. F. Serologic approaches to the study of cancer in animals and in man. *Cancer Res.* **28**: 1288, 1968.

81. GOLDSTEIN, G., KLEIN, G., PEARSON, G. and CLIFFORD, P. Direct membrane immunofluorescence reaction of Burkitt's lymphoma cells in culture. *Cancer Res.* **29**: 749, 1969.

82. KLEIN, G., GEERING, G., OLD, L. J., HENLE, G., HENLE, W. and CLIFFORD, P. Relation between Epstein-Barr viral and cell membrane immunofluorescence in Burkitt tumor cells. III. Comparison of blocking of direct membrane immunofluorescence. *J. exp. Med.* **129**: 697, 1969.

83. KLEIN, G., GEERING, G., OLD, L. J., HENLE, G., HENLE, W. and CLIFFORD, P. Comparison of the anti-EBV titer and the EBV-associated membrane reactive and precipitating antibody levels in the sera of Burkitt lymphoma and nasopharyngeal carcinoma patients and controls. *Int. J. Cancer* **5**: 185, 1970.

84. AHLSTRÖM, C. G., ANDERSSON, T., KLEIN, G. and ÅKERMAN, M. Malignant lymphoma of "Burkitt type" in Sweden. *Int. J. Cancer* **2**: 583, 1967.

85. GUNVÉN, P., KLEIN, G., HENLE, G., HENLE, W. and CLIFFORD, P. Antibodies to Epstein-Barr virus (EBV) associated membrane (MA) and viral capsid (VCA) antigens in African Burkitt lymphoma patients and controls. *Nature (Lond.)* (in press).

86. EINHORN, N., KLEIN, G. and CLIFFORD, P. Increase in antibody titer against the EBV associated membrane antigen complex in Burkitt's lymphoma and nasopharyngeal carcinoma after local irradiation. *Cancer (Philad.)* (in press).

87. YATA, J., KLEIN, G., HEWETSON, J. and GERGELY, L. Effect of metabolic inhibitors on membrane immunofluorescence reactivity of established Burkitt lymphoma cell lines. *Int. J. Cancer* **5**: 394, 1970.

88. FENYÖ, E. M., KLEIN, E., KLEIN, G. and SWIECH, K. Selection of an immunoresistant Moloney lymphoma subline with decreased concentration of tumor specific surface antigens. *J. nat. Cancer Inst.* **40**: 69, 1968.

89. HAUSCHKA, T. S., KVEDAR, B. J., GRINNEL, S. T. and AMOS, D. B. Immunoselection of polyploids from predominantly diploid cell populations. *Ann. N.Y. Acad. Sci.* **63**: 683, 1956.

90. BURKITT, D. Chemotherapy of jaw tumors, in: Burchenal, J. H. (Ed.), "Treatment of Burkitt's Tumors." UICC Monograph Series, Heidelberg, Springer Verlag, 1967, v. 8, p. 2.

91. BURKITT, D. and KYALWAZI, S. K. Spontaneous remission of African lymphoma. *Brit. J. Cancer* **21**: 14, 1967.

92. HENLE, W., HENLE, G., ZAJAC, B. A., PEARSON, G., WAUBKE, R. and SCIRBA, M. Differential reactivity of human sera with EBV-induced "early antigens." *Science* **169**: 188, 1970.

93. BREYERE, E. J. and WILLIAMS, L. B. Antigens associated with a tumor virus: Rejection of isogenic skin grafts from leukemic mice. *Science* **146**: 1055, 1964.

94. MATHÉ, G. Antigénicité nouvelle (démontrée par isogreffe) d'un fragment de peau de souris infectée par un virus leucémigène. *C. R. Acad. Sci. (Paris)* **264**: 2702, 1967.

95. PASTERNAK, G. Serologic studies on cells of Graffi virus-induced myeloid leukemia in mice. *J. nat. Cancer Inst.* **34**: 371, 1965.

96. SJÖGREN, H. O. and HELLSTRÖM, I. Induction of polyoma specific transplantation antigenicity in Moloney leukemia cells. *Exp. Cell Res.* **40**: 208, 1965.

97. STÜCK, B., OLD, L. J. and BOYSE, E. A. Antigenic conversion of established leukaemias by an unrelated leukaemogenic virus. *Nature (Lond.)* **202**: 1016, 1964.

98. SVET-MOLDAVSKY, G. J., MKHEIDZE, D. M. and LIOZNER, A. L. Phenomena associated with skin grafting. Two phenomena associated with skin grafting from tumor-bearing syngeneic donors. *J. nat. Cancer Inst.* **38**: 933, 1967.

99. BURKITT, D. Etiology of Burkitt's lymphoma—an alternative hypothesis to a vectored virus. *J. nat. Cancer Inst.* **42**: 19, 1969.

100. SOUTHAM, C. M., TANAKA, S., ARATA, T., SIMKOVIC, D., MIURA, M. and PEPTIOPULES, S. F. Enhancement of responses to chemical carcinogens by nononcogenic viruses and antimetabolites. *Progr. exp. Tumor Res. (Basel)* **11**: 194, 1969.

101. RUBIN, H. A virus in chick embryos which induces resistance in vitro to infection with Rous sarcoma virus. *Proc. nat. Acad. Sci.* **46**: 1105, 1960.

102. RICH, M. A. Virus-induced murine leukemia, in: Rich, M. A. "Experimental leukemia." Amsterdam, North Holland Publishing Co. 1968, p. 1.

103. CHURCHILL, A. E. Herpes-type virus isolated in cell culture from tumors of chickens with Marek's disease. I. Studies in cell culture. *J. nat. Cancer Inst.* **41**: 939, 1968.

104. MIZELL, M., TOPLIN, I. and ISAACS, J. J. Tumor induction in developing frog kidneys by a zonal centrifuge purified fraction of the frog herpes-type virus. *Science* **165**: 1134, 1969.

105. DE SCHRYVER, A., KLEIN, G. and DE THÉ, G. Surface antigens on lymphoblastoid cells derived from nasopharyngeal carcinoma. *Clin. exp. Immunol.* **7**: 161, 1970.

106. PREHN, R. T. The role of immune mechanisms in the biology of chemically and physically induced tumors, in: "Conceptual advances in immunology and oncology." New York, Hoeber, 1963, p. 475.

107. MUIR, C. S. and SHANMUGARATNAM, K. "Cancer of the nasopharynx." UICC Monograph series,

Copenhagen, Munksgaard, 1967, p. 1.

108. ABERCROMBIE, M. Contact inhibition: The phenomenon and its biological implications, in: "Cell tissue and organ culture." *Nat. Cancer Inst. Monograph* **26**: 249, 1966.

109. BURGER, M. M. Isolation of a receptor complex for a tumor specific agglutinin from the neoplastic cell surface. *Nature (Lond.)* **223**: 710 1969.

110. INBAR, M. and SACHS, L. Structural difference in sites on the surface membrane of normal and transformed cells. *Nature (Lond.)* **223**: 710, 1969.

111. HAKAMORI, S. I. and MURAKAMI, W. T. Glycolipids of hamster fibroblasts and derived malignant-transformed cell lines. *Proc. nat. Acad. Sci. (Wash.)* **59**: 254, 1967.

112. MORA, P. T., BRADY, R. O., BRADLEY, R. M. and McFARLAND, V. W. Gangliosides in DNA virus-transformed and spontaneously transformed tumorigenic mouse cell lines. *Proc. nat. Acad. Sci. (Wash.)* **63**: 1290, 1969.

113. KLEIN, G., BREGULA, U., WIENER, F. and HARRIS, H. The analysis of malignancy by cell fusion. I. Hybrids between tumor cells and L cell derivatives. *J. Cell Sci.* (in press).

114. RABINOWITZ, Z. and SACHS, L. The formation of variants with a reversion of properties of transformed cells. *Virology* **40**: 193, 1970.

115. MACPHERSON, I. The characteristics of animal cells transformed in vitro. *Advanc. Cancer Res.* **13**: 169, 1970.

116. POLLACK, R. E., GREEN, H. and TODARO, G. J. Growth control in cultured cells: Selection of sublines with increased sensitivity to contact inhibition and decreased tumor-producing ability. *Proc. nat. Acad. Sci. (Wash.)* **60**: 126, 1968.

117. YATA, J. and KLEIN, G. Some factors affecting membrane immunofluorescence reactivity of Burkitt lymphoma tissue culture cell lines. *Int. J. Cancer* **4**: 767, 1969.

118. EPSTEIN, M. A., ACHONG, B. G., BARR, Y. M., ZAJAC, B., HENLE, G. and HENLE, W. Morphological and virological investigations on cultured Burkitt tumor lymphoblasts (strain Raji). *J. nat. Cancer Inst.* **37**: 547, 1966.

119. DIEHL, V., HENLE, G., HENLE, W. and KOHN, G. Demonstration of a herpes group virus in cultures of peripheral leukocytes from patients with infectious mononucleosis. *J. Virology* **2**: 663, 1968.

120. HENLE, W., DIEHL, V., KOHN, G., ZUR HAUSEN, H. and HENLE, G. Herpes-type virus and chromosome marker in normal leukocytes after growth with irradiated Burkitt cells. *Science* **157**: 1064, 1967.

121. POPE, J. H., HORNE, M. K. and SCOTT, W. Identification of the filtrable leukocyte-transforming factor of QIMR-WIL cells as herpeslike virus. *Int. J. Cancer* **4**: 255, 1969.

122. GERBER, P., WHANG-PENG, J. and MONROE, J. H. Transformation and chromosome changes induced by Epstein-Barr virus in normal human leukocyte cultures. *Proc. nat. Acad. Sci. (Wash.)* **63**: 740, 1969.

123. NISHIOKA, K., TACHIBANA, T., KLEIN, G. and CLIFFORD, P. Complementological studies on tumor immunity. Measurement of Cl bound to tumor cells and immune adherence with Burkitt lymphoma cells. *Gann Monog.* **7**: 49, 1968.

124. STJERNSWÄRD, J., CLIFFORD, P., SING, S. and SVEDMYR, E. Indications of cellular immunological reactions against autochthonous tumor in cancer patients studied in vitro. *E. Afr. med. J.* **45**: 484, 1968.

125. KLEIN, G. Humoral and cell-mediated mechanisms for host defense in tumor immunity, in: Burdette, W. J. (Ed.), "Viruses inducing cancer, implications for therapy." Salt Lake City, Univ. of Utah Press, 1966, p. 323.

126. HELLSTRÖM, I. and HELLSTRÖM, K. E. Colony inhibition studies on blocking and non-blocking serum effects on cellular immunity to Moloney sarcomas. *Int. J. Cancer* **5**: 195, 1970.

127. HELLSTRÖM, I., HELLSTRÖM, K. E., EVANS, C. A., HEPPNER, G. H., PIERCE, E. G. and YANG, J. P. S. Serum-mediated protection of neoplastic cells from inhibition by lymphocytes immune to their tumor-specific antigens. *Proc. Nat. Acad. Sci. (Wash.)* **62**: 362, 1969.

128. SKIPPER, H. E. Destruction of leukemia cells in animals. Criteria associated with destruction of leukemia and solid tumor cells in animals. *Cancer Res.* **27**: 2636, 1967.

129. MATHÉ, G. Approaches to the immunological treatment of cancer in man. *Brit. med. J.* **4**: 7, 1969.

ANTIGENIC RELATIONSHIPS BETWEEN CELL MEMBRANES OF NORMAL AND SV$_{40}$ TRANSFORMED HAMSTER KIDNEY CELLS

E. KEDAR, M. WIENER, N. GOLDBLUM and D. SULITZEANU

Departments of Immunology and Virology, Hebrew University–Hadassah Medical School, Jerusalem, Israel

ABSTRACT

The antigenic relationships between normal hamster kidney cells, SV$_{40}$ induced hamster solid tumor cells, and BHK21 (non-transformed) and HK7 (SV$_{40}$ transformed) hamster cell lines were studied by means of several rabbit antisera. The antisera were prepared against membranes of hamster kidney cells, against membranes of SV$_{40}$ transformed hamster kidney cells growing *in vitro* or *in vivo* (solid tumors) and against sheep red blood cells. The experiments were performed by means of the indirect fluorescent antibody technique and with radioiodinated antibodies. To ascertain the specificity of the antisera for the cell membranes, tests were also carried out with antibodies specifically purified by absorption onto, and elution from, living cells. The antiserum to the normal kidney cell membranes stained the tubular cell membranes very strongly, but stained the other cell types only weakly. The antisera against the tumor cell membranes stained the kidney glomeruli, the solid tumor cells and both cultured cell lines intensely. It was concluded on this basis that the cultured lines were derived from glomerular cells. Three antigens or groups of antigens were clearly distinguished: Forssman antigen, present in all cell types; G (glomerular) antigen, present in the glomeruli, the cultured cell lines and the solid tumor cells; and KT antigens, present in the kidney tubules. The radioiodinated IgG fraction of the antiserum to HK7 cell membranes was tested for its ability to bind *in vitro* to HK7, BHK21, normal hamster kidney and human leukemic cells. Specifically purified, radioiodinated antibodies bound, to a higher extent, to the SV$_{40}$ transformed than to the non-SV$_{40}$ transformed hamster cells and not at all to the human cells. The immunological specificity of the interaction between labeled antibody and cells was confirmed by the observations that: a) excess, nonlabeled antiserum blocked the binding of radioactivity to the cells; and b) purified antibody preparations failed to react with human normal or leukemic cells.

INTRODUCTION

In recent years there has been a growing interest in the structure of the mammalian cell membrane. It has become quite clear by now that the cell membrane is a fairly labile structure, since its composition can change during growth *in vitro* or following viral infection and neoplastic transformation. The subject has been reviewed recently (1). The present report is concerned with some antigenic relationships between membranes of four types of hamster kidney cells: normal adult hamster kidney (NK) cells, a baby hamster kidney cell line grown *in vitro* (BHK 21), and hamster kidney cells made neoplastic by SV_{40}, propagated *in vitro* (HK7 cell line) or *in vivo* [solid tumors (ST)].

MATERIALS AND METHODS

Animals. Random bred Syrian hamsters were used for propagating the SV_{40} induced tumors, and as donors of kidneys for the preparation of normal cell membranes. Antisera were prepared in a local strain of random bred rabbits.

Cell lines. The BHK21/C13 cell line was derived from baby hamster kidney (2). These cells have oncogenic potential in hamsters, but do not synthesize SV_{40} tumor antigen (3). They were grown in Eagle's Glasgow modified medium, with 10% inactivated calf serum, 100 units of penicillin and 100 μg of streptomycin/ml.

The other cell line, HK7, is a line of hamster kidney cells transformed *in vitro* by SV_{40} (4). These cells synthesize the intranuclear tumor antigen (T) and produce tumors in hamsters, but lack infective virus. The HK7 cultures were grown in Eagle's basal medium supplemented with 10% inactivated calf serum and antibiotics, as above.

Cell suspensions. Suspensions were prepared from cells grown in culture and from cells obtained directly from tissues (kidneys and solid tumors). The cells grown in culture were harvested after three to four days of incubation. The medium was discarded and the cell layer was washed once with trisodium edetate (VERSENE®) solution prewarmed to 37 C [0.02% Versene in phosphate buffered saline (PBS) prepared without Ca^{++} and Mg^{++}]. The cells were dispersed by incubating the cultures for 10 to 20 min at 37 C in 15 ml Versene solution with intermittent shaking. Kidneys of one- to three-month-old hamsters were perfused *in situ* with borate buffered saline, pH 8.0 (BS). The cells were dispersed with a wire brush in dextrose-free Hank's solution (DF medium). Tumors (15 mm diameter at most) were cut into small pieces and the necrotic tissue was removed. The cells were dispersed by scraping the tissue with a wire brush or by rubbing it against a stainless steel sieve. Cell suspensions were partially freed of debris by passing first through a 60 mesh stainless steel sieve and then through several layers of gauze. Prior to further processing, all cells were washed three times in cold DF medium.

Cell membranes. Cell membranes were prepared from hamster kidney cells (normal membranes), from HK7 cells and from solid tumor (ST) cells by the Tris method of Warren et al. (5). The membranes were washed twice in M/15 phosphate buffer, pH 7.0, which contained 5×10^{-3} M $MgCl_2$.

Antisera. Antiserum to sheep red blood cells (ASRBC) was prepared according to Campbell et al. (6). Its hemolytic titer was 1/100,000. Antisera to NK (AN), HK7 (AHK7), ST (AST) cell membranes were obtained by injecting groups of three rabbits each with the membranes incorporated in complete Freund's adjuvant. Two or three administrations of antigen were given, at seven- or 14-day intervals, each injection consisting of 0.5 ml antigen given s.c., 0.5 ml i.m. and 0.1 ml into the footpad. Bleedings were started seven days after the last injection. Antisera were inactivated before use. The preparation of the fluorescent guinea pig anti-rabbit γ-globulin serum has been described (7).

Absorption of antisera. Appropriate dilutions of the inactivated antisera were added to living, packed cells and the mixtures were rotated slowly in a roller drum for 1 hr at 37 C or at room temperature. The cells were removed by centrifugation, and the absorption repeated once or twice, as required. AHK7 was absorbed with one or several of the following: BHK21, HK7, hamster kidney cells, ST cells and sheep red blood cells (SRBC). ASRBC and AN were absorbed with SRBC, kidney cells and solid tumor cells.

Isolation of serum globulin fractions. Whole serum globulin was isolated by precipitation with ammonium sulfate at 50% saturation. Crude γ-globulin (γGl) was precipitated with ammonium sulfate at 33% saturation. Purified IgG fraction was isolated by chromatography on DEAE-cellulose. The technique recommended by Campbell et al. was followed (8), except that the fractionation was carried out on columns.

Fluorescent antibody technique. The indirect technique was used throughout (7). Living cell suspensions, cell smears, monolayer cell cultures and frozen tissue sections were examined. Living cells were suspended in two drops of antiserum and rotated in a roller drum for 1 hr. They were washed three times in DF medium, resuspended in two drops of fluorescent antiserum and rotated in the roller drum as above. After further washing, they were suspended in glycerol phosphate buffer for microscopic examination. Cell smears were prepared in the hot room (37 C), from washed cells suspended in inactivated guinea pig serum. They were dried under a fan for 15 min

133

and kept at –20 C until used (no more than 10 days). Tumors and organs were frozen at –20 C. Two-micron sections were cut. Both fixed and nonfixed preparations were tested. Fixation was carred out at –20 C (acetone, 1 min or 10 min; ethanol, 10 min) or at room temperature (methanol, 10 min). Pooled, inactivated normal rabbit serum was used as control.

Iodination of IgG with I^{125}. The chloramine T method of Greenwood et al. was used (9). One mc of carrier-free I^{125} was generally used to iodinate 10 to 20 µg IgG. Approximately 30% of the radioactivity became bound to the protein. After removing the nonbound iodine, the preparation contained 90% of the radioactivity in bound form, with a specific activity of approximately 15 µc/µg.

Antiserum to human leukemic cells, radioiodinated by the same procedure, was a gift from Dr. Z. Bentwich, from the Department of Medicine A, Hadassah University Hospital.

Binding of radioiodinated antibodies to cells. Antibody binding experiments were carried out in the presence of 5 to 10% normal rabbit serum (NRS) in PBS, pH 7.2 to 7.4. The cell suspensions were washed three times in PBS, in 15 ml plastic tubes. To the cell sediment (1 to 20 $\times$ 10^6 cells) 1 ml of radioiodinated antibody was added: 10^4 to 10^6 count/min of the original radioactive γ-globulin, or approximately 3,000 count/min of the specifically purified antibody. The mixture was rotated on a roller drum or gently shaken on a horizontal shaker, for 60 min at room temperature. After washing three times in PBS, the radioactivity remaining in the cell sediment was determined in a well type scintillation counter. ST and NK cells were of smaller size than the cultured cells. To compensate for this, larger numbers of these cells were used in the binding tests.

Specific purification of antibodies to cell membranes. Antibodies to cell membranes were purified by absorption onto, and elution from, living cells. The elution was carried out in the presence of 1% NRS. Either the technique of Harris et al. (10) or that of Woodruff (11) was followed, with minor modifications; the elution medium (2 to 3 ml) contained 1% NRS. The elution procedure was repeated for a second time (lasting for 10 min), as this increased the yield of radioactivity by about 30%. After completing the elution, the cells were centrifuged for 10 min at 400 $\times$ g, following which the supernate (eluate) was centrifuged for 10 min at 12,000 $\times$ g, neutralized with

0.5 M, K_3PO_4 and dialyzed overnight against BS. The eluate was finally centrifuged at 12,000 $\times$ g for 20 min. Effectiveness of the elution procedure was checked by the fluorescent antibody technique. Twenty-five to 50% of the original antibodies were recovered, as judged by the titer of fluorescent staining.

Specific purification of radioiodinated antibodies to cell membranes. AHK7 was absorbed with washed SRBC, 1 ml packed cells/ml, until all hemolytic activity was removed, and with normal hamster kidney cells (2.5 $\times$ 10^8 cells/ml) until its capacity to react with these cells in the fluorescent antibody test was lost. The antiserum was then passed through a column of DEAE-cellulose and the purified IgG fraction was iodinated with I^{125} ($A^{125}HK7$). Two µg of the labeled IgG (20 $\times$ 10^6 count/min) were absorbed onto 1 to 2 $\times$ 10^8 HK7 cells. About 20% of the original radioactivity remained in the cell sediment after washing. Fifteen percent of this radioactivity was eluted from HK7 cells by the technique of Harris and 19% by that of Woodruff (purified $A^{125}HK7$). More radioactivity was eluted from ST cells (25% by the Harris and 29% by the Woodruff technique). All eluates were equally active as regards ability to bind to fresh cells. Binding could be further enhanced by repeating the absorption-elution procedure (doubly purified eluates).

Hemolytic test. All reagents were diluted in veronal buffer, pH 7.4 (12). The reaction mixture contained 0.2 ml of 2% washed SRBC, 0.2 ml of antiserum dilution, 0.2 ml of a 1/10 dilution of fresh guinea pig serum, and 0.4 ml of veronal buffer. Tests were read after 30 min incubation at 37 C.

RESULTS

Fluorescent antibody experiments

Antigenic relationships between kidney cells taken from the animal and kidney cells grown in vitro (BHK21). The results of the fluorescent antibody experiments are summarized in Tables 1 and 2. Cells grown *in vitro* gave a very strong fluorescence with AHK7. Staining was positive up to 1/128 dilution or more and at least 90% of the cells reacted. However, only 5 to 10% of the kidney cells taken from the animal were stained by AHK7 at all concentrations tested (Fig. 1). In the acetone

TABLE 1. *Summary of results of fluorescent antibody experiments*

Anti-serum used	Antiserum absorbed with	*Reciprocal of staining titer with*					
		HK7	BHK21	*Kidney*		*Tumor*	
				Smears	*Sections*	*Smears*	*Sections*
AHK7	——	256	128	256[a]	256[b]	128	256
	Kidney cells or SRBC or						
	Kidney cells + SRBC	128	32	0	32	32	32
	BHK21	32	8	16	—	64	—
	BHK21 + kidney + SRBC	16	0	0	—	4	—
	ST cells	128	128	8	—	16	—
	ST cells + SRBC	64	16	0	32	4	16
	HK7	0	0	0	—	0	—
AN	——	16	16	256	256[c]	16	16
	Kidney cells	0	0	0	0	0	0
	SRBC	—	—	32	32	0	4
ASRBC	——	64	16	64[a]	128[d]	32	128
	SRBC	0	0	0	4	0	4
	Kidney cells	—	—	32[a]	128	8	128
	Kidney or tumor cells + SRBC	—	—	0	0	0	0
	Tumor cells	—	—	64	128	8	8

Each figure represents the mean value of five tests; in no instance was there an appreciable deviation from the means.
AHK7 = Anti HK7 membrane serum, hemolytic titer 1/4000.
AN = Anti hamster kidney cell membrane serum, hemolytic titer 1/100.
ASRBC = Antisheep red blood cells serum, hemolytic titer 1/100,000.
— = Not done.
[a] Only 5 to 10% of the cells were stained.
[b] Mainly glomeruli were stained.
[c] Only tubuli were stained.
[d] Only distal tubuli were stained.

TABLE 2. *Fluorescent antibody staining by specifically purified AHK7[a]*

Treatment of AHK7	*Reciprocal of staining titers of suspensions of the following cell types*				
	HK7	BHK21	ST	*NK*	
				Suspension	*Section*
Eluted from BHK21	16	16	4	4[b]	16[c]
Eluted from HK7	64	64	16	4[b]	16[c]
Eluted from HK7, absorbed with BHK21	2	0	0	0	0

[a] AHK7 was absorbed with SRBC and NK before the elution procedure.
[b] Only a small proportion of the cells, approximately 5%, was stained.
[c] Staining was confined largely to the glomeruli, but there was also some staining in the intertubular tissue.

fixed frozen kidney sections treated with this antiserum, only the glomeruli showed intense fluorescence (Fig. 2). It seems, therefore, that the 5 to 10% fluorescent cells seen in the kidney smears were of glomerular origin. There was some fluorescence in what were

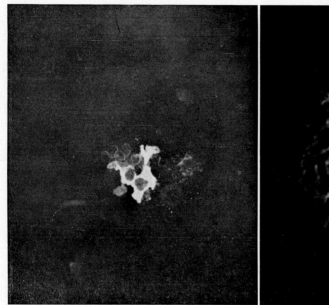

FIG. 1. Smear of hamster kidney cells fixed in acetone, stained with AHK7. Only a small proportion of the cells are fluorescent. × 190.

FIG. 2. Kidney section stained with AHK7, showing fluorescence in the glomeruli. × 190.

probably Henle's loops and in the tubular cell membranes. Ethanol fixed kidney sections also showed some staining in the intertubular capillaries.

Absorption of AHK7 with SRBC, kidney cells or both abolished its reactivity with the smeared kidney cells, indicating that most of the antibodies responsible for this reactivity were Forssman (F) antibodies. AHK7 thus absorbed reacted, however, with BHK21. This reactivity was strongly diminished by absorption with BHK21 (titer, 1/8) and was totally abolished by sequential absorption with BHK21, SRBC and kidney cells.

AN displayed a totally different type of reactivity: it stained strongly (up to 1/256) most of the smeared kidney cells. In frozen kidney sections fixed with ethanol, the fluorescence was mainly localized in the tubular cell membranes, with the glomeruli showing no fluorescence whatever. The antigens involved were designated KT (kidney tubules) antigens. They are probably kidney specific,

since AN did not stain hamster liver, spleen or heart (Sulitzeanu and Feinwax, unpublished

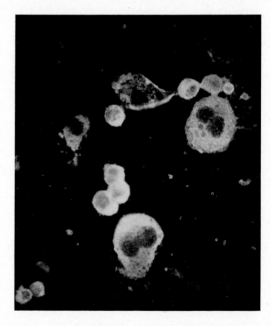

FIG. 3. Strongly fluorescent, fixed HK7 cells stained with AHK7. × 600.

136

observations). BHK21, like all the other preparations, were stained only weakly by AN, to a titer of 1/16.

Antigenic relationships between the SV_{40} transformed and non-transformed cultured cell lines. The HK7 cells fixed with acetone (1 min) gave a very intense, overall fluorescence after treatment with AHK7, up to 1/256 dilution (Fig. 3). The nucleus was not stained. When stained without fixation, as monolayers in Leighton tubes and, in particular, as cell suspensions, the fluorescence was less intense and was limited to the cell membrane. The fixed, non-transformed BHK21 cells showed a characteristic granular type of fluorescence, up to 1/128 dilution. About 90% of the cells were stained in both cases. Absorption of AHK7 with kidney cells enhanced the difference between the two cell lines: fewer BHK21 cells were stained by the absorbed AHK7, and the granular appearance of the stain became more evident. The fluorescence of the transformed HK7 cells was hardly affected by the absorption with either kidney cells, SRBC or both (Table 1). Therefore, most antibodies in AHK7 reacting with HK7 were not F antibodies. Absorption of AHK7 with BHK21 cells greatly reduced both the titer (1/8) and the intensity of the staining of BHK21 cells, while still permitting relatively good staining of the HK7 cells, up to a dilution of 1/32.

No differences were noted between the cultured cell lines on staining with AN. Both cell types showed only a weak fluorescence with this antiserum.

These experiments showed at the most some quantitative differences between the membranes of the two cultured cell lines, but no clear cut qualitative differences. This conclusion was reinforced by experiments with specifically purified AHK7 (Table 2). The antiserum used in these tests was first absorbed with SRBC and NK. Antibodies purified by absorption onto, and elution from, either BHK21, HK7 or ST were tested. The use of living cell preparations in the purification procedure ensured that only antimembrane antibodies were recovered. The protein content of the eluate from HK7 cells was 200 µg/ml, as compared to approximately 70,000 µg/ml of protein in the original antiserum. As the staining titer of the eluate was about one-fourth that of the antiserum, the purification achieved was of the order of 50- to 100-fold at least. Eluates from either HK7 or BHK21 reacted almost identically with all cells tested (Table 2). It is worth stressing, in particular, that both eluates stained the glomeruli but not the tubular cells (Fig. 4, 5), indicating that both cultured cell lines had probably originated from glomerular cells or from antigenically related cells. Eluates from ST had a lower titer, but otherwise behaved in the same manner. Fig. 6 shows two living HK7 cells stained with purified AHK7.

Antigenic relationships between cultured SV_{40} transformed cells and solid tumor cells. The solid tumor cells were much smaller than the cultured cells. Most of them showed a

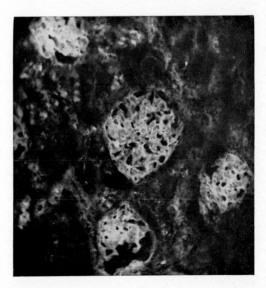

FIG. 4. Kidney section stained with specifically purified AHK7, preabsorbed with SRBC and normal kidney cells. × 190.

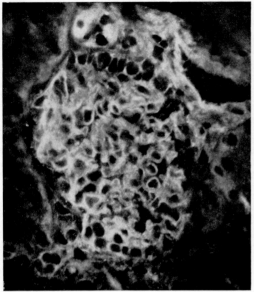

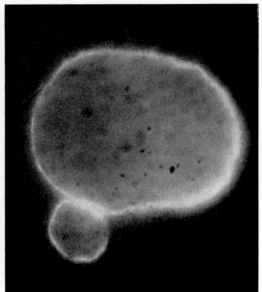

FIG. 5.   Kidney section, stained as above, enlarged to show membrane fluorescence. × 380.

FIG. 6.   Living (nonfixed) HK7 cells (one very large) stained with specifically purified AHK7, preabsorbed with SRBC and kidney cells. Only the cell membrane is fluorescent. × 1,000.

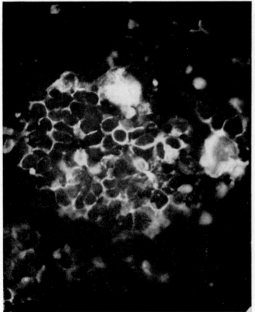

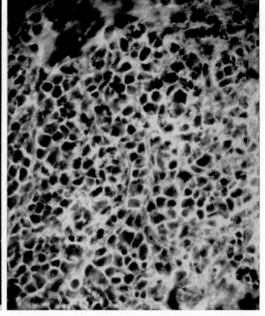

FIG. 7.   Smear of solid tumor cells, treated with AHK7. Characteristic "ring" type fluorescence. × 380.

FIG. 8.   Section of solid tumor stained with AHK7. × 380.

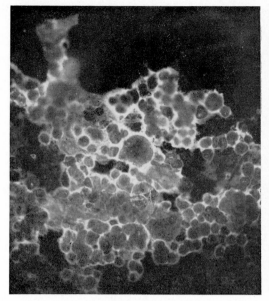

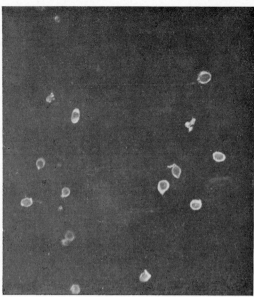

FIG. 9.   Staining of HK7 by ASRBC. × 200.

FIG. 10.   Staining of BHK21 by ASRBC. × 200.

rather weak, "ring" type fluorescence when treated with AHK7 (Fig. 7), quite unlike the intense overall fluorescence of the cultured cells (Fig. 3).

Acetone fixed, frozen solid tumor sections treated with AHK7 showed intense fluorescence in the cell membranes up to 1/256 dilution (Fig. 8). Following sequential absorption with BHK21, SRBC and NK, AHK7 failed to stain the ST cells and gave only marginal fluorescence with the HK7 cells.

On the basis of these results, the following antigens were postulated:

1)   F antigen, was present in all cell types, as shown by the following findings: a) AHK7 hemolyzed SRBC to a titer of 1/4,000. Absorption of its hemolytic activity with SRBC reduced the intensity of staining of all cell preparations tested. b) AN was hemolytic (titer 1/100), showing the presence of F antigen in normal kidney cell membranes. c) ASRBC (hemolytic titer $1/10^5$) stained strongly the HK7 and BHK21 cells fixed with methanol (Fig. 9, 10). It also stained

strongly the kidney and solid tumor sections, and less intensely the smeared kidney and tumor cells. In the kidney sections, the fluores-

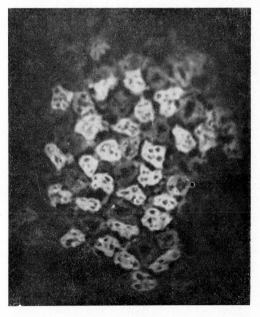

FIG. 11.   Kidney section stained with ASRBC. Fluorescence is localized in the distal tubules. × 200.

139

cence was localized in the cells of the distal tubules (Fig. 11). Staining was abolished following absorption with SRBC.

2) Antigen(s) present in the kidney glomeruli (G), in HK7, BHK21, and ST cells. G cannot be identical with F, because: a) Staining by AHK7 could be abolished by absorption with HK7 (Table 1) or BHK21 (Table 2), but was hardly affected by absorption with SRBC (Table 1). b) Staining by ASRBC could be entirely removed by absorption with SRBC (Table 1).

3) KT antigen, found mainly in the normal kidney tubules.

Experiments with radioiodinated antibodies

Binding of radioiodinated AHK7 to various cell types. As mentioned in Materials and Methods, AHK7 was first absorbed with SRBC and NK before iodination. Nonpurified and specifically purified labeled preparations were tested for their ability to bind to HK7, BHK21, ST and NK cells. The purified A^{125}HK7 was tested both in its original form and after further absorption with NK cells. Following purification, the percent A^{125}HK bound to HK7 cells increased at least two-

fold, reaching 40% binding or more with doubly purified preparations. As seen in Table 3, the cultured cells bound much more radioactivity than the kidney cells. A preferential binding of labeled antibodies to HK7, as compared to BHK21, was noted with both the singly and the doubly purified antibodies, thus confirming the results obtained in the fluorescent antibody work. Labeled normal rabbit γ-globulin (NRG) did not bind to cells to any appreciable extent—less than 3% even after "specific purification" from HK7 cells.

Solid tumor cells bound less radioactivity than HK7 cells, most likely because of their small size. As an example, 20×10^6 ST cells bound in one experiment 16% of the radioactivity from a specifically purified AHK7 preparation, while the HK7 cells bound 21%.

Binding of radioactivity to cells is specific. Antibodies radioiodinated at the fairly high specific activity used here (15 µc/µg) do not seem to have been used before as tools for analyzing the antigenic structure of the cell membrane. It appeared worthwhile, therefore, to ascertain that the binding of radioactivity to the cells is indeed specific.

TABLE 3. *Binding of nonpurified and of specifically purified AHK7 to various cell types*

Experiment no.	Preparation tested	% radioactivity bound to[a]			Radioactivity used in binding test (count/min)
		HK7	BHK21	NK	
1	A^{125}HK7	7	—	1.5	20,000
	Purified A^{125}HK7	36	—	5.5	20,000
	Purified A^{125}HK7 absorbed with NK[b]	27	18	2.2	10,000
2	Doubly purified A^{125}HK7[c]	35	26	—	3,000
	Doubly purified A^{125}HK7 absorbed with 45×10^6 BHK21	9.8	5.2	—	3,000

[a] 10×10^6 cells used in the binding tests.
[b] 1.5×10^8 NK cells were used to absorb the A^{125}HK7 preparation (1.3×10^5 count/min).
[c] Antibodies purified by two sequential absorption-elution cycles from HK7 cells.
— = Not done.

TABLE 4. *Competition between labeled and nonlabeled antibodies for binding sites on the cell membranes*

Amount of inhibitor (µg)	% radioactivity bound in the presence of		
	No inhibitor	AHK7	NRG
—	16.6		
100		6.6	13.1
1,000		2.9	9.0

TABLE 5. *Binding of purified antibodies to homologous and heterologous cells*

Purified antibodies tested	Cells used for specific purification of antibodies	% radioactivity bound to	
		HK7	LC[a]
A[125]HK7	HK7	20	2.1
A[125]LC	LC	4.5	26
A[125]LC[b]	HK7	4.0	6.1

10×10^6 cells were used in the binding test.
[a] LC = Human leukemic cells.
[b] ALC = Antiserum to human leukemic cells.

Two types of tests indicated that this was indeed so. The first was a competition experiment, in which binding was carried out in the presence of a large excess (100 to 1,000 µg) of nonlabeled AHK7 or NRG (both obtained by precipitation at 33% saturation with ammonium sulfate). Table 4 shows the results. While AHK7 globulin strongly inhibited the binding of radioactivity to the cells, NRG had only a small inhibitory effect. It was estimated that, to reduce the binding of radioactivity by 50%, about 30 µg of nonlabeled AHK7 were needed, as compared to 2,000 µg NRG. In the second test, the affinity for cells of specifically purified A[125]HK7 was compared with that of a similar preparation from an unrelated antiserum directed against human leukemic cells (A[125]LC). The results, summarized in Table 5, were clear cut: A[125]HK7 eluate bound to a high extent (20%) to HK7 cells and practically not at all to human leukocytes; it has already been shown

in Table 3 that very little bound to NK cells. On the other hand, A[125]LC bound very well to the human cells but not to the hamster cells. The activity of A[125]LC towards the hamster cells was not improved even when solid hamster tumor cells, rather than human cells, were used for the specific purification of antibodies.

DISCUSSION

The conclusions drawn from this work are based on the assumption that the antimembrane sera used (AHK7, AST and AN) contained antibodies directed largely against the cell membranes. This assumption appears justified by the finding that the fluorescent staining ability of all antisera could be entirely abolished by absorption with living cell preparations. Moreover, the results obtained with the whole antisera were confirmed by experiments with specifically purified antibodies, isolated after binding to living cells. Clearly, the purified preparations could not contain appreciable quantities of antibodies not directed to antigens on the cell membranes.

The most interesting result of this work was the finding that the antigenic constitution of BHK21, HK7 and ST cells was quite different from that of the large majority of the normal adult kidney cells. The antiserum to normal adult kidney cell membranes stained mostly the kidney tubular cells and very little the other cell types. AHK7 and AST stained mainly the glomeruli in the kidney, the ST cells and the *in vitro* grown lines, but hardly the kidney tubular cells. AHK7 stained the glomeruli even after specific purification, by elution from either HK7 or BHK21. It would seem, therefore, that BHK21, HK7 and ST cells have a common source, namely a cell derived from the glomerulus.

It was reported by Weiler (13, 14) that stilbestrol induced kidney carcinoma in the hamster lacks the normal kidney specific

141

antigen. This work led to the widely held belief that neoplastic transformation is likely to be accompanied by loss of normal cellular antigen. While this may be true, our own work suggests that Weiler's results could equally well be due to the tumor cells originating from a cell type different antigenically from the majority of the cells in the kidney.

The differences in the antigenic makeup of the transformed and non-transformed cell lines were rather small. It is well known that the transformed cells possess at least two, apparently unrelated (15) surface antigens: the tumor specific transplantation antigen (TSTA) responsible for resistance to tumor growth, and S antigen(s), detected by fluorescent antibody tests with homologous (hamster) antisera. It would have been too much to hope that the heterologous antiserum used here would reveal qualitatively and unequivocally the presence of these antigens, and a similar attempt made by Robertson and Black (16) was unsuccessful. The antisera employed by these investigators, prepared by injecting into rabbits whole cells rather than cell membranes, contained no antibodies to other membrane components except the F antigen. Our antiserum did contain antibodies to additional membrane antigens and was sufficiently discriminating to allow us to detect at least quantitative differences between the transformed and non-transformed cells: the transformed cells stained to a higher titer in the fluorescent antibody test and bound more radioactivity from the radioiodinated preparations. Also, the overall fluorescence of the HK7 membranes contrasted with the granular appearance of the stained BHK21 cells.

The F antigen was encountered in all cells tested. The appearance of this antigen in hamster kidney cells has been studied by Fogel and Sachs (17, 18) and by O'Neill (19). There is agreement between these investigators concerning the presence of F antigen in trans-

formed BHK21 cells and its absence in the non-transformed line. However, in contrast to Fogel and Sachs, who could only detect F antigen in hamster embryo cells after two days in culture, O'Neill demonstrated its presence in cells taken directly from the embryo. One might have concluded from the above investigations that an apparently embryonic antigen had reappeared in a cell line after neoplastic transformation, in agreement with Prehn's hypothesis (20), according to which tumor specific antigens might in fact be embryonic antigens. In our experience, however, the non-transformed BHK21 line we studied also contained the F antigen. The fluorescent staining properties of this line were sufficiently different from those of the transformed cells to make contamination of the cultures an unlikely explanation. Furthermore, even the normal hamster kidney cells appeared to contain F antigen. It must be concluded, therefore, that the appearance of F antigen in the cultured or transformed cells is due to an increase in the amount of an antigen already present and not, as Robertson and Black propose, to the loss of a blocking group attached to the Forssman moiety (16).

The potentially high sensitivity of radioiodinated antibodies in detecting cell surface antigens has been little explored so far. Sparks et al. (21) were able to demonstrate isoantibodies after first set skin grafts, using an indirect labeled anti-globulin test. We have shown in this work that specifically purified radioiodinated antibodies with reasonably high specific activity can be prepared, with a high degree of specificity for the neoplastic cell membrane. The purification procedure increased the percent of radioactive AHK7 bound to cells by a factor of 2, and repeating the purification yielded preparations binding better than the nonpurified antiserum by a factor of 4. It had been originally hoped to attain higher specific activities by iodinating the antibodies after specific purification by the absorption-elution technique. However, iodination of eluates purified by chromatography on DEAE-cellulose did not yield radioactive preparations with high binding activity. In fact, these preparations reacted with the HK7 cells to the same extent as the nonpurified labeled IgG. This was probably due to the fact, confirmed in experiments not reported here, that the elution technique extracts from the cells nonantibody proteins, which are not retained by the ion exchanger and cannot, therefore, be separated from antibodies.

It is expected that the labeled antibodies will be particularly useful in the fractionation of the cell membrane antigens, as reagents by means of which the fractionation procedure can be followed.

We wish to thank Dr. J. Boss for helping with the interpretation of histological sections, Dr. M. Margalith for instruction and advice on cell cultivation and Mrs. E. Feinwax for preparing the antiserum to normal cell membranes.

This work could not have been carried out without the generous support of the Concern Foundation of Los Angeles, the Sam Lautenberg Fellowship and the R. Kunin and S. Lunenfeld Fund.

REFERENCES

1. FRANKS, D. Antigens as markers on cultured mammalian cells. *Biol. Rev.* **43**: 17, 1968.
2. MACPHERSON, I. and STOKER, M. Polyoma transformation of hamster cell clones—an investigation of genetic factors affecting cell competence. *Virology* **16**: 147, 1962.
3. RAPP, F., KHERA, K. S. and MELNICK, J. L. Resistance of BHK21 hamster cells to SV$_{40}$ Papovavirus. *Nature (Lond.)* **201**: 1349, 1964.
4. ASHKENAZI, A. Action of 5-iodo-2-deoxyuridine (IUDR) on *in vitro* transformation of hamster kidney cells by SV$_{40}$ virus. *Israel J. med. Sci.* **1**: 1012, 1965.
5. WARREN, L., GLICK, M. C. and NASS, M. K. Membranes of animal cells. I. Methods of isolation of the surface membrane. *J. cell comp. Physiol.* **68**: 269, 1966.
6. CAMPBELL, D. H., GARVEY, J. S., CREMER, N. E. and SUSSDORF, D. H. "Methods in immunology." New York, W. A. Benjamin Inc., 1963, p. 101.
7. SULITZEANU, D., SLAVIN, M., KARAMAN, H. and GOLDMAN, W. Antigenic components of rat connective tissue. II. Fluorescent antibody studies with antisera to connective tissue antigens. *Brit. J. exp. Path.* **48**: 159, 1967.
8. CAMPBELL, D. H., GARVEY, J. S., CREMER, N. E. and SUSSDORF, D. H. "Methods in immunology." New York, W. A. Benjamin Inc., 1963, p. 122.
9. GREENWOOD, F. C., HUNTER, W. M. and GLOVER, J. S. The preparation of I^{131}-labelled human growth hormone of high specific radioactivity. *Biochem. J.* **89**: 114, 1963.
10. HARRIS, T. N., OGBURN, C. A., HARRIS, S. and Farber, M. B. Preparation by elution from specific aggregates of the isoantibody causing rejection of transferred rabbit lymph node cells. *Transplantation* **1**: 261, 1963.
11. WOODRUFF, M. F. A. Purification of antilymphocytic antibody. *Nature (Lond.)* **217**: 821, 1968.
12. CAMPBELL, D. H., GARVEY, J. S., CREMER, N. E. and Sussdorf, D. H. "Methods in immunology." New York, W. A. Benjamin Inc., 1963, p. 246.
13. WEILER, E. Antigenic differences between normal hamster kidney and stilboestrol induced kidney carcinoma: complement fixation reactions with cytoplasmic particles. *Brit. J. Cancer* **10**: 553, 1956.
14. WEILER, E. Antigenic differences between normal hamster kidney and stilboestrol induced kidney carcinoma: histological demonstration by means of fluorescing antibodies. *Brit. J. Cancer* **10**: 560, 1956.
15. TEVETHIA, S. S., DIAMANDOPOULOS, G. TH., RAPP, F. and ENDERS, J. F. Lack of relationship between virus-specific surface and transplantation antigens in hamster cells transformed by simian papovavirus SV$_{40}$. *J. Immunol.* **101**: 1192, 1968.
16. ROBERTSON, H. T. and BLACK, P. H. Changes in surface antigens of SV$_{40}$ virus transformed cells. *Proc. Soc. exp. Biol. (N. Y.)* **130**: 363, 1969.
17. FOGEL, M. and SACHS, L. Studies on the antigenic composition of hamster tumors induced by polyoma virus and of normal hamster tissues in vivo and in vitro. *J. nat. Cancer Inst.* **29**: 239, 1962.
18. FOGEL, M. and SACHS, L. The induction of Forssman antigen synthesis in hamster and mouse cells in tissue culture, as detected by the fluorescent antibody technique. *Exp. Cell Res.* **34**: 448, 1964.
19. O'NEILL, C. H. An association between viral transformation and Forssman antigen detected by immune adherence in cultured BHK21 cells. *J. Cell Sci.* **3**: 405, 1968.
20. PREHN, R. T. The significance of tumor-distinctive histocompatibility antigens, in: Trentin J.J. (Ed.), "Cross reacting antigens and neoantigens." Baltimore, Williams and Wilkins, 1967, p. 105.
21. SPARKS, F. C., TING, C. C., HAMMOND, W. G. and HERBERMAN, R. B. An isotopic antiglobulin technique for measuring antibodies to cell-surface antigens. *J. Immunol.* **102**: 842, 1969.

TUMOR-SPECIFIC ANTIGENS IN 2-ACETYLAMINOFLUORENE-INDUCED RAT HEPATOMAS AND RELATED TUMORS

R. W. BALDWIN and M. J. EMBLETON

British Empire Cancer Campaign Research Laboratories, University of Nottingham, England

ABSTRACT

Hepatomas and ear duct carcinomas induced by 2-acetylaminofluorene were shown to be generally lacking in immunogenicity as assessed by their capacity to induce resistance against transplanted tumor cells in syngeneic rats. Where resistance could be induced, this was only weak as measured by the maximum tumor cell inoculum rejected. The low immunogenicity of these tumors was also reflected by their inability to reproducibly induce tumor-specific humoral antibody responses detectable by membrane immunofluorescence reactions. These results contrast with the more uniform expression of tumor-specific antigens on aminoazo dye and diethylnitrosamine-induced rat hepatomas.

INTRODUCTION

Chemically-induced tumors frequently possess new antigens termed tumor-specific transplantation antigens because of their capacity to elicit rejection responses against transplanted tumor cells in syngeneic hosts (1–3). These antigens are also recognized by the autochthonous host (4, 5), and as new cellular determinants on neoplastic cells may be expressions of carcinogen-induced genetic change. Tumors induced by different carcinogens vary markedly in antigenicity, which may reflect quantitative or qualitative differences in the expression of tumor-specific antigen. This is exemplified by the low immunogenicity of murine sarcomas induced by plastic films (6) compared with those induced by 3-methylcholanthrene (4). Similarly, diethylnitrosamine-induced hepatomas in the guinea pig are im-

munogenic (7), whereas tumor-specific antigen was not detected in murine lung adenocarcinomas induced by the same carcinogen (8). These differences may be interpreted as reflecting the degree of cellular derangement induced by chemical carcinogens since most antigenic tumors have been obtained with highly tissue-reactive carcinogens. Alternatively, weak antigenicity may result from modification of tumor antigen expression during tumor development through external immunological pressures (9).

Rat hepatomas induced by aminoazo dyes are immunogenic, (10) and these carcinogens, like the polycyclic hydrocarbons, react with cellular macromolecules (11). In contrast, rat mammary adenocarcinomas induced by 2-acetylaminofluorene (AAF), which has a biochemical reactivity similar to that of the carcinogenic aminoazo dyes (11), are generally lacking in immunogenicity (12). It may be argued, however, that tumors arising in different tissues are not directly comparable, and the present studies were initiated to establish whether hepatomas induced by AAF carry cell surface-expressed tumor-specific antigens. This was determined from the capacity of these hepatomas to elicit tumor-specific immune responses in syngeneic rats measured by the induction of host resistance. Also, the tumor-specific humoral antibody response was examined by membrane immunofluorescence reactions, since this method can detect cell surface tumor antigens on carcinogen-induced rat hepatomas (13) and sarcomas (14) as well as mammary carcinomas arising without deliberate inducement (15). Hepatomas induced by diethylnitrosamine (DENA) were also tested for tumor antigenicity, since this carcinogen, like AAF, interacts with tissue components (11). In addition, the spectrum of AAF-induced tumors tested was increased by examining ear duct carcinomas and nephroblastomas.

MATERIALS AND METHODS

Induction of tumors. Wistar rats of both sexes were fed a powdered diet (MRC41B) containing 0.04% w/w AAF (Aldrich Chemical Co. Inc., Milwaukee, Wisconsin) with water ad lib. Liver tumors, classified histologically as hepatocellular carcinomas, arose in 10 rats with latent induction periods between 41 and 67 weeks. Three squamous cell carcinomas arising in association with glands of the external ear duct were also obtained in rats fed the AAF diet for 52 to 55 weeks. The pathogenesis of these tumors has been described (16). Two nephroblastomas were also obtained from rats on AAF diet for 24 weeks and 46 weeks, respectively.

DENA (bp 174 C) was administered continuously at a level of 0.006% v/v in drinking water to rats on a normal cubed diet (MRC 41B). Under these conditions, seventeen rats developed hepatocellular carcinomas with latent periods between 19 and 25 weeks.

Immunization against tumors. Details of the syngeneic Wistar rats used in these studies and

the methods of immunization by excision of tumor grafts or implantation of heavily-irradiated tumor have been described elsewhere (10, 12). For immunization with irradiated tumor, trocar graft pieces attenuated by Co^{60} γ-irradiation (15,000 R) were implanted s.c. at two- to four-weekly intervals, as dictated by the tumor growth potential. Control rats were similarly treated with irradiated normal liver, kidney and spleen grafts. To measure the immune response evoked by a growing tumor, subcutaneous grafts implanted as superficially as possible were allowed to develop until they attained an average diameter of between 1.0 and 1.5 cm (two to four weeks). They were then surgically excised complete with the overlying skin. Control rats received similar surgical treatments.

Animals immunized by these two procedures, together with the appropriate controls, were challenged s.c. with defined numbers of viable tumor cells, brought into suspension by trypsinization (10, 12), seven to 14 days after the final immunization treatment. Initial challenges were usually given at a dose of 10^3 to 10^4 cells, then increasingly higher doses were administered at intervals of four to six weeks until progressive tumor growth was obtained in the controls. For each challenge, a group of untreated controls was generally included. In tests with AAF-induced tumors, rats received whole body Co^{60} γ-irradiation (400 R) 24 hr before tumor inoculation. Since this suppresses any primary immune response to the tumor without markedly affecting the secondary immune response in immunized hosts, sensitivity was increased, allowing weak levels of resistance to be detected.

Membrane immunofluorescence. Tumor-specific immune sera were obtained from rats immunized against individual tumors by graft excision or repeated implantation of irradiated tumor. Isoantisera were obtained from Slonaker rats repeatedly allografted with a transplanted hepatoma (D23) of Wistar origin. The indirect membrane immunofluorescence test was performed on viable tumor cells in suspension, as previously described (13, 15). Fluorescence indexes (FI) were calculated from the proportions of unstained cells in samples exposed to test and normal sera (13).

RESULTS

Immunogenicity of hepatomas induced by AAF and DENA. Tumor-specific transplantation antigens were detected in three of the

TABLE 1. *Immune response to irradiated grafts of AAF-induced rat hepatomas*

Immunizing tumor and transfer generations	No. of irradiated tumor implants for sequential immunization	Challenge tumor	Cell dose[a]	Growth of tumor challenge inocula					
				Treated rats		Normal tissue controls		Untreated controls	
				Tumor takes	Latent period[b]	Tumor takes	Latent period	Tumor takes	Latent period
AAF23/1–3	5	AAF23/6	5×10^4	1/4	43	0/4	—	1/4	58
		AAF23/7	10^5	3/3	20	3/3	20	5/5	13
AAF28/4–5	4	AAF28/6	10^5	0/5	—	0/3	—	0/4	—
		AAF28/7	5×10^5	5/5	35	3/3	35	5/5	35
AAF29/1–2	5	AAF29/3	10^4	0/3	—	0/4	—	0/4	—
		AAF29/4	5×10^4	3/3	56	1/4	70	3/4	42
AAF35/1–3	4	AAF35/6	4×10^5	2/3	8	2/5	8	1/6	8
		AAF35/7	10^6	1/1	28	3/3	28	4/4	28
AAF42/1–3	4	AAF42/3	10^3	0/6	—	1/4	12	1/4	54
		AAF42/4	10^4	3/6	34	2/3	27	4/4	20
		AAF42/6	2×10^4	3/3	24	—	—	4/4	24
AAF47/1–3	4	AAF47/3	5×10^4	0/5	—	0/5	—	0/6	—
		AAF47/4	2×10^5	3/4	35	2/2	28	4/6	35
AAF50/1–5	5	AAF50/6	5×10^4	0/3	—	2/3	50	3/4	71
		AAF50/7	10^5	0/3	—	—	—	5/5	49
AAF51/1–2	4	AAF51/2	10^4	0/4	—	0/4	—	0/4	—
		AAF51/3	5×10^4	2/4	53	0/4	—	4/5	63
		AAF51/4	5×10^5	2/2	15	4/4	8	4/4	8
AAF53/2–3	4	AAF53/4	5×10^4	0/5	—	3/5	22	3/5	22
		AAF53/5	10^5	2/5	5	2/2	5	3/4	26

[a] Rats received 400 R whole body γ-irradiation 24 hr before challenge
[b] Time in days when tumors were first palpable

nine AAF-induced rat hepatomas (AAF42, AAF50 and AAF53) by the capacity of heavily irradiated (15,000 R) grafts to induce resistance against a subsequent challenge with cells of the immunizing tumor (Table 1). These tumors were weakly immunogenic, treated rats rejecting challenges with only low numbers of cells of the immunizing tumor. Thus, following repeated immunization with hepatoma AAF42, 3/6 rats rejected an inoculum of 10^4 tumor cells which was just sufficient to produce progressive growth in untreated controls or rats treated with irradiated normal tissues. This resistance completely broke down against a subsequent challenge with 2×10^4 tumor cells. Comparably, rats immunized against hepatomas AAF50 or AAF53 rejected challenges with 10^5 cells of the immunizing tumor, this being only twice greater than the dose necessary to obtain

progressive tumor growth in controls. With the six other AAF-induced hepatomas, no resistance could be demonstrated against the minimum challenge inoculum needed for progressive tumor growth in the controls. In these experiments, tumors developed in both test and control rats, and there was no difference in the time required to produce palpable growths or in their rate of development.

Previous studies with aminoazo dye-induced hepatomas established that resistance can be induced with tumor inactivated by γ-irradiation (10), and doses in excess of 50,000 R are required to produce inactivation of cell surface expressed tumor-specific antigens demonstrable by membrane immunofluorescence (Baldwin, unpublished findings). Nevertheless, the low immunogenicity of AAF-hepatomas could possibly reflect the radiosensitivity of their tumor-specific antigens,

TABLE 2. *Immune response following excision of subcutaneous grafts of AAF-induced rat hepatomas*

| Immunizing tumor and transfer generation | Challenge tumor | Cell dose[a] | Growth of tumor challenge inocula | | | | | |
| | | | Treated rats | | Mock excision controls | | Untreated controls | |
			Tumor takes	Latent[b] period	Tumor takes	Latent period	Tumor takes	Latent period
AAF23/2	AAF23/6	5×10^4	0/4	—	1/3	50	1/4	58
	AAF23/7	10^5	4/4	25	2/2	20	4/4	20
AAF28/2	AAF28/5	5×10^4	1/6	42	0/4	—	0/4	—
	AAF28/6	10^5	0/5	—	0/4	—	0/4	—
	AAF28/7	5×10^5	4/4	35	4/4	35	5/5	35
AAF29/1	AAF29/3	10^4	0/6	—	0/3	—	—	—
	AAF29/4	5×10^4	5/6	49	3/3	42	2/4	42
AAF42/1	AAF42/2	10^3	0/4	—	0/4	—	—	—
	AAF42/3	10^4	3/4	19	4/4	26	4/4	19
AAF45/2	AAF45/4	5×10^5	0/4	—	0/4	—	0/4	—
	AAF45/5	10^6	4/4	19	2/4	19	1/5	68

[a,b] See footnotes to Table 1.

TABLE 3. *Induction of immunity to DENA-induced rat hepatomas*

| Immunizing tumor and transfer generations | Immunization procedure | Challenge tumor | Cell dose | Growth of tumor challenge inocula | | | | | |
| | | | | Treated rats | | Control rats | | Untreated controls | |
				Tumor takes	Latent period[a]	Tumor takes	Latent period	Tumor takes	Latent period
DENA 1/1–2	Irradiated tumor	DENA1/3	2×10^5	0/3	—	—	—	3/3	31
		DENA1/4	4×10^5	2/3	21	—	—	3/3	37
DENA 3/1–5	Irradiated tumor	DENA3/1	2×10^5	0/8	—	0/8	—	0/4	—
		DENA3/2	5×10^5	3/8	106	0/8	—	0/5	—
		DENA3/3	10^6	3/5	25	4/8	39	1/4	25
DENA3/1	Excision	DENA3/2	10^5	1/5	19	3/4	14	—	—
		DENA3/3	5×10^5	1/3	75	—	—	5/5	25
DENA 13/1–2	Irradiated tumor	DENA13/4	5×10^5	2/5	29	2/6	29	3/5	29
		DENA13/7	10^6	1/3	22	4/4	22	5/5	15
DENA 13/2	Excision	DENA13/3	2×10^5	0/4	—	1/4	36	1/5	36
		DENA13/4	5×10^5	2/4	26	3/3	26	4/4	36
		DENA13/6	10^6	0/2	—	—	—	5/6	15

[a] Time in days when tumors were first palpable

and to examine this, the immune response evoked following total extirpation of developing subcutaneous hepatoma grafts was determined (Table 2). None of the five hepatomas tested in this manner induced any detectable resistance, tumors developing in almost all treated rats following challenge with the minimum cell dose necessary for consistent growth in untreated and sham-operated rats. Moreover, there was no significant difference in the latent period for tumor development or the rate of tumor growth in treated and control groups. It is concluded, therefore, that AAF-induced rat hepatomas, unlike those induced with aminoazo dyes (10) are generally lacking in tumor-specific transplantation antigens.

Tests with diethylnitrosamine-induced hepatomas were less satisfactory because of their inconsistent growth on transplantation; only three of eleven hepatomas grew from low cell inocula. The other tumors required trocar graft implants to ensure growth, and frequently these were slowly developing. Moreover, some examples could not be maintained by serial transplantation. Resistance against challenge inocula of between 1 and 2×10^5 cells of the immunizing tumor was demonstrated following immunization against hepatomas DENA1 and DENA3 by graft excision or treatment with irradiated tumor (Table 3). Combined tests with hepatoma DENA13 following immunization by both procedures indicated that

$4/5$ treated rats rejected challenge with 10^6 tumor cells whereas this dose grew in almost all control rats.

Immunogenicity of AAF-induced ear duct carcinomas and nephroblastomas. Oral administration of AAF results in the induction of mainly hepatomas and mammary adenocarcinomas, but a few tumors arise at other sites and these were also tested for tumor-specific antigenicity. Three squamous cell carcinomas were obtained arising in sebaceous glands (Zymbal's glands) associated with the external auditory duct. On subcutaneous transplantation, these tumors developed as well-encapsulated growths still retaining the capacity for wax secretion. With two examples, reproducible growth was obtained from inocula of 5×10^4 tumor cells, but the third tumor (AAF36) only grew consistently from trocar implants. Two other tumors arising in the kidney and classified histologically as nephroblastomas grew less consistently, and inocula of the order of 10^6 cells or trocar graft implants were necessary.

The tumor-immune response evoked by

TABLE 4. *Immune response to irradiated grafts of AAF-induced ear duct carcinomas and nephroblastomas*

Immunizing tumor and transfer generations	No. of irradiated tumor implants for sequential immunization	Challenge tumor	Cell dose[a]	Growth of tumor challenge inocula					
				Treated rats		Normal tissue controls		Untreated controls	
				Tumor takes	Latent period[b]	Tumor takes	Latent period	Tumor takes	Latent period
Ear duct carcinoma AAF26/2–4	5	AAF26/6	10^4	1/5	21	1/5	13	0/4	—
		AAF26/7	5×10^4	1/4	21	4/4	21	4/4	21
		AAF26/8	10^5	3/3	8	—	—	3/3	8
AAF36/1–4	4	AAF36/8	10^5	0/5	—	0/4	—	0/4	—
		AAF36/9	5×10^5	0/5	—	0/4	—	0/4	—
		AAF36/10	Graft	5/5	8	4/4	8	4/4	8
AAF49/1–3	4	AAF49/3	10^4	0/4	—	0/4	—	0/4	—
		AAF49/5	5×10^4	4/4	8	4/4	8	4/4	8
Nephroblastoma AAF40/1–4	4	AAF40/7	5×10^4	0/5	—	0/5	—	0/4	—
		AAF40/8	2×10^5	4/5	22	1/5	29	2/5	29
		AAF40/10	10^6	1/1	15	4/4	15	5/5	15

[a,b] See footnotes to Table 1.

TABLE 5. *Immune response following excision of subcutaneous grafts of AAF-induced ear duct carcinomas and nephroblastomas*

Immunizing tumor and transfer generations	Challenge tumor	Cell dose[a]	Treated rats		Mock excision controls		Untreated controls	
			Tumor takes	Latent period[b]	Tumor takes	Latent period	Tumor takes	Latent period
Ear duct	AAF36/8	2×10^5	0/6	—	0/4	—	0/4	—
carcinoma	AAF36/9	10^6	0/6	—	0/4	—	0/4	—
AAF36/1	AAF36/10	Graft	6/6	8	3/3	8	5/5	8
AAF49/1	AAF49/2	10^4	0/5	—	0/4	—	—	—
	AAF49/3	5×10^4	5/5	23	4/4	14	4/4	23
Nephro-	AAF40/7	10^5	1/5	34	0/3	—	0/4	—
blastoma	AAF40/8	2×10^5	2/4	22	—	—	2/5	29
AAF40/1	AAF40/10	10^6	2/2	15	—	—	5/5	15
AAF32/1	AAF32/4	10^5	1/5	43	0/3	—	0/4	—
	AAF32/6	10^6	1/4	50	2/3	15	1/4	15
	AAF32/7	Graft	3/3	23	1/1	27	2/4	30

[a,b] See footnotes to Table 1.

repeated implantation of irradiated grafts of these tumors is summarized in Table 4. Resistance was demonstrable in rats immunized with ear duct carcinoma AAF26, and a challenge with 5×10^4 tumor cells, which grew in all controls, was rejected by all but one animal. This resistance broke down against a subsequent challenge with 10^5 tumor cells. No resistance in treated rats was detectable against the other two ear duct carcinomas or the nephroblastomas. Excision of subcutaneously growing tumor failed to produce resistance against two ear duct carcinomas (AAF36 and AAF49) or the nephroblastomas (Table 5).

Membrane immunofluorescence tests. Cell surface-expressed isoantigens were demonstrable on all the AAF- and DENA-induced tumors, as indicated by their reactions with Slonaker-anti-Wistar isoantiserum giving FI between 0.60 and 1.00 (Table 6). Immunofluorescence reactions of these tumors with sera from syngeneic rats immunized by graft excision or implantation of irradiated tumor were essentially the same and the data have been combined. Only one AAF-induced hepatoma (AAF53) consistently gave positive reactions with sera from rats immunized against this tumor (mean FI 0.42 ± 0.03, $P < 0.05$), and, significantly, this was immunogenic in transplantation tests (Table 1). All the other AAF-induced hepatomas, including the weakly immunogenic AAF42, showed almost complete lack of reactivity with sera from treated rats (FI 0.05 to 0.22). FI of 0.19 to 0.28 (mean 0.25 ± 0.04) were obtained with hepatoma DENA3 and sera from rats immunized against this tumor, which represents a positive reaction ($P < 0.05$). Negative FI (0.03 to 0.24, mean 0.10 ± 0.07) were obtained in tests with the other immunogenic hepatoma DENA13 and serum from immune donors. Comparably, immunofluorescence tests with AAF-induced ear duct carcinomas and nephroblastomas and serum from treated rats were also negative (FI 0.00 to 0.06).

None of the sera from rats immunized against one tumor reacted positively with

149

TABLE 6. *Membrane immunofluorescence tests with AAF- and DENA-induced rat tumors*

| Tumor target cells of | FI with sera from rats immunized with | | | | | | | | | | | | | | FI with Slonaker anti-hepatoma D23 isoantiserum |
| | Hepatoma | | | | | | | | | | Ear duct carcinoma | | Nephroblastoma | | |
	AAF23	AAF29	AAF35	AAF42	AAF44	AAF45	AAF51	AAF53	DENA3	DENA13	AAF26	AAF49	AAF32	AAF40	
Immunizing tumor	0.06	0.00, 0.03 0.06, 0.08 0.32	0.00 0.05	0.04, 0.08 0.36	0.19, 0.25	0.15	0.08, 0.13 0.32	0.36, 0.42 0.43, 0.46	0.19, 0.27 0.28	0.03, 0.06 0.10, 0.13 0.16, 0.24, 0.24	0.01, 0.02 0.02	0.00, 0.04	0.00, 0.02 0.06	0.00, 0.01	0.90 to 1.00
Homologous tumors[a]	—	0.01, 0.06 0.07	0.05	0.01, 0.03 0.09	0.00, 0.03 0.03, 0.16	0.05	0.00, 0.06 0.10	0.00, 0.00 0.05, 0.07 0.10	0.00	0.00, 0.10	0.00, 0.02	0.01, 0.01 0.01	0.00, 0.16	—	0.60 to 0.96

a Values represent tests with individual tumors of the same type induced by the same carcinogens.

cells of other homologous tumors induced by the same carcinogen (Table 6). Included in these results are cross-tests with hepatoma AAF53-immune sera which reacted positively with cells of the immunizing tumor (FI 0.42 ± 0.03), but showed no reactivity with cells of five other AAF-induced hepatomas (FI 0.00 to 0.01).

DISCUSSION

These results indicate that AAF-induced hepatomas are not consistently immunogenic since only three of the ten examples tested possessed the capacity to induce resistance against transplanted tumor cells in syngeneic recipients. Moreover, the immunogenicity of these examples was weak as measured by the ratio of the maximum tumor cell inoculum rejected by immunized rats compared with the minimum number of cells necessary for growth in controls. The weak immunogenicity of these hepatomas was also shown by the essentially negative membrane immunofluorescence data; only one (AAF53) of the eight tumors examined gave positive FI. This compares with the regular tumor-specific humoral antibody response detected by membrane immunofluorescence tests with aminoazo dye-induced hepatomas (13), reflecting the capacity of these tumors to induce tumor rejection responses (10). AAF-induced squamous cell carcinomas arising in glands of the external ear duct also were generally lacking in immunogenicity, only one of these possessing the capacity to elicit weak tumor rejection reactions, and two nephroblastomas were completely inactive.

These findings, together with previous studies of mammary adenocarcinomas (12), indicate that tumors induced by AAF in several tissues generally lack demonstrable immunogenicity. Because of the limitations of the transplantation methods, this probably reflects a low degree of expression of tumor-specific antigen on these tumors rather than a total absence of such antigens. Attempts to resolve this question using membrane immunofluorescence methods were unsuccessful since, although the technique proved capable of detecting cell surface expressed tumor-specific antigens on hepatoma AAF53, its sensitivity was not as great as that obtained in tumor rejection tests. This difference in sensitivity is illustrated by tests on ear duct carcinoma AAF26 which evoked tumor-specific immunity (Table 4) whereas sera from immunized rats gave negative immunofluorescence reactions (Table 6).

Compared with the present results on AAF-induced hepatomas, histologically similar tumors induced in the same strain of rats with 4-dimethylaminoazobenzene (DAB) are uniformly immunogenic (10). Both these carcinogens have basically similar mechanisms of action, as indicated by their metabolic conversion to reactive N-hydroxylated derivatives (17) and their interaction with cellular macromolecules (11). Although most tumors found to be immunogenic have been induced by potent carcinogens, it is unlikely that the expression of tumor-specific antigen can be related simply to the degree of cellular derangement induced by the carcinogen during neoplastic transformation. Another feature which may be important in tumor antigen expression is the degree of differentiation of the tumor, since hepatomas induced by AAF are similar to minimal deviation hepatomas characterized by essentially normal enzyme profiles (18). Similarly, both AAF-induced mammary and ear duct carcinomas retain a degree of normal tissue function as indicated by their capacity for milk and wax secretion, respectively.

It has been postulated that the immune status of the host is an important factor influencing the degree of tumor antigenicity.

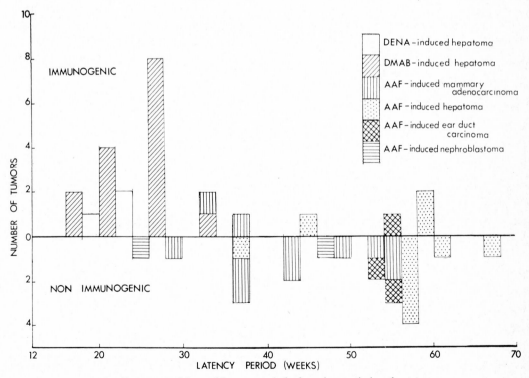

FIG. 1.   Immunogenicity and latency period of carcinogen-induced rat tumors.

151

This is supported by the finding that 3-methylcholanthrene-induced tumors arise more rapidly in animals immunologically suppressed by treatment with antilymphocyte serum and have a greater antigenicity (19, 20). It has been demonstrated, however, that DAB and AAF have comparable immunosuppressive activities, at least as measured by their acute influence on the immune response to sheep erythrocytes (21). It is not likely, therefore, that carcinogen-induced modification of host immune status influences the antigenicity of hepatomas induced by these carcinogens. Conversely, it has been argued that tumor antigenicity is related to the duration of the latency period after carcinogen administration, reflecting immunoselection by the host against antigenic tumor cell populations (9). In this respect, the immunogenic DAB-induced hepatomas have much shorter induction periods than the AAF-induced hepatomas (Fig. 1). Although tests with DENA-induced hepatomas were not so comprehensive, three immunogenic examples also had latent periods comparable with those of the DAB-induced hepatomas. Moreover, the weakly-immunogenic AAF-induced ear duct carcinomas had latent periods similar to those of the hepatomas and mammary carcinomas induced by this carcinogen. In general, therefore, the present studies with several tumor types induced by AAF support the concept of an interrelationship between tumor antigen expression and latent induction period.

The skilful assistance of Mrs. M. E. Marshall and Mrs. C. Wright is gratefully acknowledged. We are indebted to Dr. D. D. Eley for making available Co60-irradiation facilities.

Supported by research grants from the British Empire Cancer Campaign for Research and the Medical Research Council.

REFERENCES

1. OLD, L. J. and BOYSE, E. A. Immunology of experimental tumors. *Ann. Rev. Med.* **15**: 167, 1964.

2. GREEN, H. N., ANTHONY, H. M., BALDWIN, R. W. and WESTROP, J. W. "An immunological approach to cancer." London, Butterworth, 1967, p. 165.

3. PASTERNAK, G. Immunologische Eigenschaften chemisch und physikalisch induzierter Tumoren. *Arch. Geschwulstforsch.* **29**: 113, 1967.

4. KLEIN, G., SJÖGREN, H. O., KLEIN, E. and HELLSTRÖM, K. E. Demonstration of resistance against methylcholanthrene-induced sarcomas in the primary autochthonous host. *Cancer Res.* **20**: 1561, 1960.

5. ALEXANDER, P. Immunotherapy of cancer: experiments with primary tumours and syngeneic tumour grafts. *Progr. exp. Tumor Res. (Basel)* **10**: 22, 1968.

6. KLEIN, G., SJÖGREN, H. O. and KLEIN, E. Demonstration of host resistance against sarcomas induced by implantation of cellophane films in isologous (syngeneic) recipients. *Cancer Res.* **23**: 84, 1963.

7. ZBAR, B., WEPSIC, H. T., RAPP, H. J., BORSOS, T., KRONMAN, B. S. and CHURCHILL, W. H. Antigenic specificity of hepatomas induced in strain-2 guinea pigs by diethylnitrosamine. *J. nat. Cancer Inst.* **43**: 833, 1969.

8. PASTERNAK, G., HOFFMANN, F. and GRAFFI, A. Growth of diethylnitrosamine-induced lung tumours in syngeneic mice specifically pretreated with X-ray killed tumour tissue. *Folia Biol. (Praha)* **12**: 299, 1966.

9. PREHN, R. T. The significance of tumor-distinctive histocompatibility antigens, in: Trentin, J. J. (Ed.) "Cross-reacting antigens and neoantigens." Baltimore, Williams and Wilkins Co., 1967, p. 105.

10. BALDWIN, R. W. and BARKER, C. R. Tumour-specific antigenicity of aminoazo dye-induced rat hepatomas. *Int. J. Cancer* **2**: 355, 1967.

11. MILLER, E. C. and MILLER, J. A. Mechanisms of chemical carcinogenesis: nature of proximate carcinogens and interactions with macromolecules. *Pharmacol. Rev.* **18**: 805, 1966.

12. BALDWIN, R. W. and EMBLETON, M. J. Immunology of 2-acetylaminofluorene-induced rat mammary adenocarcinomas. *Int. J. Cancer* **4**: 47, 1969.

13. BALDWIN, R. W. and BARKER, C. R. Demonstration of tumour-specific humoral antibody against aminoazo dye-induced rat hepatomata. *Brit. J. Cancer* **21**: 793, 1967.

14. BALDWIN, R. W. and PIMM, M. V. Humoral antibody response against tumour-specific antigens on 3-methylcholanthrene-induced rat sarcomas. *Ann. Rep. Brit. Emp. Cancer Campaign* **47**: 266, 1969.

15. BALDWIN, R. W. and EMBLETON, M. J. Immunology of spontaneous rat mammary adenocarcinomas, in: Severi, L. (Ed.), "Immunity and tolerance in oncogenesis." *IV Perugia Quadrennial Int. Conf. on Cancer, 1969* (in press).

16. BALDWIN, R. W., CUNNINGHAM, G. J., SMITH, W. R. D. and SURTEES, S. J. Carcinogenic action of 4-acetamidostilbene and the N-hydroxy derivative in the rat. *Brit. J. Cancer* **22**: 133, 1968.

17. MILLER, J. A. and MILLER, E. C. The metabolic

activation of carcinogenic aromatic amines and amides. *Progr. exp. Tumor Res. (Basel)* **11**: 273, 1969.

18. MORRIS, H. P. Studies on the development, biochemistry and biology of experimental hepatomas. *Advanc. Cancer Res.* **9**: 227, 1965.

19. BALNER, H. and DERSJANT, H. Increased oncogenic effect of methylcholanthrene after treatment with anti-lymphocyte serum. *Nature (Lond.)* **224**: 376, 1969.

20. JOHNSON, S. The effect of thymectomy and of the dose of 3-methylcholanthrene on the induction and antigenic properties of sarcomas in C57BL mice. *Brit. J. Cancer* **22**: 93, 1968.

21. BALDWIN, R. W. and GLAVES, D. Immunodepressive action of carcinogenic aminoazo dyes. *Ann. Rep. Brit. Emp. Cancer Campaign* **46**: 236, 1968.

THE INDUCTION OF PRECIPITATING ANTIBODIES TO THE MAMMARY TUMOR VIRUS IN SEVERAL INBRED MOUSE STRAINS

JO HILGERS, J. H. DAAMS and P. BENTVELZEN

MTV Research Unit, Antoni van Leeuwenhoekhuis, The Netherlands Cancer Institute, Amsterdam, and Radiobiological Institute TNO, Rijswijk (Z.H.), The Netherlands

ABSTRACT

After hyperimmunization with purified Bittner mammary tumor virus (MTV-S) preparations isolated from BALB/cfC3H mammary tumors, employing Freund's adjuvant, mice of strains C57BL, O20, BALB/c, GR, C3Hf, C3H, RIIIf, and RIII developed precipitating antibodies to several MTV-associated antigens, as detected by double immunodiffusion using a microtechnique. At least some sera from every mouse strain precipitated one or more of the following antigens: the complete virion, a soluble virus membrane antigen, and the internal antigen termed s_1. Polyvalent, highly absorbed rabbit antisera to purified MTV-S, gave reactions of identity with these three different mouse precipitation lines. The appearance of antibodies in C3H mice, which are neonatally infected with MTV-S may indicate that these animals are not fully tolerant to the virus. The appearance of antibodies in C3Hf and GR mice, which are hereditarily infected with other variants of MTV (MTV-L and MTV-P), might reflect a true breaking of tolerance to these MTV strains, as also suggested by the cross-reaction of these antibodies with purified MTV-P particles.

In the early stages of investigation on the mouse mammary tumor virus (MTV), the antigenicity of this agent to other species was clearly demonstrated (1–3). Until recently, however, it was seriously doubted whether MTV is antigenic to its host species, the mouse (4–6).

Nevertheless, already in 1945, Andervont (7) reported an indication that females of the resistant mouse strain I could passively immunize their offspring to the virus. Precipitating antibodies to MTV-associated antigens have now been demonstrated in mice by Blair et al. (8), Nowinski et al. (9) and Fink et al. (10), and the production of neutralizing mouse antibodies has also been described (11).

The aim of the present investigation was to study more systematically the production of antibodies to MTV in several mouse strains, with attention to the problem of tolerance and the nature of the antigens involved.

MATERIALS AND METHODS

Mice. The following highly inbred mouse strains were used: C57BL/LiA and O20/A, which do not carry a manifest MTV; C3Hf/A, which carries the low-oncogenic MTV-L; C3H/HeA, which carries the highly oncogenic MTV-S; RIII/SeA and GR/A which carry the lesser oncogenic

MTV-P; and BALB/c AnDeA, which proved to carry an unsuspected MTV, designated MTV-O (Daams, unpublished results). For the nomenclature of the various MTV-strains, see Bentvelzen and Daams (12).

Virus preparations. B particles, which represent the MTV virions (13, 14), were isolated and purified from BALB/cfC3H mammary tumors according to the technique of Calafat and Hageman (15). The virus stock contained approximately 1 mg wet wt of virus/1 ml of a buffer, consisting of 2 M McIlvaine's phosphate-citrate buffer + 0.61% NaCl + 0.04% bovine serum albumin (BSA). The virus was stored in ampoules of liquid nitrogen until use. A preparation of MTV-s_1, purified in Sephadex-G200 was kindly provided by Dr. R. C. Nowinski. Gross leukemia virus and an extract from strain SJL/J leukemia were a gift of Dr. L. J. Old.

Immunization. Adult mice, between two and five months of age, were injected i.p. with approximately 5 µg purified virus and emulsified in 0.1 ml of complete Freund's adjuvant + 0.4 ml phosphate buffered saline (PBS). One week later, the same amount of virus was injected, but now emulsified in incomplete Freund's adjuvant. Thereafter, virus without adjuvant was injected twice at weekly intervals. Every two to three months, the mice were given a booster injection of 20 µg of virus emulsified in complete Freund's adjuvant.

In a second group of adult female mice, the purified virus was disrupted with ether and the same amounts of virus were injected after disruption of the particles (2 mg B particles in 2 ml buffer were stirred for 1 hr at room temperature with 40 ml ether, with continuous aspiration of the evaporating ether through a Pasteur pipette connected to a waterpump).

Blood was taken by orbital puncture one to three weeks after each booster treatment; the sera were absorbed with approximately 1 mg BSA/ml for 1 hr at 37 C.

Immunodiffusion. Mouse sera were tested against stock solutions of B particles with the micro-Ouchterlony test of Wadsworth (16) and Crowle (17, 18), as applied to MTV by Fink et al. (10). The wells of plastic template, which was superimposed on a standard microscopic slide covered with a 0.2 mm thick layer of 0.75% agarose, could contain 30 µl of the reagents. The slides were incubated for 48 hr in a humidified box at 4 C. Thereafter, the templates were removed and the slides soaked for at least 1 hr in a cadmium-barbital buffer (250 mg cadmium-acetate in 1 liter barbital buffer, pH 8.4, LKB Stockholm, Cat. # 3276-VB). Each slide was photographed with a Polaroid CU 5 camera.

As a reference for the mouse sera, a highly absorbed rabbit antiserum to purified B particles (19) was used.

The virus was placed in the wells either complete or disrupted. Disruption for this purpose was achieved by either treatment with ether or by freezing and thawing three to six times.

RESULTS

Antibodies to complete MTV particles were detected in sera from immunized mice of every strain studied. As already described by Blair et al. (20, 21) and Daams (19), the corresponding precipitation line originates near the antigen well and is strongly curved towards this reservoir (Fig. 1).

It was found that the best way to produce this line is to use freshly isolated B particles, and to add 0.04% BSA to the agarose. If BSA is omitted, as in Fig. 1, some particles are disrupted during the diffusion process, and another line further away from the antigen well develops.

The line produced by mouse antibodies near the antigen well was seen to fuse with a similar line produced by rabbit antiserum (Fig. 2), which indicates that both sera con-

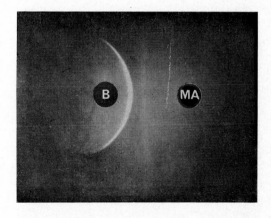

FIG. 1. Precipitation of B particles by mouse antiserum. B, freshly isolated B particles; MA, RIII mouse anti-MTV antiserum.

155

tain antibodies directed at the MTV particle. Mouse sera, which reacted with MTV-S virions also precipitated B particles isolated from GR strain mammary tumors (MTV-P), indicating that both MTV strains have antigenic determinants at their surface in common which can be detected by mouse antisera.

When the virus was completely disrupted by freezing and thawing six times, no preci-

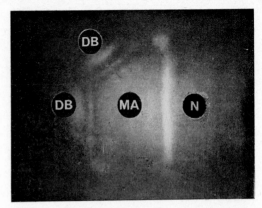

FIG. 4. Reaction of mouse anti-MTV antiserum with MTV nucleoids. MA, RIII-mouse strain anti-MTV antiserum; DB, dissociated B particles, thawed and frozen twice; N, nucleoids isolated from B particles.

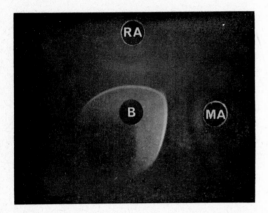

FIG. 2. Reaction of identity with mouse and rabbit anti-MTV antisera producing the virion precipitation line. B, freshly isolated B particles; RA, rabbit anti-MTV antiserum; MA, RIII mouse anti-MTV antiserum.

pitation line near the antigen well was formed, but another line was produced near the antiserum reservoir. Tests with rabbit antiserum indicated that this line represents a soluble membrane antigen (19). When the particles were treated somewhat more mildly, by freezing and thawing three times or by shaking with ether, some sera produced another line, which was almost straight and was located approximately halfway between the antigen and antiserum wells (as in Fig. 1). This line

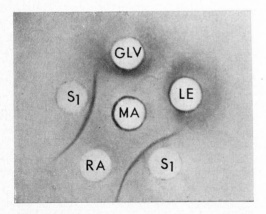

FIG. 3. Reaction of identity with mouse and rabbit anti-MTV antisera producing the s_1 precipitation line. MA, 020 mouse strain anti-MTV antiserum; RA, rabbit anti-MTV antiserum; s_1, MTV-s_1 purified on Sephadex; GLV, purified Gross leukemia virus; LE, SJL/J mouse leukemia extract.

TABLE 1. *Number of sera from different mouse strains[a] which detected MTV-antigens after the first booster with complete virus particles*

Strain	Number of sera tested	MTV-antigens[b]		
		P	NS	MS
C3H	3	0	0	0
C3Hf	4	4	0	0
GR	4	4	0	0
BALB/c	2	0	0	0
O20	3	2	0	1
C57BL	3	1	0	0
RIII	4	3	0	3

[a] Male animals were used.
[b] P (particle) = the virion and the assumed intact nucleoid; NS (nucleoid soluble) = the s_1 antigen and also the one often appearing near it; and MS (membrane soluble) = the soluble membrane antigen.

TABLE 2. *Number of sera from different mouse[a] strains which detected MTV-antigens after the second booster with complete virus particles*

| Strain | Sera obtained seven days after the second booster | | | Sera obtained 14 days after the second booster | | | Sera obtained 21 days after the second booster | | |
| | Number of sera tested | MTV-antigens | | Number of sera tested | MTV-antigens | | Number of sera tested | MTV-antigens | |
		NS	MS		NS	MS		NS	MS
C3H	3	0	1	3	0	1	2	0	1
C3Hf	4	0	0	4	0	0	4	1	0
GR	3	0	2	4	0	4	2	0	1
BALB/c	2	0	0	1	0	1	1	0	0
O20	3	0	1	3	0	1	3	0	1
C57BL	3	0	1	2	0	2	3	0	0
RIII	3	0	3	3	2[b]	3	3	2[b]	3

[a] Male animals were used.
[b] Two sera reacted with both NS and MS antigens.

represents the MTV-s_1 antigen (9, 22) because it is identical with the line produced by purified s_1 antigen from Dr. Nowinski. It also fused with a similar line produced by a rabbit anti-MTV antiserum. There was no reaction with Gross leukemia virus nor with an extract from mouse strain SJL/J leukemia (Fig. 3). Sometimes two lines appeared at the site of the s_1 line; it has not been established whether two different antigens are responsible for these lines, as in the case of rabbit anti-MTV antiserum (19).

Nucleoids isolated from B particles by Dr. Hageman according to the technique of Calafat and Hageman (23) produced a particularly strong s_1 line with a RIII-strain anti-MTV-antiserum (Fig. 4). It has been found, sporadically, that if B particles, which are not freshly isolated, are used in Ouchterlony tests, another precipitation line is produced near the antigen well, less curved towards this well than the fresh virion line. It is assumed that this line represents the intact nucleoid of the virus.

Tables 1 and 2 present the number of sera of the different mouse strains which detected the various MTV antigens. The results with sera taken 21 days after the first booster with complete particles are presented in Table 1.

Only sera from C3H and BALB/c gave no reaction at all. Most of the other sera reacted only with P antigens, presumably the virion. The RIII sera gave the strongest reactions with the P antigen and, except for one O20 serum, they were the only ones which reacted with the MS antigen of the disrupted virus.

Table 2 shows the results with sera taken seven, 14 and 21 days after the second booster with complete virions; these sera were not tested against complete virus particles. It appears that the best results were obtained with sera taken 14 days after boosting. After this second booster a positive reaction was found in all mouse strains studied. After a third and

TABLE 3. *Number of sera from different mouse[a] strains which detected MTV-antigens after immunization with ether-treated virus particles*

| Strain | Number of sera tested | MTV-antigens | |
		NS	MS
C3H	4	2	2
C3Hf	3	1	3
GR	4	2	0
BALB/c	4	3	1
C57Bl	3	3	0
RIIIf	3	3	1

[a] Female animals were used.

fourth booster, each mouse strain gave many positive reactions, and C3H and BALB/c mice showed positive reactions also with complete virions.

Table 3 shows the results with sera taken from mice immunized with ether-treated MTV. These animals were not boosted. In contrast to the experiment with whole virus, these mice reacted without a booster stimulation. The fact that in this experiment females were used might offer an explanation for this difference. It is noted that in this experiment most sera reacted with the NS antigens, whereas when whole virus was employed, only RIII sera gave this reaction.

DISCUSSION

Blair et al. (8, 21) observed the production of antibodies to the whole MTV virion in immunized C3H, C3Hf, BALB/c, and I mice. Nowinski et al. (9) detected antibodies to the s_1 antigen in sera of hyperimmunized I strain mice. Fink et al. (10) reported the induction of precipitating antibodies to two MTV-associated antigens in BALB/c and C3Hf animals; they did not discuss the nature of the antigens detected by their sera. From our data, it becomes obvious that at least some mice of all strains tested so far can produce antibodies to one or more of the following: the whole virus particle, the s_1 antigen, a membrane antigen, and some other MTV-specific antigens. This finding demonstrates the immunogenicity of MTV in its host species, the mouse.

Until now, spur formation could not be observed in fusion experiments with mouse vs. rabbit anti-MTV sera. This might well indicate that the antibodies in both groups of sera were directed against the same antigenic determinants of the various antigens.

Our mouse antisera here produced five lines with MTV, while rabbit antisera may produce up to seven (19). It could be that further boosting is needed, especially of the mice immunized with disrupted virus, to increase the

number of lines. Another possibility is that mice are tolerant to some group-specific MTV antigens, which can however be detected by heterologous antisera. The latter situation, existing in the case of some other RNA oncogenic viruses, is a basic aspect of the theory of Huebner and Todaro (24) on genetically transmitted C-type RNA tumor viruses. There is considerable evidence that B-type RNA tumor viruses (MTV) are genetically transmitted (12, 25–28).

Our results with C3H-strain sera confirm the earlier finding of Blair et al. (8), that despite neonatal infection with MTV-S, antibodies may be produced after challenge with the same virus. On the basis of mammary tumor transplantation experiments, Morton and associates (29–31) concluded that neonatally infected mice are truly tolerant to MTV. However, Bentvelzen et al. (32) found precipitating antibodies to MTV in mammary tumor bearing C3H mice. They also found that inoculation of MTV-S together with complete Freund's adjuvant into neonatally infected mice leads to an enhancement of mammary tumor development. This suggests the existence of some "underground" immunity to MTV (32, 33) both at the cellular and the humoral level in these mice.

Heppner (34) found that sera from one neonatally infected mouse could abrogate to some extent the cytotoxic effect of lymphocytes of another mouse towards mammary tumor cells, as detected by the colony-inhibition test. Although Heppner pays more attention to the much stronger immune reactions to noncross-reacting antigens of mammary tumors, her findings again indicate the existence of both cellular and humoral immunity to a cross-reacting antigen, most likely MTV.

Yunis et al. (35) found that an injection of adult C3H spleen cells into neonatally thymectomized C3H mice can elicit considerable resistance to mammary tumor development, as compared to injection of C3Hf spleen cells or of thymus cells of both strains. This can be explained by the transfer of adoptive immunity to MTV by C3H spleen cells. It is interesting that in C3H mice we here observed not only immunity to the virion, as might be expected on the basis of the findings mentioned above, but also to inner components of the virus, such as s_1.

In the GR strain, another variant of MTV (MTV-P) is transmitted before birth to the offspring either by the male (27) or through the ovum (36). This mode of transmission, which is different from the milk transmission in the C3H strain, is highly dependent upon the host genome (25–27). It has been assumed, therefore, that MTV-P is transmitted for all practical effects as a genetical factor of the GR host, as has been postulated for the Gross leukemia virus in AKR mice (24, 37, 38), and such prenatal infection might lead to true tolerance. So far no sign of immunity to MTV-P has been observed in GR mice (32), but the tolerance-postulate has not yet been rigorously tested by a hyperimmunization scheme, as was done for MTV-S in this study. GR mice rapidly produce antibodies to MTV-S, which also react with MTV-P. It is suggested, accordingly, that immunization with MTV-S may lead to a break in tolerance to MTV-P; it has also been observed that inoculations of MTV-S into GR mice can bring about significant delay in mammary tumor development, which may well be immunological in nature (32, 33).

We are much indebted to Miss Margreet Ojemann and Dr. Theodora Ionescu for valuable technical assistance; to Dr. Philomena Hageman for providing purified B particles and for highly stimulating discussions; and to Professor O. Mühlbock and Dr. Ph. Rümke for their great interest.

REFERENCES

1. ANDERVONT, H. B. and BRYAN, W. R. Properties of the mouse mammary tumor agent. *J. nat. Cancer Inst.* **5**: 143, 1944.
2. GREEN, R. G., MOOSEY, M. M. and BITTNER, J. J. Antigenic character of the cancer milk agent in mice. *Proc. Soc. exp. Biol.* (*N.Y.*) **61**: 115, 1946.
3. BITTNER, J. J. and IMAGAWA, D. T. Effect of the source of the mouse mammary tumor agent (MTA) upon neutralization of the agent with antisera. *Cancer Res.* **15**: 464, 1955.
4. BITTNER, J. J. Biologic assay and serial passage of the mouse mammary tumor agent in mammary tumors from mothers and their hybrid progeny, in: Ciba Foundation Symposium "Tumor viruses of murine origin." Boston, Little, Brown and Co., 1962, p. 55.
5. SQUARTINI, F. Tumours arising from vertical transmission, in: Handbook of Experimental Pharmacology XVI/13. Berlin, Springer Verlag, 1966, p. 1.
6. ANDREWES, C. and PEREIRA, H. G. "Viruses of Vertebrates." London, Baillière, Tindall and Cassell, 1967, p. 139.
7. ANDERVONT, H. B. Susceptibility of young and adult mice to the mammary tumor agent. *J. nat. Cancer Inst.* **5**: 397, 1945.
8. BLAIR, P. B., LAVRIN, D. H., DEZFULIAN, M. and WEISS, D. W. Immunology of the mouse mammary tumor virus (MTV): Identification in vitro of mouse antibodies against MTV. *Cancer Res.* **26**: 647, 1966.
9. NOWINSKI, R. C., OLD, L. J., MOORE, D. H., GEERING, G. and BOYSE, E. A. A soluble antigen of the mammary tumor virus. *Virology* **31**: 1, 1967.
10. FINK, M. A., FELLER, W. F. and SIBAL, L. R. Methods for detection of antibody to the mammary tumor virus. *J. nat. Cancer Inst.* **41**: 1395, 1968.
11. BLAIR, P. B. Immunology of the mouse mammary tumor virus (MTV): Neutralization of MTV by mouse antiserum. *Cancer Res.* **28**: 148, 1968.
12. BENTVELZEN, P. and DAAMS, J. H. Hereditary infections with mammary tumor viruses in mice. *J. nat. Cancer Inst.* **43**: 1025, 1969.
13. BERNHARD, W. Electron microscopy of tumor cells and tumor viruses: A review. *Cancer Res.* **18**: 491, 1958.
14. HAGEMAN, P. C., LINKS, J. and BENTVELZEN, P. Biological properties of B particles from C3H and C3Hf mouse milk. *J. nat. Cancer Inst.* **40**: 1319, 1968.
15. CALAFAT, J. and HAGEMAN, P. Some remarks on the morphology of B particles and their isolation from mammary tumors. *Virology* **36**: 308, 1968.
16. WADSWORTH, C. A slide microtechnique for the analysis of immune precipitates in gel. *Int. Arch. Allergy* **10**: 355, 1957.
17. CROWLE, A. J. A simplified micro double-diffusion agar precipitin technique. *J. Lab. clin. Med.* **52**: 784, 1958.
18. CROWLE, A. J. Enhancement by various cations of the double-diffusion precipitin test. *Int. Arch. Allergy* **16**: 113, 1960.
19. DAAMS, J. H. Immunofluorescence studies on the biology of the mouse mammary tumor virus, in: Severi, L. (Ed.), "Immunity and tolerance ino ncogenesis," *IV Peungia Quadrienuial Int. Conf.,* 1969 (in press).
20. BLAIR, P. B., WEISS, D. W. and PITELKA, D. R. Immunology of the mouse mammary tumor

virus (MTV): Correlation of the immunodiffusion precipitate line with the type B virus particles. *J. nat. Cancer Inst.* **37**: 261, 1966.

21. Blair, P. B., Smoller, C., Bonhag, R. S. and Weiss, D. W. Immunology of the mouse mammary tumor virus (MTV): Electron microscopic studies of interaction between MTV and specific antibody in immunodiffusion. *J. nat. Cancer Inst.* **40**: 1325, 1968.

22. Nowinski, R. C., Old, L. J., Boyse, E. A., de Harven, E. and Geering, G. Group specific viral antigens in the milk and tissues of mice naturally infected with mammary tumor virus or Gross leukemia virus. *Virology* **34**: 617, 1968.

23. Calafat, J. and Hageman, P. The structure of the mammary tumor virus. *Virology* **38**: 364, 1969.

24. Huebner, R. J. and Todaro, G. Oncogenes of RNA oncogenic viruses as determinants of cancer. *Proc. nat. Acad. Sci.* (*Wash.*) **64**: 1087, 1969.

25. Bentvelzen, P., Timmermans, A., Daams, J. H. and Gugten, A. van der. Genetic transmission of mammary tumor viruses in mice: possible implications for murine leukemia. *Bibl. haemat.* **31**: 101, 1968.

26. Bentvelzen, P. "Genetical control of the vertical transmission of the Mühlbock mammary tumor virus in the GR mouse strain." Amsterdam, Hollandia, 1968.

27. Mühlbock, O. and Bentvelzen, P. The transmission of the mammary tumor viruses, in: Pollard, M. (Ed.), "Perspectives in virology." New York, Academic Press, 1967, v. 6, p. 75.

28. Daams, J. H., Timmermans, A., Gugten, A. van der, and Bentvelzen, P. Genetical resistance of mouse strain C57Bl to mammary tumor viruses. II. Resistance by means of a repressed, related provirus. *Genetica* **38**: 400, 1968.

29. Morton, D. L. Acquired immunological tolerance to spontaneous mammary adenocarcinomas following neonatal infection with mammary tumor agent (MTA). *Proc. Amer. Ass. Cancer Res.* **5**: 46, 1965.

30. Morton, D. L. Acquired immunological tolerance and carcinogenesis by the mammary tumor virus. I. Influence of neonatal infection with the mammary tumor virus on the growth of spontaneous mammary adenocarcinomas. *J. nat. Cancer Inst.* **42**: 311, 1969.

31. Morton, D. L., Goldman, L. and Wood, D. A. Acquired immunological tolerance and carcinogenesis by the mammary tumor virus. II. Immune responses influencing growth of spontaneous mammary adenocarcinomas. *J. nat. Cancer Inst.* **42**: 321, 1969.

32. Bentvelzen, P., Gugten, A. van der, Hilgers, J. and Daams, J. H. Breakthrough in tolerance to eggborne mammary tumor viruses, in: Severi, L. (Ed.), "Immunity and tolerance in oncogenesis," *IV Penugia Quadniennial Int. Conf. 1969.* 1970, p. 525.

33. Gugten, A. van der and Bentvelzen, P. Interference between two strains of the mouse mammary tumor virus in the GR mouse strain. *Europ. J. Cancer* **5**: 361, 1969.

34. Heppner, G. H. Studies in serum-mediated inhibition of cellular immunity to spontaneous mouse mammary tumors. *Int. J. Cancer* **4**: 608, 1969.

35. Yunis, E. J., Martinez, C., Smith, J., Stutman, O. and Good, R. A. Spontaneous mammary adenocarcinoma in mice: Influence of thymectomy and reconstitution with thymus grafts or spleen cells. *Cancer Res.* **29**: 174, 1969.

36. Zeilmaker, G. H. Transmission of mammary tumor virus by female GR mice: Results of egg transplantation. *Int. J. Cancer* **4**: 261, 1969.

37. Gross, L. "Oncogenic viruses." New York, Pergamon Press, 1961.

38. Law, L. W. Transmission studies of a leukemogenic virus, MLV, in mice. *Nat. Cancer Inst. Monogr.* **22**: 267, 1966.

IMMUNOLOGICAL ASPECTS OF THE RELATIONSHIP BETWEEN HOST AND ONCOGENIC VIRUS IN THE MOUSE MAMMARY TUMOR SYSTEM

PHYLLIS B. BLAIR

Department of Bacteriology and Immunology, and Cancer Research Genetics Laboratory, University of California, Berkeley, California, USA

ABSTRACT

There is conclusive evidence that the mouse can respond immunologically to the antigens of the mammary tumor virus (MTV), both those of the virion itself and those expressed on the cells that the virus infects. However, the neonatally infected mouse is essentially tolerant to these viral antigens. Specific antibody production and cell associated immune reactions can sometimes be induced in MTV-infected mice by immunization with MTV antigens, but the presence of any immunologic reactivity against MTV in the normal neonatally infected mouse has been difficult to demonstrate. The literature substantiating these conclusions is reviewed.

INTRODUCTION

In the mouse, tumors of the mammary gland frequently occur as the result of infection with an oncogenic virus, the mouse mammary tumor virus (MTV). The MTV shares many morphological and biologic characteristics with viruses of the avian leukosis complex, including the Rous sarcoma virus, and the mouse leukemia viruses; together, these agents form the important group of myxovirus-like RNA-containing oncogenic viruses.

The induction of mammary tumors by MTV provides an ideal model for the study of virus-host interaction in neoplasia. In contrast to many viruses studied in the laboratory, MTV occurs naturally in the experimental animal population, and the role of the investigator is limited to the selection of animals for breeding. Infection of the young occurs naturally (usually through the milk), and leads, in selected strains of mice, to high tumor incidence.

An extensive literature, dating from the early decades of this century, deals with the many influences involved in the final production of a mammary tumor in an MTV-infected female mouse. This literature has been reviewed by several authors (1–6). Within the past decade, the immunologic response of the mouse to MTV and to MTV-induced mammary tumors has been intensively investigated; these investigations are the subject of this review. Emphasis has been placed on immunologic studies carried out in the past several years; a general discussion of earlier studies in this area can be found in the 1968 review by Blair (6).

Expression of MTV-associated antigens on

161

mammary tumor cells. Principally as a result of the extensive studies of Weiss and his associates (7–11), and of Morton and his colleagues (12, 13), it is now well recognized that the prevalent antigenicity expressed in MTV-induced mammary tumors is derived from antigens associated with the presence of the virus in these tumor cells. Such studies not only demonstrated conclusively the presence of such antigenicity but also have demonstrated that it is already expressed in the preneoplastic lesions of the mammary gland (the hyperplastic alveolar nodules) and in normal mammary parenchyma (7–9).

This MTV-associated antigenicity is, as expected, cross-reactive between tumors induced by the same virus (9, 12). The experiments so far published provide little information on whether the detected antigen or antigens are components of the mature virus, expressed as the virion buds through the cell surface, or are antigens induced in the mammary cells as a result of the viral infection, since most of them have involved immunization with tissues or extracts which contained viable MTV. Thus, it is possible that infection of host cells occurred, and the resulting immune response was directed against antigens induced as a result of the infection. Nevertheless, mature virus is present in the mammary tumor cells, and it is theoretically possible that an immunologic response directed only against virion antigens could result in destruction of the tumor cell population. Some positive evidence for this has been obtained in recent experiments. Protection against implants of mammary tumors was elicited by immunization with formalin-treated (and probably inactivated) preparations of purified MTV virions (14). Immunization with MTV preparations inactivated with either formalin or H_2O_2 were effective in causing a delay in the spontaneous development of mammary tumors in mice neonatally infected with MTV, presumably because of an immune response

developing against virion antigens (15).

Further experimentation will be necessary to determine if the MTV-associated antigens expressed on mammary tumor cells represent solely antigens of the virion, solely new cellular antigens induced by the virus, or a mixture of both. Extraction and characterization of these antigens is being undertaken; Nishioka and his collaborators have reported an extensive series of experiments dealing with the characteristics of a mammary tumor cell surface antigen which can be detected by hyperimmune C3H mouse serum (16, 17). The tumor antigen could be extracted from the cells with 0.2% deoxycholate, and, in a number of tests, these authors note that there is considerable similarity between the tumor antigen and the mouse histocompatibility antigens, from the point of view of chemical properties and of cellular localization.

Expression of tumor-specific antigens on mammary tumor cells. There is clear evidence that at least some mammary tumors possess, in addition to MTV-associated antigenicity, a characteristic antigenicity which does not cross-react with that found in other mammary tumors (and thus presumably is not MTV-associated), but which is similar to the tumor-specific antigenicity usually associated with tumors induced by the chemical carcinogens. Three independent observations of this type of antigenicity have now been reported (18–22).

There has been speculation (23, 24) that the tumor-specific antigens in these tumors may represent the re-expression of embryonic antigens, as has been demonstrated in other tumor systems. An attempt to demonstrate this in BALB/cfC3H females was essentially negative. Females were immunized with embryonic tissues or tissue extracts and then observed for the spontaneous development of tumors; essentially no differences were observed between the control and the experimental groups (24). It is to be noted, however, that these negative results do not preclude the possibility that more rigorous immunization procedures, or the use of the response to iso-grafts instead of spontaneous tumor devel-opment as a measure of host response, might produce positive results.

Weiss (23) has suggested that some of these tumor-specific antigens may be organ-specific antigens. Normally, the mouse is tolerant to such antigens, but if they are sequestered from the immunological recognition mechanisms by the partially privileged nature of the mam-mary fat pad (25), they might well function as tumor-specific antigens after immunization and challenge.

CELL-ASSOCIATED IMMUNITY

Attempts to immunize mice against challenge implants of MTV-infected mammary tumors, or to prevent the spontaneous development of these tumors by various immunization procedures have been carried out throughout this century, in some cases with success, in other cases without (for review of the early literature, see ref. 6).

Since the prevalent antigenicity expressed in MTV-induced mammary tumors is derived from antigens associated with the presence of the virus in the tumor cells, the most dramatic demonstrations of mammary tumor antigenicity are found in experimental situa-tions in which mice not previously exposed to the virus (and not neonatally tolerant to it) are immunized with viral or tumor-cell anti-gens and then challenged with isografts of MTV-infected mammary tumors. Experi-ments of this type have been carried out by a number of workers (7–9, 12, 26–28). A con-siderable host response to MTV-associated antigens in tumor cells can also be demon-strated frequently on primary exposure of MTV-free mice to isogenic MTV-infected mammary tumor tissue (9, 13, 29, 30) or to leukemias possessing MTV-associated anti-genicity (31).

Mice free of MTV can usually be immu-nized readily against MTV-associated antigens, and are thereafter either less susceptible to, or completely resistant against, challenge im-plants of MTV-infected mammary tumor tissue. A number of tissues and immunization procedures have been used by different in-vestigators, such as multiple injections of extracts of lactating mammary gland tissue (12, 27) or MTV virion preparations (14), or pretreatment with an implant of MTV-infect-ed mammary tissue (7–9).

There are also a number of reports in the literature describing the immunogenicity of MTV-positive mammary tumors in isogenic MTV-infected hosts. This immunogenicity may be expressed in test mice by resistance to challenge tumor implants (32–35), by en-hancement of tumor growth after immuniza-tion (36), and sometimes by both (37–40). Some success has also been reported in de-creasing the incidence of spontaneous mam-mary tumors by immunization (41), although immunization procedures may also enhance the development of such neoplasms (42). It also has been possible to alter the growth of tumors already developed in the autochtho-nous host (11, 43). In most cases, it is not possible to determine if these experiments are detecting the presence of tumor-specific anti-gens or if the tolerance to MTV antigens usually found in MTV-infected mice was either incomplete or broken by the immuniza-tion procedures employed.

Adoptive transfer of immunity to MTV-induced mammary tumors. Resistance to mam-mary tumor growth has successfully been transferred from an immunized host to a normal recipient in a number of experiments (12, 14, 26, 31, 44).

Müller (44) reported that spleen or lymph node cells from MTV-infected mice could, when inoculated into normal recipients, affect the growth of subsequent challenge implants of the tumor. In some experiments, tumor inhibition resulted and in others acceleration of tumor growth occurred; an important variable was the time interval between inoculation of the sensitizing tumors into the donors and the harvesting of the lymphoid cells. Serum from these sensitized donors also affected the growth of challenge tumor inocula in recipient mice, as will be described in the next section.

Burton et al. (14) reported that peritoneal cells from BALB/c mice which had been immunized by four i.p. inoculations of purified MTV virions (either intact or treated with formalin) could inhibit the growth of MTV-infected BALB/cfC3H mammary tumor cells if incubated with the tumor cell suspension in vitro prior to inoculation into a normal BALB/c host. Morton and his associates (12) reported that spleen cells from immune MTV-free mice could cause, when transferred to a normal recipient, the rejection of a subsequent implant of mammary tumor tissue. Spleen cells from normal MTV-free mice, similarly transferred, could also either completely or partially inhibit the growth of challenge mammary tumor implants. In contrast, spleen cells from MTV-infected mice did not inhibit the growth of the challenge implants in the recipients.

In an experiment carried out by Nowinski and associates (31), an MTV-infected BALB/cfDBA mammary tumor was mixed with peritoneal cells and inoculated into normal BALB/c females. If the peritoneal cells were obtained from mice that had been immunized by inoculation of a leukemia possessing ML antigenicity, the development of the mammary tumor transplants was considerably delayed over that observed in control animals, in which the tumor cells were mixed with peritoneal cells obtained from mice immunized with a leukemia not possessing antigenicity cross-reactive with MTV.

In vitro *demonstration of cell-associated immunity*. Heppner and Pierce (18) demon-strated, using the colony inhibition technique developed by the Hellströms (45), that lymph node cells taken from animals bearing autochthonous MTV-induced mammary tumors could react in vitro against cells of that tumor. They also immunized MTV-free BALB/c females by the s.c. implantation of BALB/cfC3H mammary tumor cells (followed by excision of the resulting tumor); lymph node cells from these animals were reactive in vitro against the tumor used for immunization in 12 of 13 experiments. The specificity of the response was demonstrated by control experiments, in which six of seven tests utilizing lymph node cells from the immunized BALB/c females gave no evidence of inhibition in tests with methylcholanthrene-induced sarcomas.

Heppner and Pierce (18), and later Heppner (19) observed, as might be predicted from the in vivo experiments in MTV-infected mice, that such animals bearing autochthonous tumors apparently produced a cell-associated immune response directed against non-cross-reacting, tumor-specific antigens, rather than a response against cross-reacting, MTV-associated antigens; although lymph node cells from most of the autochthonous mice tested were capable of inhibiting colony formation of the autochthonous tumor cells in vitro, none of them were capable of reacting against another isogenic MTV-induced mammary tumor. Similarly, if mice neonatally infected with MTV were immunized with one of the mammary tumors, the lymph node cells from these animals could inhibit colony formation by cells of that tumor, but not by cells of another tumor. If, however, the lymphocyte donors were immunized BALB/c females not previously exposed to MTV, the lymphocytes were capable of inhibiting the colony formation not only of cells of the immunizing tumor but also of cells of other mammary tumors. We would predict this on the basis of the previously reported in vivo experiments, most of which utilized mice of the C3H strain and its hybrids. However, an unexpected observation was the fact that although an immune response to cross-reacting tumor antigens (presumably MTV-associated) was detected in some of the immunized BALB/c females, it was not detected in all of them. Heppner and Pierce reported, for example, that lymph node cells from immunized BALB/c mice were reactive against the tumor used for immunization in 12 of 13 experiments, but, when these lymph node cells were tested against another mammary tumor, significant inhibition of the tumor cells was demonstrated in only seven of the 13 experiments. These results suggest that the expression of MTV antigens in tumor tissue may be influenced by the host genotype.

HUMORAL IMMUNE RESPONSE

Production of humoral antibodies against MTV virions. Early attempts to detect an immunological reaction of the mouse against MTV virions were negative (for review, see ref. 6). Within the past decade, however, the ability of the mouse to produce antibodies capable of precipitating (46) or neutralizing (47) the MTV virion have been reported, and these results have been amply confirmed (14, 48–50). Mouse antibodies were first detected in some of the sera obtained from C3H and C3Hf mice immunized with extracts or implants of MTV-containing tissue, or challenged with isogenic MTV-containing mammary tumor tissue, or both (46), but they have since been found in mice immunized by a variety of procedures.

The antisera of the immunized C3H and C3Hf mice described above reacted in immunodiffusion with the antigens of the MTV virion coat, and precipitated the virion (46). Immunized mice can also react against the soluble MTV antigenicity which is present in MTV infected milk samples and which can be released from MTV virions by treatment with ether; this MTV-associated soluble antigenicity was first identified by Lezhneva (51)

and later characterized by Nowinski and associates (48).

Nowinski et al. (48) produced mouse antisera against MTV antigens by immunizing mice with transplants of mammary tumor tissue of ML + leukemias. Hybrid (BALB/c × DBA/2) mice were immunized with a histocompatible, transplanted DBA/2 leukemia known to possess ML antigenicity, and mice of the I strain were immunized by the implantation of histoincompatible MTV-infected DBA/2 mammary tumor tissue; sera from both groups of mice reacted in immunodiffusion with MTV soluble antigen released by ether treatment from an MTV virion preparation. Both of these mouse antisera gave reactions of identity with rabbit anti-MTV serum in immunodiffusion tests with mammary tumor extracts.

To produce mouse antisera reactive against MTV, Fink and her associates (49) used immunization procedures that had been successfully applied to the production of antibodies against various mouse leukemia antigens. Purified virus was emulsified in complete Freund's adjuvant and inoculated i.p. into MTV-free BALB/c or C3H/fB mice. At least 28 days later a single booster injection without adjuvant was inoculated s.c. Sera from both groups of mice reacted positively with MTV in immunodiffusion, detecting more than one antigen. The MTV virions used as antigen in the immunodiffusion tests were pretreated with tween-ether; thus, at least one of the antigens detected was probably MTV soluble antigen. The C3H/fB serum was also tested in the hemagglutination assay for MTV developed by this group (52); it was positive to a titer of 1:8. The serum could also neutralize MTV bioactivity, as demonstrated by use of the nodulogenic assay for MTV developed by Nandi (53).

Mouse antibodies against MTV can also be produced by a series of i.p. injections, given either with or without adjuvant. Burton et al.

(14) reported that adult BALB/c mice given partially purified preparations of MTV virions on days 1, 4, 8 and 22 produced antibodies against the MTV virion which could be detected in serum collected on day 29; the sera were tested in immunodiffusion. Similarly, serum from strain I mice immunized by four i.p. injections of MTV virions contained antibodies which reacted in immunodiffusion with the agent and also neutralized its biologic activity (47). Variations of this protocol have been used routinely to produce antibodies against MTV in adult males and females of the I strain, adult BALB/c females, and adult hybrid females resulting from the mating of C57BL females with either BALB/c or I males. Antibodies have been produced in these mice using MTV partially purified by differential centrifugation from tumor extracts, or by sucrose density gradient centrifugation from milk. In most experiments, at least four injections of antigen have been necessary before antibodies could be detected in immunodiffusion (Blair, unpublished observations). In addition, antibodies have been evoked in BALB/c females by the inoculation of irradiated isogenic MTV-infected mammary tumor cells.

Bentvelzen and associates (50) recently summarized their findings from an extensive series of experiments searching for antibodies against MTV in mice of various strains; they used an immunodiffusion procedure for testing the sera, reacting the sera against MTV virions. A series of seven injections of MTV, most of them including complete Freund's adjuvant, were used for immunization. Antisera were successfully produced in mice of the C3Hf, C3H, RIII, C57BL, 020, BALB/c and GR strains. The Dutch workers note (54) that it is easiest to produce antibodies in mice of the C57BL strain, which is also the strain most resistant to infection with MTV.

Bentvelzen and associates (50) also report that the antibodies produced in the various strains of mice examined will react with MTV virions from a variety of sources and possessing widely differing oncogenic potential and biologic activity; these results are in agreement with those of Blair (55) who has found, using rabbit antisera, that antigenic similarity exists between the virions of all sources of MTV tested. It was also noted by the Bentvelzen group that it was possible to induce in mice of the RIII strain antibodies to the MTV soluble antigen characterized by Nowinski and associates (48).

Although antibodies against MTV can be evoked even in mice neonatally infected with the virus by various immunization procedures, including the implantation of isogenic MTV-infected mammary tumor tissue, the first attempts to detect antibodies against MTV in normal mice in which mammary tumors develop spontaneously with high frequency were unsuccessful. Attempts have been made to detect such antibodies in immunodiffusion (46), and by reaction of ferritin-conjugated serum with MTV-infected tumor cells (56). Bentvelzen and his colleagues (50) have now reported that antibodies which precipitate the virion in immunodiffusion could be detected in the sera of eight of 24 mammary-tumor-bearing C3H mice. They postulate that since, as shown by Moore (57), many virions are found in the blood of tumor-bearing mice, this release of virus can be regarded as a booster injection, leading to antibody production. On the other hand, these authors also report that antibodies could not be found in the sera of any of 65 normal C3H mice that were tested. In addition, there are obvious strain differences in immunological reactivity to MTV; although these workers were able to detect antibodies in the sera of C3H tumor-bearing mice, they were unable to find similar antibodies in any of 125 mammary-tumor-bearing GR animals.

Production of humoral antibodies against MTV-infected cells. The mouse is also fully capable of producing antibodies which react with MTV-associated antigens expressed on the surface of tumor cells.

Humoral antibodies are readily produced in immunized MTV-free mice; they have been detected in cytotoxicity tests (58), in the antiglobulin consumption test (59), and by the colony inhibition technique (19).

Stuck and associates (58) reported that several DBA leukemias contained an antigen (designated ML) which cross-reacts with an antigen in MTV-infected mammary tissue (possible MTV itself); this antigen could be demonstrated in cytotoxic tests utilizing mouse antisera. C57BL mice were immunized against histoincompatible leukemias of DBA/2 mice; after appropriate absorption with normal DBA tissues, the resulting antisera were found to contain antibodies against the leukemic cells which could be absorbed by MTV-containing tissues but not by the appropriate controls. Workers from this laboratory have suggested that the DBA/2 strain may contain a leukemogenic variant of MTV (31) which is responsible for the detected antigenicity.

Another *in vitro* test which has been used for the detection of mouse antibodies against MTV-infected mammary tumor cells is the antiglobulin consumption test, adapted to the mammary tumor system by Holmes and Morton (59). This test is based on the same principle as complement fixation, but instead of utilizing complement as an indication of antigen-antibody reaction, the indicator used is antiserum against mouse globulin. The antimouse globulin is added to a tumor cell suspension which has been mixed with the test antiserum and then washed. If mouse antiserum has bound to the tumor cells, the antimouse globulin will then be bound to it; its loss from the supernatant fluid is then measured in a second reaction involving sensitized red blood cells. Using this test, Holmes and Morton found that MTV-free C3Hf mice

produced humoral antibodies against MTV-associated antigens on mammary tumor cells after immunization with histoincompatible MTV-induced mammary tumors.

Other workers have demonstrated that production of humoral antibodies against cellular antigens is not limited to the MTV-free mouse; the MTV-infected mouse can also produce antibodies reactive against MTV-infected mammary tumor cells, and, further, the antigenicity detected may also be cross-reacting.

The indirect fluorescent antibody technique has been used by Müller (44) to demonstrate antibodies against MTV-induced CBA mammary tumor cells in MTV-infected CBA mice inoculated with mammary tumor cell suspensions. The antisera detected a surface antigen on the tumor cells. The antigenicity detected cross-reacted with other CBA mammary tumors; these tumors were capable of absorbing out the reactive antibodies. Sera from both mice with progressively growing tumors and mice injected with killed tumor cells contained such antibodies.

In a series of papers published in 1969, Nishioka and his associates demonstrated that C3H mice hyperimmunized with cell suspensions from a transplanted C3H mammary tumor produced serum antibodies which could be detected by cytotoxic tests carried out *in vivo* (60) and *in vitro* (61) and by an immune adherence test using human erythrocytes as the marker (16). The antigenicity detected was cross-reacting; the serum reacted not only with the inducing neoplasm in cytotoxicity tests, but also with a series of spontaneous C3H mammary tumors, a mammary tumor of the A strain (also MTV-infected), and the Ehrlich ascites tumor, a mammary tumor maintained in ascitic form in ddD mice. The serum did not react with unrelated tumors, such as a mouse hepatoma and sarcoma 180. The authors feel that there is a good association of the detected antigen with

167

the presence of MTV. However, they also reported that the serum did not react in cytotoxicity tests with presumably normal mammary cells obtained from pregnant MTV-infected C3H mice. Thus, the antigen appears to be mainly, if not entirely, associated with MTV-infected mammary neoplastic cells.

In the immune adherence test, which these workers used extensively in their studies (16), antigen present on the surface of the tumor cell was seen to react with specific antibody in the presence of complement to form an antigen-antibody-complement complex which will result in the adherence of the indicator human red blood cells to the tumor cell surface. The test is especially useful because it can be used to detect surface antigenicity on nonliving cells, and thus the Nishioka group has been able to investigate the nature of the antigen in extraction and solubility studies.

Effect of humoral antibodies on tumor development and growth. In a number of experiments, it has been demonstrated that serum antibodies produced by the immunized mouse can affect the survival of tumor isografts (27, 37, 44, 60) and it is suspected that they may influence the development of spontaneous tumors (42, 50).

Attia and Weiss (37) reported that large quantities of sera from immunized MTV-infected strain A mice produced enhancement of tumor isografts in normal isogenic animals; tumor implants placed in the normal recipients 6 hr after the inoculation of the enhancing serum grew more rapidly than did similar implants in mice pretreated with control serum. Dezfulian et al. (27) reported that BALB/c mice immunized with three i.p. injections of BALB/cfC3H milk possess a serum factor, presumably enhancing antibody, which, when administered to normal BALB/c females a few hours prior to the injection of a challenge inoculum of BALB/cfC3H mammary tumor cells, resulted in the increased growth of the cells as compared to that which occurred in females given serum from donors immunized with MTV-free BALB/c milk.

Müller (44) found that the sera of immunized CBA mice (which reacted with tumor cells in the indirect fluorescent antibody test) also caused either growth enhancement or growth inhibition when injected into test mice together with challenge tumor cells. Interestingly, the specific inhibitory effect of the serum could be abolished by prior absorption with mammary tumor cells, but the enhancing activity could be suppressed by absorption either with tumor cells or with normal liver, spleen or kidney cells. The effect of the serum (enhancement or inhibition) varied with the time after immunization at which the serum was collected.

Nishioka and associates (60) demonstrated that the sera from hyperimmune C3H mice, which was shown to be reactive against mammary tumor cells in the *in vitro* cytotoxicity and immune adherence tests, could also inhibit the growth of mammary tumor cells when the cells were mixed *in vitro* with the serum and then injected i.p. into C3H test animals. Control serum taken from normal or tumor-bearing C3H mice did not have any such inhibitory effect.

Bentvelzen and associates (50) have reported observations which suggest to them that enhancing antibodies may be involved in the development of mammary tumors in BALB/cfC3H mice. They observed that the spontaneous development of tumors in BALB/cfC3H females was accelerated by approximately two months if the mice were immunized with MTV virions given in Freund's adjuvant. A similar enhancement of the development of spontaneous tumors after immunization was reported by Hirsch and Iversen (42). In neither experiment were the sera of the mice examined for the actual presence of enhancing antibodies and the evidence thus remains suggestive.

There have been two reports suggesting that the "immunized" female mouse may transmit resistance factors, presumably antibodies, to her offspring.

Andervont reported in 1945 (62) that the MTV-injected, young, susceptible, hybrid offspring of females of the I strain which had been given MTV in adult life did not develop mammary tumors, although similar young, MTV-injected control hybrids whose strain I mothers had not been exposed to MTV in adulthood did develop tumors. It can be speculated that the females given MTV when they were adult developed an antibody response to the virus, and transmitted these antibodies to their offspring.

More recently, Bentvelzen has detected a similar phenomenon in C57BL animals (63). These females when infected with MTV propagate the virus poorly, and they do not transmit significant quantities of MTV in their milk. Further, such animals apparently do transmit *in utero* a factor which can protect their offspring against infection with the virus. Bentvelzen detected this in experiments in which he permitted the (C57BL × BALB/c) hybrid offspring of the MTV-infected C57BL females to nurse only briefly on fully infected BALB/cfC3H females during the first day of life. Although the BALB/cfC3H females thus transmitted some virus to the newborn mice, as shown in control experiments, these did not show evidence of MTV infection (i.e., they did not develop mammary tumors) in adult life. Bentvelzen noted that ordinary C57BL females do not transmit the protective factor; it is only transmitted by those previously exposed to MTV. He also noted that BALB/cfC3H females did not transmit such a protective factor to their hybrid offspring when tested under the same conditions of limited access of the newborn to MTV.

Interaction of immune cells and cell products with tumor cells in vitro. Given the appropriate immunization procedures, it is possible to demonstrate inhibition of tumor growth or acceleration of tumor growth, and it is also possible to show that adoptively transferred lymphoid cells or passively transferred serum from immunized donors may have similar effects of acceleration or inhibition on the growth of tumor cell populations in recipient animals. These results illustrate the complexity of the immune response in the immunized animal, and point out that the actual effect observed in *in vivo* experiments (challenge tumor growth or challenge tumor inhibition) represents only the final result of a complex interaction of immunologic and physiologic mechanisms. An elegant demonstration of the interaction of the various elements of the immune response has been presented by Heppner (19), who has used the colony inhibition technique to study the interactions of immune cells and their products with tumor cells *in vitro*.

As described above, Heppner and Pierce (18) demonstrated that lymph node cells taken from mice bearing autochthonous and progressively growing MTV-induced mammary tumors, or from mice immunized with such tumors, could inhibit the *in vitro* growth of cells of that tumor. Heppner then reported (19) that she could detect in various BALB/c and BALB/cfC3H mice serum factors (presumably antibody) which could interfere with the ability of the immune lymphocytes to inhibit *in vitro* colony formation by the tumor cells. The same specificity which characterized the reactivity of the immune lymphocytes also characterized the ability of the serum factors to inhibit the reaction. Serum from an animal bearing an autochthonous mammary tumor could protect that tumor from immune attack *in vitro*, but could not protect another tumor. Similarly, serum from immunized MTV-infected mice could protect cells from the immunizing tumor but not those from another tumor. In contrast to the observations on the frequent cross-reactivity against MTV-positive tumors of lymphocytes taken from immunized MTV-free mice, the serum from MTV-free immunized mice did not protect other tumor cell populations against colony inhibition by immune lymphocytes; however, only a limited number of tests were made.

Heppner suggests that this protective action of serum, which has been demonstrated to occur in a number of other tumor systems by the Hellströms and their associates (45), represents an *in vitro* demonstration of an *in vivo* mechanism which permits the progressive growth of a tumor cell population in an animal whose lymphocytes are demonstrably reactive against the tumor cells. It is well established in other systems, mainly involving differences in histocompatibility antigenicity, that enhancing antibody may interfere with the ability of the lymphocytes to make contact with, and destroy, the tumor cells. The *in vitro* observations on the effectiveness of serum from tumor-bearing animals in interfering with the destructive capabilities of the lymphocytes from the same animal may thus be a parallel of what happens *in vivo*.

IMMUNOLOGIC UNRESPONSIVENESS

Induction of tolerance to MTV antigens by neonatal exposure. A cell-associated immunologic response (based on rejection of tissue grafts) against MTV-associated antigens in mammary tumor tissue can easily be demonstrated in mice which were not exposed to MTV at birth, but not in similar animals neonatally infected with the virus. It has been postulated that neonatal infection with MTV results in the development of immunologic tolerance to MTV and to MTV-associated antigens expressed on mammary tissue (10, 13).

Early attempts to detect tumor-specific or tumor-associated antigens in MTV-infected mammary tumors were negative, and in fact, mammary tumors frequently were used as controls in experiments demonstrating the tumor-specific antigenicity of cancers induced by chemical carcinogens. In these early experiments, however, the mammary tumors were transplanted into mice neonatally infected with MTV. Several workers have now observed that MTV-infected tumors can be transplanted more readily into MTV-infected mice than into isogenic MTV-free hosts, and that MTV-free animals can be immunized more readily against MTV-infected tumors than can MTV-infected mice. As discussed above, these experiments demonstrate that mammary tumors induced by MTV do contain antigenicity associated with the presence of the virus; they also demonstrate that mice neonatally infected with MTV are at least partially tolerant to this antigenicity, and thus are more difficult to immunize than are MTV-free mice.

Weiss and his associates have demonstrated that C3Hf mice can be immunized against challenge implants of isogenic MTV-infected mammary tumor tissue under conditions where MTV-infected C3H animals cannot (8, 10), and that MTV-free BALB/c mice can be immunized against challenge implants of isogenic MTV-infected mammary tumor tissue whereas MTV-infected BALB/cfC3H cannot (27). Further, in both strains of mice, primary implants of isogenic MTV-infected mammary tumor tissue grew better in the MTV-infected host than in the MTV-free host (10, 11, 27). Not only MTV-infected tumors but also MTV infected preneoplastic mammary tissue grows better in the isogenic MTV-infected host (8, 10, 11).

Morton (13) has reported similar data indicating that neonatally infected mice are immunologically tolerant to MTV-associated antigens. Adult reciprocal hybrids between C57BL and C3H mice were implanted with C3H mammary carcinomas; the MTV-infected hybrids were uniformly more susceptible to the tumor than were the reciprocal MTV-free hybrids. This effect was observed only in the immunologically mature hosts; when newborn, MTV-free and MTV-infected mice were equally susceptible to the tumor cell suspensions. Morton also demonstrated that he could produce resistant hosts by foster-nursing to eliminate infection with the virus, or could produce susceptible ones by injecting the young mice with MTV.

Immunologic tolerance to MTV-associated antigens has also been demonstrated by transplantation of the DBA/2 leukemias which possess the ML antigen. Transplants of these leukemias grow progressively in MTV-infected compatible hosts but not in MTV-free hosts (31, 64).

The lessened reactivity of mice neonatally infected with MTV towards MTV-associated antigens is readily demonstrated in tumor immunization and challenge experiments, in which the mouse's cell-associated immune responses are tested. This has been corroborated in the *in vitro* colony inhibition technique; although the lymphocytes from immunized MTV-infected mice are capable of reacting against tumor-specific antigens, they do not react against MTV-associated antigens (19). However, even though neonatally infected animals do not respond to MTV antigens of tissue implants with an effective cell-mediated immunity, humoral antibodies capable of reacting with the MTV virion in immunodiffusion can be detected in their sera. These antibodies are readily detected in immunized neonatally infected mice, and can also be found occasionally in females bearing autochthonous mammary tumors.

Similar results demonstrating a lack of, or a slow development of, cell-mediated immunity to virus-associated antigens which is not paralleled by the lack of a humoral antibody response in the neonatally infected "tolerant" animal have been reported by others for oncogenic viruses such as mouse leukemia virus and polyoma (65, 66). The lack of cell-mediated immune reactivity is not absolute,

but, significantly, this deficiency is more pronounced than any observed in the humoral antibody response.

The apparent partial tolerance of the neonatally infected mouse to virus-associated antigens has several possible explanations. For example, tolerance to virion antigens may be "broken" more readily than tolerance to virus-induced tissue antigens, either spontaneously or during immunization. Mature virion antigens may not be available to immunologically competent cells during development, so that tolerance is not induced or not maintained, whereas cells altered by the viral genome, and possessing distinctive antigenicity, may be present early and commonly. It is evident, in addition, that the various tests are measuring different virus-associated antigens.

Experimental manipulation of the host's immune response. The recognition that mammary tumors induced by MTV possess new antigens, at least some of which are determined by the inducing virus, has led to several attempts to alter the development of the tumors by immunological manipulation of the infected mouse.

Thymectomy, usually carried out during the neonatal period, has been used to depress immunologic reactivity by several investigators (67–74). One might expect that mammary tumors, since they contain tumor-specific and tumor-associated antigenicity, would develop more readily in thymectomized animals. However, neonatal thymectomy has been found by at least some workers to have an inhibiting effect upon the development of MTV-induced lesions in the mammary gland. In MTV-infected BALB/c females, thymectomy within the first three days after birth significantly reduced the incidence of mice which develop hyperplastic alveolar nodules during exogenous hormonal stimulation (69, 70) and both lengthened the latent period before tumor development and decreased the

171

final tumor incidence in virgin females (69). In multiparous females of the BALB/cfC3H strain, neonatal thymectomy significantly lengthened the latent period before tumor development, but the final tumor incidence was the same in thymectomized and control females (70); in multiparous BALB/cfRIII females, neonatal thymectomy also lengthened the latent period, but did not decrease final tumor incidence (69). In the C3H strain, thymectomy at three days of age reduced the incidence of both hyperplastic alveolar nodules and mammary tumors (73).

Thus, contrary to expectation, there appears to be considerable agreement that neonatal thymectomy can inhibit the development of both hyperplastic alveolar nodules and mammary tumors in the MTV-infected mouse. These results parallel the effect of thymectomy on the development of virus-induced leukemias in the mouse, but in the latter case, removal of the target tissue of the oncogenic virus is assumed to be at least partially the cause of the decrease in tumor incidence.

Martinez (67) suggested that the inhibiting effect of thymectomy could be due to an alteration in the hormonal milieu, to the necessity of the thymus for the growth and multiplication of MTV, or to a relationship between oncogenesis and the immunologic responsiveness of the host. All three of these possibilities have been examined experimentally.

Heppner et al. investigated the possibility that thymectomy may interfere with infection or with the multiplication of MTV, and did not find evidence for this. Biologically active virus could be recovered from the blood of both thymectomized and control mice (71), and neonatal thymectomy did not inhibit the secretion of MTV virions in the milk of lactating females (72). Further, the offspring of thymectomized BALB/cfC3H mothers were just as likely as those of control BALB/cfC3H mothers to be infected with MTV (72). Thus,

there is no gross diminution in the propagation and transmission of MTV in thymectomized females; the techniques used, however, would not have detected minor variations in the replication of the virus.

Sakakura and Nishizuka (73) suggest that endocrinologic mechanisms may be involved; lobuloalveolar development of the normal mammary gland in C3H and (C3H × 129) hybrid females maintained as virgins and in those subjected to exogenous hormone administration was reduced in thymectomized as compared to control mice. They noted that the ovaries and the uterus were smaller in the thymectomized subjects, and that the ovaries had essentially no follicles. Nishizuka and Sakakura (75) have since shown that a similar arrest of ovarian function occurs in (C57BL × A) hybrids, that most of the thymectomized females are sterile and have abnormal estrus cycles, and that the effect on the ovary is noted only if thymectomy is carried out before the mice are a week of age. Thymectomized males, on the other hand, appeared normal; no effect on the testis was noted, and the animals were fertile. Grafts of thymus tissue restored ovarian function in the females if implanted shortly after thymectomy but not if implantation was delayed for 40 days. It would appear that the ovarian arrest resulting from thymectomy in the C3H strain and in the hybrids tested can easily account for the decrease in mammary tumor incidence noted, since MTV-induced mammary tumors develop in mice only in an adequate hormonal milieu (76).

The situation may be different in the BALB/cfC3H mice studied by Heppner (72). She found that mammary gland development was normal in thymectomized mice of this strain, and she suggested that the reason why thymectomized BALB/cfC3H females ultimately develop a normal incidence of mammary tumors, whereas thymectomized C3H mice do not, may reside with genotype differences.

Some of the effects of thymectomy upon the development of mammary tumors may well be related to the role of the thymus in immunologic responsiveness. Although tumors developed at a later age in thymectomized BALB/cfC3H females, more tumors per mouse and faster growing tumors were found in the thymectomized mice than in the controls (70), as would be expected in immunologically depressed hosts. Further, if MTV infection was delayed until the mice were about three months old, more preneoplastic lesions developed in the mammary glands of the neonatally thymectomized females than developed either in the controls or in thymectomized females infected at a younger age (71).

There is clear evidence that the thymectomized mouse is capable of responding immunologically against antigens expressed in mammary tumor cells. Equal numbers of lymphocytes from immunized donors were equally effective in inhibiting the development of colonies of cells from the sensitizing tumor in the *in vitro* colony inhibition technique regardless of whether the donors had been thymectomized or not (72). However, the thymectomized animals had a smaller total population of lymphocytes than the sham-operated controls. Thus, although thymectomized mice are capable of producing an immunological response against antigens in mammary tumors, this cell-associated immune response is quantitatively less than that of normal mice.

Heppner (72) has also observed that the serum from thymectomized mice after immunization is not capable of protecting tumor cells from the inhibition of colony formation occurring after exposure to immune lymphocytes in the colony inhibition technique. This is in contrast to the effect of serum obtained from immunized intact donors. Heppner suggests that enhancing antibodies may play a role in natural mammary tumor development, and, since actual development of a tumor may thus result from an interplay between cell associated immunity and enhancing antibody response, the observed greater resistance of thymectomized mice to mammary tumor development may occur because the diminished cellular immune response of the thymectomized mouse may still be very effective in the absence of an enhancing antibody response.

The development of MTV-induced mammary tumors in infected mice is also drastically reduced by treatment with another immunologic depressant, antilymphocyte serum (ALS) (77). A series of eleven i.p. injections of ALS (0.25 ml/ injection) was administered by us to MTV-infected BALB/cfC3H females three weeks after the mice had produced either their first or second litters. Some of the animals received allografts of DBA/2 skin to determine the extent of the immune depression induced by the serum; recovery from the depression, as measured by rejection of the allografts, occurred four to six weeks after the beginning of treatment. In the various experiments, several types of BALB/cfC3H control mice were used, including untreated females, splenectomized females and females given eleven injections of normal rabbit serum (NRS).

Some of the animals were sacrificed ten weeks *post partum* and examined for the presence of hyperplastic alveolar nodules in their mammary glands. In primiparous animals, no difference in nodule incidence was observed between the ALS-treated and the NRS-treated groups. However, in multiparous females, fewer ALS-treated mice had developed nodules (13/23 or 57%) than had NRS-treated mice (10/13 or 77%).

Development of mammary tumors in the ALS-treated mice was both delayed and depressed. The first mammary tumors had appeared in all control groups by 20 weeks *post partum*, but the ALS-treated mice remained tumor-free for another 10 to 12 weeks.

173

In addition, significantly fewer tumors developed in the ALS-treated mice than in the controls; whereas 21 of 42 mice in the various control groups had developed tumors by 36 to 40 weeks *post partum*, only two of the 16 ALS-treated mice developed mammary tumors within this time.

Treatment of the host mouse with ALS or with antithymocyte serum (ATS) also has a depressant effect upon the survival and growth of transplants of normal mammary gland. In four serial transplant generations of BALB/c mammary gland in BALB/c young adult virgin females, 50 to 85% of the transplants survived and grew in the NRS-treated controls, whereas only 33 to 55% of the transplants grew in the ALS- or the ATS-treated mice (Blair and Lappé, unpublished results).

Thus, the results of treatment of mice with antilymphocyte serum are remarkably similar to those obtained following neonatal thymectomy. Both procedures cause immunologic depression, both have some effect on the growth or development of the normal mammary gland, and both either reduce or delay the development of MTV-induced neoplastic and preneoplastic lesions in the mammary gland.

Both of these methods of inducing immunological depression, as well as a third, sublethal X-irradiation, have also been used in attempts to alter the receptiveness of the host to implants of MTV-induced mammary tumors (12, 72, 78–80). The effect of these treatments on the growth of tumor isografts has been mixed.

Heppner (72) reported that thymectomized animals accepted tumor isografts less readily as adults than did the controls if they were infected with MTV when young, but that if MTV infection was delayed, isografts grew equally well in thymectomized and in control mice.

Fisher and associates (79) reported that C3HB mice treated with ALS accepted transplants of C3H mammary tumor tissue more readily than did NRS-treated controls. Woodruff and Smith, on the other hand, reported that ALS inhibited the growth of mammary tumor transplants in strain A mice (80).

Morton and associates (12) and Prehn (78) found that sublethal X-irradiation of MTV-free mice prior to the inoculation of isografts of MTV-induced mammary tumor tissue resulted in an increase in the growth of the isografts over that seen in unirradiated control mice. This observation is in agreement with the expectation based on the known immunosuppressive effect of this treatment, although it is in contrast to the results noted for the effect of immunosuppressive treatments on spontaneous mammary tumor formation. Both authors reported that irradiation of the host did not increase the growth of these tumors if the hosts were neonatally infected with MTV, and Prehn suggested that the tumors might actually be growing less readily in the irradiated MTV-infected hosts.

Although the number of these experiments is limited, and the various observations are not entirely consistent, it would seem that the response of the mouse to an immunologic depressant is dependent upon whether or not the mouse is infected with MTV. If the treated animals are not infected with the virus, they accept isografts of MTV-infected mammary tumors more readily than do control mice. On the other hand, if the treated animals are infected with the virus, they usually accept mammary tumor isografts less readily than do similar MTV-infected controls. The response appears to be specific for mammary tumor transplants, since transplants of other types of tumors grow more readily in the depressed animals (80).

Attempts to enhance the general immunological reactivity of mice and thereby to affect the development of mammary tumors have been more limited than attempts to depress reactivity.

Weiss and his associates have used a nontoxic methanol-insoluble fraction of phenol-killed, acetone-washed, attenuated tubercle bacilli of the BCG strain to heighten resistance of laboratory animals to a variety of pathogens and tumors; they have found that treatment of mice with this material prior to the inoculation of MTV-induced mammary tumor isografts markedly retards the development of the isografts compared to that seen in control animals (10). Injection of this immunologic activator into breeding MTV-infected C3H females during the first few months of life has been shown to decrease their subsequent development of spontaneous mammary tumors during adult life (10). The number of preneoplastic hyperplastic alveolar nodules (the precursors of mammary tumors) which develop in the mammary glands of hormonally stimulated mice can also be decreased by pretreatment with this immunological activator, suggesting that at least part if not all of its role in preventing the development of mammary tumors may lie in the development of a heightened response of the host to newly arisen variants in the mammary parenchyma.

HOST-VIRUS INTERACTION

Influence of mouse genotype upon the expression of MTV biologic potential. Comparison of spontaneous tumor incidence between different inbred strains does not differentiate the specific effect of genotype from that of the characteristic biological activity of the MTV agent present. However, hybridization experiments, in which the maternal influence is kept constant and genetic differences are introduced by the use of fathers from various strains have shown that genotype can play a large role in determining the incidence of MTV-induced mammary tumors. Mice of several strains foster-nursed on a single virus-possessing strain show different incidences of mammary tumors, which can be attributed to genetic factors of the host.

There is general agreement upon a theory of multiple gene inheritance (for review see ref. 6). Several pathways for genetic expression in tumor development are possible, such as susceptibility of the mammary tissue to the oncogenic virus, alterations in hormonal milieu, effects on the propagation and transmission of the MTV, and variations in immunological responsiveness to MTV and MTV-associated antigens.

Effect of the host upon propagation and transmission of MTV. When MTV is introduced into a strain such as BALB/c, which is genetically susceptible to mammary tumor development, a high incidence of tumors will result in that and in succeeding generations. On the other hand, similar introduction of the virus into a genetically resistant strain such as the C57BL or I results in only a low percentage of tumors, and within a few generations the virus is undetectable. A number of genetic factors are involved, and, interestingly, the hybrids resulting from a cross of two MTV-resistant strains may be more susceptible to MTV infection than either parent strain. For example, $(C57BL \times I^s)F_1$ mice are susceptible to infection with MTV, and the hyperplastic alveolar nodules which develop in such infected mice possess a high tumorigenic potential (81, 82).

Even within susceptible strains of mice, the genotype of the host may greatly influence the propagation of MTV. The conventional tumorigenic strains of MTV are routinely transmitted to the next generation via the milk, regardless of the genotype of the infected mouse. Transmission by the male, however, can occur in rare circumstances, such as in some sublines of C3H mice; the number of strains in which male transmission of this type of MTV occurs is limited, and within these strains not all male mice can transmit the virus (83).

In GR mice, the plaque-forming MTV carried by this strain is routinely transmitted not only through the milk but also through the germ cells. However, when this virus is transferred to mice of another genotype, it is thereafter transmitted only via the milk in the new strain.

Similarly, a representative low-tumorigenic variant of MTV, the nodule-inducing-virus (NIV) found in C3Hf mice, is transmitted within one mouse strain at conception, but in mice of another genotype, it is transmitted only through the milk. This is a very interesting example, and will be considered here in some detail. Specifically, in mice of the C3H genotype, the variant is transmitted by either parent at conception, but apparently not through the milk. MTV antigenicity, as measured by immunodiffusion, is difficult to detect in the milk of C3Hf mice (48 and Blair, unpublished observations), although some MTV virions are present (84). In mice of the BALB/c genotype, on the other hand, the variant is readily transmitted through the milk, and it is not transmitted by either parent at conception (85). Further, MTV antigenicity is easily detected in the milk of the infected BALB/c females and MTV virions can readily be isolated from milk samples (Blair, unpublished observations). In addition, hyperplastic alveolar nodules are easily induced by this virus in BALB/c, but not in C3Hf, females, when the animals are subjected to hormonal stimulation. Other characteristics of the virus, such as the low tumorigenic potential of the nodules that it induces (85), appear to be the same in mice of either genotype.

It is exceedingly difficult to transfer this variant of MTV from the C3Hf mouse to another strain. Attempts to transfer the virus from C3Hf animals using techniques successful with conventional strains of MTV have been unsuccessful. A few years ago it was successfully transferred to BALB/c mice by a double transplantation experiment; BALB/c mammary tissue was transplanted into a (C3Hf × BALB/c) hybrid mouse infected with the variant; in this host, the tissue became infected and, as a result, developed hyperplastic alveolar nodules. The nodules were then transplanted into BALB/c females, and one of the outgrowths which survived and grew transmitted the virus to its BALB/c hosts. After that, the virus multiplied in the BALB/c, and could be transmitted normally through the mother's milk to the next generation.

Since then, a number of additional attempts have been made at the Cancer Research Genetics Laboratory to transfer NIV from the C3Hf mouse to the BALB/c, all of them unsuccessful. Recent results of Medina (86) indicate that this difficulty lies not in the first step of the transfer (infection of BALB/c mammary tissue while it resides in an NIV-infected hybrid host), but rather in the second step (infection of the BALB/c host carrying the NIV-infected BALB/c mammary tissue). Transplanted virus-free BALB/c hyperplastic alveolar nodule outgrowth tissue could be infected with NIV by maintenance in an infected hybrid, as evidenced by alteration in tumorigenic potential of the outgrowth and by the presence of typical type B virus particles in the infected tissue. However, after the infected tissue was returned to BALB/c hosts, no evidence of infection of the hosts or their offspring could be detected (86).

Recently, Bentvelzen and his associates have undertaken an extensive analysis of this host-virus relationship, and they have described in a series of communications a number of genes in different strains which control various aspects of viral transmission, propagation, and oncogenesis (15, 50, 54, 87–89).

Effect of the host upon the replication of MTV in mammary tissues. The production of MTV type B virus particles in infected mammary glands and tumors is influenced by the genotype of the infected mouse. Hairstone and associates (90) reported, as part of a survey of the relative number of B particles in the tumors of mice of eight different strains, that the highest numbers of virus particles were found in the tumors of MTV-infected BALB/c mice, with lesser numbers present in the tumors of mice of the A strain infected with the same MTV. This morphological observation agrees with observations on the relative abundance of MTV antigens in these tumors; in general, type B particles and MTV-associated antigen are more abundant in the tumors and milk of infected BALB/c mice than in the tumors and milk of infected mice of other genotypes (Blair, unpublished observations).

More examples of this phenomenon, involving mice infected with the low tumorigenic variants of MTV, have been observed by Hageman and Calafat (cited in ref. 87). Hybrid offspring of C3Hf mice mated with C57BL or with 020 mice had no type B particles in their mammary tumors, whereas the mammary tumors of hybrid offspring of C3Hf mice mated with BALB/c mice contained many type B particles. Similarly, mammary tumors of the (C3Hf × BALB/c) hybrid mice contained many more type B particles than did those of C3Hf mice.

Effect upon MTV infection of the host's immunologic responsiveness. Mice of different genotype possess, of course, different capabilities for immunologic response against test antigens (63). As is to be expected, therefore, mice of different strains have different levels of immunologic response to MTV and to MTV-associated antigens. In general, strains of mice which are the most resistant to infection with MTV are also the ones in which it is easiest to produce circulating antibodies to MTV by immunization. For example, the C57BL strain is more resistant to MTV infection than the C3Hf, 020 or BALB/c strains (87), and, although all four strains will produce antibodies to MTV if immunized with high doses of MTV antigen, only the C57BL still produces detectable antibody if

low doses of antigen are used (54, 63). Similarly, the I strain is very resistant to MTV infection, whereas the BALB/c strain is susceptible, and similar immunization procedures evoke a higher incidence of antibody response in I than in BALB/c mice (Blair, unpublished observations). The strains most resistant to MTV infection, the C57BL and the I, are also the two strains which are capable of transmitting to their offspring resistance factors, presumably antibody, which interfere with MTV infection in the offspring (62, 63).

General effects of MTV upon the infected mouse. The characteristic lesions resulting from MTV infection are mammary tumors. Typically, these structures are adenocarcinomas, either type A or type B. The tumors appear in the adult female many months after the neonatal introduction of MTV via the mother's milk. Prior to the development of tumors, preneoplastic lesions can be detected in the mammary gland tissue. Depending upon the strain of the inducing virus, these may be either hyperplastic alveolar nodules or flat ductal growths called plaques; foci of neoplastic cells eventually develop in some of these lesions.

With the exception of the lesions in the mammary gland, very little effect of the virus upon the host has been reported so far (for review, see ref. 6). There is some indication that MTV may influence the hormonal milieu of the mouse, and that it may alter the sensitivity of normal mammary gland to hormones. MTV may also decrease the life expectancy of the infected mouse. Recently, however, it has been observed that BALB/c mice infected with MTV exhibit impairment in general immunologic reactivity as they age (Lappé and Blair, in preparation). There is thus a close immunologic relationship between virus and host.

Immunologic depression induced by infection with MTV. The immunologic responsiveness of the MTV-infected mouse decreases as the animal ages. This has been demonstrated for both humoral antibody production, by measuring hemagglutinin production to sheep red blood cells, and cell-associated immunologic reactivity, by measuring allograft survival (Lappé and Blair, in preparation).

MTV-free BALB/c and MTV-infected BALB/cfC3H virgin females were age-matched and immunized with several injections of sheep red blood cells when they were six, eight, or 12 months old. The sera were tested at several intervals after immunization by a standard hemagglutination assay. There was a stepwise decline in peak serum titer production with age in the MTV-infected females which was not observed in the MTV-free females. Further, in each age group the MTV-infected females developed lower peak serum titers than did the MTV-free females, and, in the two older age groups, the differences were statistically significant. These differences were not observed in an earlier study, measuring the humoral antibody response to crystalline bovine serum albumin and to sheep red blood cells in younger females of these strains (9).

Cell-associated immunologic responsiveness was tested in other groups of MTV-free BALB/c and MTV-infected BALB/cfC3H virgin females at two, four, eight to ten, 12 and 16 months by comparing the length of survival of skin allografts from the DBA strain, which shares the same H-2 locus. In each age group, the allografts survived longer on the MTV-infected females than they did on the MTV-free females, and, as observed in the study on humoral antibody response, the differences were significant in the older age groups. There was a stepwise decline in immunologic reactivity with age in the MTV-infected females, indicated by the steadily increasing time intervals required for the females to reject the skin allografts.

Thus, the MTV-infected females of this strain develop a progressive deficiency in immunologic reactivity, and they become significantly less responsive than MTV-free mice to antigenic stimulation when they reach 10 to 12 months of age. It is at this age that mammary tumors begin to develop in the MTV-infected BALB/cfC3H virgin female, and it is interesting to speculate that this progressive immunologic deficiency may be involved etiologically in the appearance of the MTV-induced tumors. Experiments are in progress to determine if MTV infection in other strains induces similar immunologic deficiencies, and if the temporal association between the decrease in immunologic reactivity and the development of MTV-induced neoplasia is causal or coincidental.

Biologic effects of different strains of MTV. Many characteristics of tumor development in infected mice are dependent upon the strain of the inducing virus. Several different strains of MTV have been recognized and characterized during recent decades (for review, see ref. 6). Most of these strains have been transmitted vertically within inbred strains of mice for 40 years or more, without experimental manipulation. They can be characterized as belonging to one group of viruses on the basis of the well-documented cross-reactivity in virion coat antigenicity, and by the fact that they induce related hyperplastic or neoplastic lesions in the mammary gland of the mouse.

In addition to these similarities, the various strains of MTV also have a number of distinctive biological characteristics. For example, strains of MTV differ in tumorigenic potential, which can be demonstrated by comparison of the differences in tumor incidence produced in genetically identical infected mice, by differences in the average age at which the tumors develop, or by differences in the potential to complete the neoplastic transformation exhibited by the induced hyperplastic lesions. MTV may also be characterized on the basis of the type of lesions which they induce in the mammary parenchyma. Further, they can be differentiated by the mode of transmission from one generation to the next, such as through the milk or at the time of conception; however, as has been noted the characteristic mode of transmission is partly determined by the genotype of the infected mouse.

Although, theoretically, each strain of MTV carried by a different strain of mouse might be considered to be a variant, with potentially distinguishable characteristics, it has been observed repeatedly that the various strains of MTV can be grouped into three general classes, based on their effect upon the infected host.

MTV carried by many of the mouse strains developed in the United States during the early decades of this century are quite similar in their biological characteristics. Strains such as DBA, C3H and CBA were developed in the United States by Little and by Strong from crosses of related stocks, and therefore the MTV possessed by these strains may have a common origin. Characteristically, the MTV carried in these strains of mice have a fairly high tumorigenic potential (with some demonstrated differences), and they induce hyperplastic or preneoplastic lesions in the mammary gland which are designated, on the basis of their morphology, as hyperplastic alveolar nodules. These nodules, when transplanted, exhibit a high potential for the development of neoplastic foci. Mammary tumors induced by this group of MTV are characteristically hormone-independent and progressive in growth from their first appearance. Members of this group of MTV have been called by a variety of names, including Bittner agent, mammary tumor agent, mammary tumor incitor, and, of course, MTV. Historically, this group represents the conventional or standard MTV, and, for this reason, has recently been designated MTV-S (50).

The second group of MTV share a European origin. The RIII strain of mice was developed in Paris by Dobrovolskaia-Zavadskaia, and it is apparently unrelated to the strains developed in the United States. The GR strain of mice was developed in Holland, and is also apparently unrelated to those developed in the United States. The MTV carried by these two strains, as well as that carried by a third strain of mice, the DD (which originated in Germany and was developed in Japan), share several biologic characteristics, and it is possible that these three MTV strains are of close ancestry. Characteristically, these MTV induce plaques in the mammary parenchyma which can be distinguished from hyperplastic alveolar nodules on the basis of morphology and hormonal responsiveness. The tumors induced by these MTV are hormonally responsive; they grow slowly and frequently regress, with perhaps several episodes of growth and regression before they become progressively growing neoplasms. It is important to emphasize that these tumor growth patterns are controlled mainly by the inducing strain of MTV, not by the genotype of the infected mouse, as foster-nursing experiments have clearly shown. This group of plaque-forming viruses has recently been designated MTV-P (50).

The third group of viruses consists of MTV that, like the standard MTV, induce hyperplastic alveolar nodules in the mammary gland. These nodules, however, have only a limited potential to produce foci of neoplastic cells, and, as a result, the tumorigenic potential of viruses in this group is low. Members of this group of MTV are frequently found in mouse strains in association with a standard tumorigenic MTV, and they are not detected until the more tumorigenic virus is removed by foster-nursing; obviously, the less tumorigenic variant can only be detected by this procedure if it is transmitted at conception and if the tumorigenic variant is transmitted only through the milk. One example of a virus in

179

this group has been well documented, and there is suggestive evidence that similar low-tumorigenic MTV variants may exist in other mouse strains in association with the conventional tumorigenic MTV. The C3H sublines derived from Heston's colony possess, in addition to the standard MTV, a low-tumorigenic variant which is transmitted via germ cells rather than through the milk, and therefore remains in the C3Hf sublines produced by foster-nursing. This MTV variant has been designated NIV by members of the Cancer Research Genetics Laboratory in Berkeley, who have extensively studied it (for review, see ref. 6), and it is also called MTV-L (50).

Antigenic diversity of MTV strains. Within the past few years, evidence has been presented which indicates that some of the strains of MTV may be characterized by a type-specific antigenicity, in addition to the already demonstrated cross-reacting antigenicity. This is not unexpected, but, because of technical problems, the evidence has been difficult to obtain.

This type-specific antigenicity was first demonstrated in neoplastic and preneoplastic mammary tissue cells in tumor immunity experiments carried out by Weiss and his associates (7, 8). Mice of the C3Hf subline are not infected with biologically active MTV, and they could be considered "MTV-free" hosts in Weiss' tumor transplantation experiments. However, these mice are infected with the variant of MTV designated NIV, which possesses a low tumorigenic potential. The experiments demonstrated that these NIV-infected mice could respond well immunologically to MTV-associated antigens; the immunogenicity detected is apparently related to an antigen associated with MTV but not with NIV.

These initial observations on type-specific MTV antigenicity have recently been confirmed and extended (91). Not only the MTV carried by the C3H strain, but also that carried by the A strain induces in mammary tissue a type-specific antigenicity which is not elicited by the C3Hf-NIV variant of MTV; no type-specific differences in antigenicity between the C3H and the A MTV were detected in these experiments. In other experiments, suggestive but not statistically significant evidence was obtained indicating that mice infected with the RIII MTV may not be tolerant to at least one MTV-associated antigen induced by the A and C3H MTV; thus the RIII MTV may also lack the type-specific antigenicity carried by the agent of the C3H and the A strains. Further experimentation is necessary to establish this point. It is certainly provocative to note, however, that the detected type-specific MTV-associated antigenicity corresponds so far to that which might be predicted on the basis of the classification of the strains of MTV according to their biological characteristics. Similar expressions of type-specific antigenicity in infected tissues have been reported for other groups of related viruses such as the mouse leukemia virus and the polyoma virus (92, 93).

Early attempts to detect directly type-specific antigenicity on MTV virions were unsuccessful. For example, absorption experiments reported by Tanaka and Moore (56) did not detect any antigenic differences between the virions of the MTV carried by their RIII subline and the agent resembling NIV which is present in RIIIf mice. Early attempts to demonstrate possible differences between MTV strains in immunodiffusion experiments were also unsuccessful; in fact, as has been amply demonstrated, a dominant characteristic of MTV virions from various sources is their antigenic cross-reactivity, with regard to the antigenicity of both the intact B particle (55, 94) and the soluble components which are released by ether treatment of MTV preparations and which are found naturally in milk (55, 95).

Type-specific antigenicity of the virion can be demonstrated, however, in immunodiffusion, if the technical problems of variations in antigen and antibody titer can be overcome, using spur analysis or absorption experiments. Using a battery of rabbit antisera and a spur analysis procedure, it has been possible to detect on the virions of MTV derived from the C3H and the DBA strains an antigenicity which was not present on the virions of the NIV variant derived from the C3Hf strain or the MTV variant isolated from wild house mice and now carried in BALB/c females (55). These spur analysis results have been confirmed by absorption experiments, and they are currently being extended. Preliminary results indicate that considerable antigenic diversity exists among MTV strains derived from different sources. Some of the differences detected appear to represent qualitative differences in antigenicity; others may represent quantitative differences in the expression of similar antigens on the virion coat (Blair, unpublished observations).

SUMMARY AND CONCLUSIONS

Relationship between host and virus in the natural state: Recapitulation. There is thus no doubt but that the mouse can respond immunologically, as well as otherwise, to the antigens of MTV, both those of the virion and those expressed on the cells that the virus infects. There is also evidence that the virus can profoundly influence the host, such as by its depressant effect upon general immunological reactivity. Most of the data which substantiate these conclusions were, of course, obtained from experimental situations. It thus seems appropriate to summarize at this point what we know, and what we can guess, about the relationship that exists between the host mouse and the infecting virus in the natural state.

Certainly the most important observation is that the neonatally infected mouse is at least partially tolerant to the antigens of the virus, and to the virus-associated antigens present in infected cells. On the other hand, the MTV-infected mouse is certainly capable of responding immunologically to MTV-associated antigenicity; this has been thoroughly demonstrated by a number of workers during the past decade, and the pertinent literature has been cited above. The situation can be summarized as follows: Although humoral antibody production can be elicited in MTV-infected hosts against MTV virion antigens and against MTV-associated cellular antigens, and although some protection (presumably cell-associated immunity) against spontaneous tumor development or against challenge implants of isogenic mammary tissue can also occasionally be induced by immunization, the presence of any immunologic reactivity against MTV in the normal neonatally infected mouse has been exceedingly difficult to demonstrate. Serum antibodies against MTV virions have been reported in one-third of a sample of C3H females bearing spontaneously developed mammary tumors (50); however, this observation represents the exception rather than the rule. There is some evidence that an MTV-infected female mouse which is genetically resistant to MTV may transmit to her offspring resistance factors, presumably antibody, which interfere with the infection of the offspring by MTV (62, 63), but genetically susceptible mice apparently do not generally produce such resistance factors.

Adoptive transfer of lymphoid cells and passive transfer of serum antibody from immunized MTV-infected mice have demonstrated that protection against the development of challenge isografts of mammary tumor can frequently be afforded. Nevertheless, the demonstration of reactive cells and serum in the normal MTV-infected host is largely limited to the observations of Heppner and Pierce (18) and Heppner (19), and the antigens involved here were not MTV-associated but rather non-cross-reacting antigens, as are those found in tumors induced by chemical carcinogens.

Prospects for immunotherapy. It is important to note that it is relatively easy, by immunization, to elicit a humoral antibody response against MTV-associated antigens in the neonatally infected, and therefore tolerant, mouse but that it is very difficult to induce a cell-associated immune response against these antigens. And, indeed, many attempts to immunize MTV-infected mice against mammary tumors have resulted in acceleration of tumor growth rather than repression. Since the dominant component in immunological protection against solid tissues containing foreign antigens is cell-associated and not humoral, any attempt to use immunization to protect against development of these tumors, or to aid in the defense against already developed tumors, either in this virus-induced tumor system or in others for which this may serve as a model, is likely to fail unless careful attention is given to the mode of immunization and the elimination thereby of unwanted humoral antibody responses. Immunotherapy in cancer research needs at this time not attention to the question of the presence or absence of tumor-associated antigens (already well demonstrated in many animal and human systems), but rather attention to the basic problem of how to evoke cell-associated immunological responses by immunization with membrane-bound antigens.

Despite this somewhat gloomy note, there is considerable room for optimism in the realm of specific immunotherapy in cancer research. The potential for interference with tumor development in a model system such as we are considering here lies in two main areas. Since it is a common observation with the naturally occurring oncogenic viruses that infection of the host occurs at a very early age, with the resulting development of tolerance to the virus-associated antigens in the host, methods of breaking immunologic tolerance to these antigens offer a useful approach to immunotherapy. Since tolerance can frequently be broken by immunization with similar but not completely cross-reacting antigens (96), and since in all of the RNA oncogenic virus systems so far studied, antigenically distinct but partially cross-reacting virus strains exist, it seems possible that appropriate immunization with inactivated similar but not identical virus strains might well induce an immunologic response in the host which would be effective against its own virus-induced neoplasm.

It is most heartening that recent evidence clearly demonstrates that MTV-induced tumors contain not only virus-associated antigenicity but also tumor-specific antigenicity. If this observation is found to be true for other virus-induced tumors, exploitation of the potential ability of the host to respond to these antigens (to which it is probably not neonatally tolerant) may be a useful tool in immunotherapy. This may be accomplished specifically, by immunization with the antigens of the individual's own tumor, or nonspecifically. Indeed, nonspecific stimulation of the host's general immunological reactivity is a primary candidate for successful immunotherapy. A number of studies, especially those using various preparations and extracts of the tubercle bacillus, offer hope in this area (23).

Supported by research grant PRA-37 from the American Cancer Society, Inc., and CA-05388 from the National Cancer Institute, U.S. Public Health Service.

REFERENCES

1. DMOCHOWSKI, L. The milk agent in the origin of mammary tumors in mice. *Advanc. Cancer Res.* **1**: 103, 1953.
2. ANDERVONT, H. B. Problems concerning the tumor viruses, in: Burnet, F. M. and Stanley, W. M. (Eds.), "The viruses." New York, Academic Press, 1959, v. 3, p. 307.
3. DEOME, K. B. The mouse mammary tumor virus. *Fed. Proc.* **21**: 15, 1962.
4. GROSS, L. "Oncogenic viruses." New York, Pergamon Press, 1961.
5. NANDI, S. Interactions among hormonal, viral,

and genetic factors in mouse mammary tumori-genesis. *Canad. Cancer Conf.* **6**: 69, 1966.

6. BLAIR, P. B. The mammary tumor virus (MTV). *Curr. Top. Microbiol. Immunol.* **45**: 1, 1968.

7. LAVRIN, D. H., BLAIR, P. B. and WEISS, D. W. Immunology of spontaneous mammary carcinomas in mice. III. Immunogenicity of C3H preneoplastic hyperplastic alveolar nodules in C3Hf hosts. *Cancer Res.* **26**: 293, 1966.

8. LAVRIN, D. H., BLAIR, P. B. and WEISS, D. W. Immunology of spontaneous carcinomas in mice. IV. Association of the mammary tumor virus with the immunogenicity of C3H nodules and tumors. *Cancer Res.* **26**: 929, 1966.

9. DEZFULIAN, M., LAVRIN, D. H., SHEN, A., BLAIR, P. B. and WEISS, D. W. Immunology of spontaneous mammary carcinomas in mice: Studies on the nature of the protective antigens, in: "Carcinogenesis: A broad critique." Baltimore, Williams and Wilkins Co., 1967, p. 365.

10. WEISS, D. W., LAVRIN, D. H., DEZFULIAN, M., VAAGE, J. and BLAIR, P. B. Studies on the immunology of spontaneous mammary carcinomas of mice, in: Burdette, W. J., (Ed.), "Viruses inducing cancer—implications for therapy." Salt Lake City, University of Utah Press, 1966, p. 138.

11. WEISS, D. W. Immunology of spontaneous tumors, in: *Proceedings of the Fifth Berkely Symposium on Mathematical Statistics and Probability*. Berkeley, University of California Press, 1967.

12. MORTON, D. L., GOLDMAN, L. and WOOD, D. A. Acquired immunological tolerance and carcinogenesis by the mammary tumor virus. II. Immune responses influencing growth of spontaneous mammary adenocarcinomas. *J. nat. Cancer Inst.* **42**: 321, 1969.

13. MORTON, D. L. Acquired immunological tolerance and carcinogenesis by the mammary tumor virus. I. Influence of neonatal infection with the mammary tumor virus on the growth of spontaneous mammary adenocarcinomas. *J. nat. Cancer Inst.* **42**: 311, 1969.

14. BURTON, D. S., BLAIR, P. B. and WEISS, D. W. Protection against mammary tumors in mice by immunization with purified mammary tumor virus preparations. *Cancer Res.* **29**: 971, 1969.

15. VAN DER GUGTEN, A. and BENTVELZEN, P. Interference between two strains of the mouse mammary tumor virus in the GR mouse strain. *Europ. J. Cancer* **5**: 361, 1969.

16. NISHIOKA, K., IRIE, R. F., KAWANA, T. and TAKEUCHI, S. Immunological studies on mouse mammary tumors. III. Surface antigens reacting with tumor-specific antibodies in immune adherence. *Int. J. Cancer* **4**: 139, 1969.

17. IRIE, R. F., NISHIOKA, K., TACHIBANA, T. and TAKEUCHI, S. Immunological studies on mouse mammary tumors. IV. Extraction and solubilization of transplantation antigen of mouse mammary tumor. *Int. J. Cancer* **4**: 150, 1969.

18. HEPPNER, G. H. and PIERCE, G. In vitro demonstration of tumor-specific antigens in spontaneous mammary tumors of mice. *Int. J. Cancer* **4**: 212, 1969.

19. HEPPNER, G. H. Studies on serum-mediated inhi-bition of cellular immunity to spontaneous mouse mammary tumors. *Int. J. Cancer* **4**: 608, 1969.

20. VAAGE, J. Non-cross-reacting resistance to virus induced mouse mammary tumours in virus infected C3H mice. *Nature (Lond.)* **218**: 101, 1968.

21. VAAGE, J. Nonvirus-associated antigens in virus induced mouse mammary tumors. *Cancer Res.* **28**: 2477, 1968.

22. MORTON, D. L., MILLER, G. F. and WOOD, D. A. Demonstration of tumor-specific immunity against antigens unrelated to the mammary tumor virus in spontaneous mammary adenocarcinomas. *J. nat. Cancer Inst.* **42**: 289, 1969.

23. WEISS, D. W. Immunologic parameters of host-tumor relationships: spontaneous mammary neoplasia of the inbred mouse as a model. *Cancer Res.* **29**: 2368, 1969.

24. BLAIR, P. B. Search for cross-reacting antigenicity between MTV-induced mammary tumors and embryonic antigens: Effect of immunization on development of spontaneous mammary tumors. *Cancer Res.* **30**: 1199, 1970.

25. MORETTI, R. L. and BLAIR, P. B. The male histocompatibility antigen in mouse mammary tissue: I. Growth of the male mammary gland in female mice. *Transplantation* **4**: 596, 1966.

26. ATTIA, M. A., DEOME, K. B. and WEISS, D. W. Immunology of spontaneous mammary carcinomas in mice. II. Resistance to a rapidly and a slowly developing tumor. *Cancer Res.* **25**: 451, 1965.

27. DEZFULIAN, M., ZEE, T., DEOME, K. B., BLAIR, P. B. and WEISS, D. W. Role of the mammary tumor virus in the immunogenicity of spontaneous mammary carcinomas of BALB/c mice and in the responsiveness of the hosts. *Cancer Res.* **28**: 1759, 1968.

28. SUIT, H. D. and SILOBRCIC, V. Tumor specific antigen(s) in a spontaneous mammary carcinoma of C3H mice. II. Active immunization of MTA-free mice. *J. nat. Cancer Inst.* **39**: 1121, 1967.

29. BARRETT, M. K., DERINGER, M. K. and DUNN, T. B. Influence of the mammary tumor agent on the longevity of hosts bearing a transplanted tumor. *J. nat. Cancer Inst.* **13**: 109, 1952.

30. MUNDY, J. and WILLIAMS, P. C. Tumour incidence and tumour-free sublines in BR6 mice. *Brit. J. Cancer* **15**: 561, 1961.

31. NOWINSKI, R., BOYSE, E. A., OLD, L. J. and CARSWELL, E. A. Influence of mammary tumor virus infection on the acceptance or rejection of transplanted ML+ leukemias. *Proc. Soc. exp. Biol. (N.Y.)* **127**: 20, 1968.

32. HIRSCH, H. M., BITTNER, J. J., COLE, H. and IVERSEN, I. Can the inbred mouse be immunized against its own tumor? *Cancer Res.* **18**: 344, 1958.

33. KOLDOVSKY, P. The question of the universality of tumour antigen in isologous and homologous relationships. *Folia biol. (Praha)* **7**: 162, 1961.

34. MARTINEZ, C., AUST, J. B., BITTNER, J. J. and GOOD, R. A. Continuous growth of isotransplants of a mammary tumor associated with the development of immunity in mice. *Cancer Res.* **17**: 205, 1957.

35. RIGGINS, R. S. and PILCH, Y. H. Immunity to spontaneous and methylcholanthrene-induced tumors in inbred mice. *Cancer Res.* **24**: 1994, 1964.

36. MÜLLER, M. and WELKER, E. R. Akzeleration von Mammakarzinomtransplantaten bei CBA/ Bln-Mäusen durch Vorbehandlung mit kleinen Dosen vitaler isologer Tumorzellen. *Acta biol. med. germ.* **15**: 147, 1965.

37. ATTIA, M. A. and WEISS, D. W. Immunology of spontaneous mammary carcinomas in mice. V. Acquired tumor resistance and enhancement in strain A mice infected with mammary tumor virus. *Cancer Res.* **26**: 1787, 1966.

38. MARTINEZ, C., AUST, J. B. and BITTNER, J. J. Growth of an inbred stock mammary adenocarcinoma after transplantation at different times following prior inoculation. *Cancer Res.* **16**: 1023, 1956.

39. MÜLLER, M. and WELCKER, E. R. Wachstumsverzögerung und Akzeleration von Mammatumortransplantaten des Mäusestammes CBA/ Bln durch Vorbehandlung der Empfänger mit vitalen Tumorzellen oder Milch zweier Mäusestämme. *Acta biol. med. germ.* **16**: 558, 1966.

40. WEISS, D. W., FAULKIN, J. R. and DeOME, K. B. Acquisition of heightened resistance and susceptibility to spontaneous mouse mammary carcinomas in the original host. *Cancer Res.* **24**: 732, 1964.

41. NUTINI, L. G., PRINCE, J. E., DUARTE, A. G., JUHASZ, R. and COOK, E. S. Influence of tumor fractions on incidence of spontaneous mammary tumors in C3H/HeJ mice. *Proc. Soc. exp. Biol.* (*N.Y.*) **112**: 315, 1963.

42. HIRSCH, H. M. and IVERSEN, I. Accelerated development of spontaneous mammary tumors in mice pretreated with mammary tumor tissue and adjuvant. *Cancer Res.* **21**: 752, 1961.

43. VAAGE, J. and WEISS, D. W. Immunization against spontaneous and autografted mouse mammary carcinomas in the autochthonous C3H/Crgl mouse. *Cancer Res.* **29**: 1920, 1969.

44. MÜLLER, M. Immunologic interactions between isologous or F_1 hybrid hosts and spontaneous mammary tumors in CBA/Bln mice. *Cancer Res.* **27**: 2272, 1967.

45. HELLSTRÖM, I., HELLSTRÖM, K. E., EVANS, C. A., HEPPNER, G. H., PIERCE, G. E. and YANG, J. P. S. Serum-mediated protection of neoplastic cells from inhibition by lymphocytes immune to their tumor-specific antigens. *Proc. nat. Acad. Sci.* (*Wash.*) **62**: 362, 1969.

46. BLAIR, P. B., LAVRIN, D. H., DEZFULIAN, M. and WEISS, D. W. Immunology of the mouse mammary tumor virus (MTV): Identification *in vitro* of mouse antibodies against MTV. *Cancer Res.* **26**: 647, 1966.

47. BLAIR, P. B. Immunology of the mouse mammary tumor virus (MTV): Neutralization of MTV by mouse antiserum. *Cancer Res.* **28**: 148, 1968.

48. NOWINSKI, R. C., OLD, L. J., MOORE, D. H., GEERING, G. and BOYSE, E. A. A soluble antigen of the mammary tumor virus. *Virology* **31**: 1, 1967.

49. FINK, M. A., FELLER, W. F. and SIBAL, L. R. Methods for detection of antibody to the mammary tumor virus. *J. nat. Cancer Inst.* **41**: 1395, 1968.

50. BENTVELZEN, P., VAN DER GUGTEN, A., HILGERS, J. and DAAMS, J. H. Break-through in tolerance to eggborne mammary tumour viruses in mice, in: Severi, L. (Ed.), "Immunity and tolerance in oucogenesis." *Proc. Fourth Perugia Quadrennial International Conference on Cancer, 1969* (in press).

51. LEZHNEVA, O. M. A comparative study of the antigenic structure of the lactating mammary gland of high and low cancer strain mice. *Prob. Oncol.* (*N.Y.*) **7**: 62, 1961.

52. SIBAL, L. R., FELLER, W. F., FINK, M. A., KOHLER, B. E., HALL, W. T. and BOND, H. E. Mammary tumor virus antigen: sensitive immuno-assay. *Science* **164**: 76, 1969.

53. NANDI, S. New method for detection of mouse mammary tumor virus. II. Effect of administration of lactating mammary tissue extracts on incidence of hyperplastic mammary nodules in BALB/c Crgl mice. *J. nat. Cancer Inst.* **31**: 75, 1963.

54. VAN DER GUGTEN, A., DAAMS, J. H. and BENTVELZEN, P. Genetical resistance of inbred strain C57BL mice against mammary tumor inciting viruses. I. Immunological resistance. *Genetica* **38**: 402, 1968.

55. BLAIR, P. B. Immunology of the mouse mammary tumor virus (MTV): Comparison of the antigenicity of MTV obtained from several strains of mice. *Cancer Res.* **30**: 625, 1970.

56. TANAKA, H. and MOORE, D. H. Electron microscopic localization of viral antigens in mouse mammary tumors by ferritin-labeled antibody. 1. The homologous systems. *Virology* **33**: 197, 1967.

57. MOORE, D. H. Quantitative studies of bloodborne MTV-bio-activity. *Proc. Amer. Ass. Cancer Res.* **10**: 61, 1969.

58. STUCK, B., BOYSE, E. A., OLD, L. J. and CARSWELL, E. A. ML: A new antigen found in leukaemias and mammary tumors of the mouse. *Nature* (*Lond.*) **203**: 1033, 1964.

59. HOLMES, E. C. and MORTON, D. L. Detection of antibodies against the mammary tumor virus with the antiglobulin consumption test. *J. nat. Cancer Inst.* **42**: 733, 1969.

60. NISHIOKA, K., IRIE, R. F., INOUE, M., CHANG, S. and TAKEUCHI, S. Immunological studies on mouse mammary tumors. I. Induction of resistance to tumor isograft in C3H/He mice. *Int. J. Cancer* **4**: 121, 1969.

61. TAKEUCHI, S., IRIE, R. F., INOUE, M., IRIE, K., Izumi, R. and NISHIOKA, K. Immunological studies on mouse mammary tumors. II. Characterization of tumor-specific antibodies against mouse mammary tumors. *Int. J. Cancer* **4**: 130, 1969.

62. ANDERVONT, H. B. Susceptibility of young and of adult mice to the mammary-tumor agent. *J. nat. Cancer Inst.* **5**: 397, 1945.

63. BENTVELZEN, P. Resistance to small amounts of Bittner mammary tumor virus in offspring of female mice with the virus. *J. nat. Cancer Inst.* **41**: 757, 1968.

64. OLD, L. J. and BOYSE, E. A. Antigens of tumors and leukemias induced by viruses. *Fed. Proc.* **24**: 1009, 1965.

65. HABEL, K. The relationship between polyoma virus multiplication, immunologic competence, and resistance to tumor challenge in the mouse. *Ann. N.Y. Acad. Sci.* **101**: 173, 1962.

66. KLEIN, E. and KLEIN, G. Antibody response and leukemia development in mice inoculated neonatally with the Moloney virus. *Cancer Res.* **25**: 851, 1965.

67. MARTINEZ, C. Effect of early thymectomy on development of mammary tumors in mice. *Nature (Lond.)* **203**: 1188, 1964.

68. LAW, L. W. Studies of thymic function with emphasis on the role of the thymus in oncogenesis. *Cancer Res.* **26**: 551, 1966.

69. SQUARTINI, F., OLIVI, M. and BOLLIS, G. B. Thymic dependence of mouse mammary tumor virus and mouse mammary tumors, in: Severi, L. (Ed.), "Immunity and tolerance in oncogenesis." *Proc. Fourth Perugia Quadrennial International Conference on Cancer, 1969* (in press).

70. HEPPNER, G. H., WOOD, P. C. and WEISS, D. W. Studies on the role of the thymus in viral tumorigenesis. I. Effect of thymectomy on induction of hyperplastic alveolar nodules and mammary tumors in BALB/cfC3H mice. *Israel J. med. Sci.* **4**: 1195, 1968.

71. HEPPNER, G. H., WOOD, P. C. and WEISS, D. W. Studies on the role of the thymus in viral tumorigenesis. II. Effect of thymectomy on induction of hyperplastic alveolar nodules in BALB/c mice infected with mammary tumor virus at various ages. *Israel J. med. Sci.* **4**: 1204, 1968.

72. HEPPNER, G. H. Neonatal thymectomy and mouse mammary tumorigenesis, in: Severi, L. (Ed.), "Immunity and tolerance in oncogenesis." *Proc. Fourth Perugia Quadrennial International Conference on Cancer, 1969* (in press).

73. SAKAKURA, T. and NISHIZUKA, Y. Effect of thymectomy on mammary tumorigenesis, noduligenesis, and mammogenesis in the mouse. *Gann* **58**: 441, 1967.

74. YUNIS, E. J., MARTINEZ, C., SMITH, J., STUTMAN, O. and GOOD, R. A. Spontaneous mammary adenocarcinoma in mice: Influence of thymectomy and reconstitution with thymus grafts or spleen cells. *Cancer Res.* **29**: 174, 1969.

75. NISHIZUKA, Y. and SAKAKURA, T. Thymus and reproduction: sex-linked dysgenesia of the gonad after neonatal thymectomy in mice. *Science* **166**: 753, 1969.

76. BERN, H. A. and NANDI, S. Recent studies of the hormonal influence in mouse mammary tumorigenesis. *Progr. exp. Tumor Res. (Basel)* **2**: 90, 1961.

77. LAPPE, M. A. and BLAIR, P. B. Interference with mammary tumorigenesis by antilymphocyte serum. *Proc. Amer. Ass. Cancer Res.* **11**: 47, 1970.

78. PREHN, R. T. Influence of X irradiation and the milk agent on growth of transplanted mouse mammary tumors. *J. nat. Cancer Inst.* **43**: 1215, 1969.

79. FISHER, B., SOLIMAN, O. and FISHER, E. R. Effect of antilymphocyte serum on parameters of

80. WOODRUFF, M. and SMITH, L. H. Cytotoxic efficiency and effect on tumor growth of heterospecific antilymphocytic and antitumor sera. *Nature (Lond.)* **225**: 377, 1970.

81. DEOME, K. B. and NANDI, S. The mammary-tumor system in mice, a brief review, in: Burdette, W. J. (Ed.), "Viruses inducing cancer—implications for therapy." Salt Lake City, University of Utah Press, 1966, p. 127.

82. NANDI, S., HANDIN, M., ROBINSON, A., PITELKA, D. R. and WEBBER, L. E. Susceptibility of mammary tissues of "genetically resistant" strains of mice to mammary tumor virus. *J. nat. Cancer Inst.* **36**: 783, 1966.

83. ANDERVONT, H. B. and DUNN, T. B. Influences of heredity and the mammary tumor agent on the occurrence of mammary tumors in hybrid mice. *J. nat. Cancer Inst.* **14**: 317, 1953.

84. HAGEMAN, P. C., LINKS, J. and BENTVELZEN, P. Biological properties of B particles from C3H and C3Hf mouse milk. *J. nat. Cancer Inst.* **40**: 1319, 1968.

85. DEOME, K. B., YOUNG, L. and NANDI, S. Comparison of the behavior of nodule-inducing virus (NIV) in C3Hf (F) and BALB/c (C) mice. *Proc. Amer. Ass. Cancer Res.* **8**: 13, 1967.

86. MEDINA, D. Oncogenic agents in the neoplastic transformation in preneoplastic BALB/c nodule outgrowth lines. Ph.D. thesis, University of California, Berkeley, 1969.

87. BENTVELZEN, P. and DAAMS, J. H. Hereditary infections with mammary tumor viruses in mice. *J. nat. Cancer Inst.* **43**: 1025, 1969.

88. DAAMS, J. H., TIMMERMANS, A., VAN DER GUGTEN, A. and BENTVELZEN, P. Genetical resistance of inbred strain C57BL mice against mammary tumour inciting virus. II. Resistance by means of a repressed provirus. *Genetica* **38**: 400, 1968.

89. BENTVELZEN, P. "Genetical control of the vertical transmission of the Mühlbock mammary tumor virus in the GR mouse strain." Amsterdam, Hollandia Publ. House, 1968.

90. HAIRSTONE, M. A., SHEFFIELD, J. B. and MOORE, D. H. Study of B particles in the mammary tumors of different mouse strains. *J. nat. Cancer Inst.* **33**: 825, 1964.

91. BLAIR, P. B. Antigens of tumors and hyperplastic lesions induced by the mouse mammary tumor virus (MTV). Search for antigenic similarities and differences in hyperplastic and neoplastic mammary tissues induced by MTV derived from different strains of mice, in: Severi, L. (Ed.), "Immunity and tolerance in oncogenesis." *Proc Fourth Perugia Quadrennial International Conference on Cancer, 1969* (in press).

92. OLD, L. J., BOYSE, E. A. and STOCKERT, E. Typing of mouse leukemias by serological methods. *Nature (Lond.)* **201**: 777, 1964.

93. HARE, J. D. Transplant immunity to polyoma virus induced tumors. I. Correlations with biological properties of virus strains. *Proc. Soc. exp. Biol. (N.Y.)* **115**: 805, 1964.

94. BLAIR, P. B. Immunology of the mouse mammary tumor virus (MTV): A qualitative *in*

vitro assay for MTV. *Nature (Lond.)* **208**: 165, 1965.

95. NOWINSKI, R. C., OLD, L. J., BOYSE, E. A., DE HARVEN, E. and GEERING, G. Group-specific viral antigens in the milk and tissue of mice naturally infected with mammary tumor virus or Gross leukemia virus. *Virology* **34**: 617, 1968.

96. CINADER, B. Perspectives and prospects of immunotherapy. Autoantibodies and acquired immunological tolerance. *Canad. Cancer Conf.* **5**: 279, 1963.

STUDIES ON THE IMMUNOGENICITY OF PRENEOPLASTIC AND NEOPLASTIC MAMMARY TISSUES OF BALB/c MICE FREE OF THE MAMMARY TUMOR VIRUS

DAVID W. WEISS, ADA SULITZEANU, LARRY YOUNG,
MICHAEL ADELBERG and YORAM SEGEV*

Department of Immunology, Hebrew University–Hadassah Medical School, Jerusalem, Israel

ABSTRACT

A study was undertaken of the immunogenicity in isogenic animals of preneoplastic and neoplastic mammary tissues of BALB/c mice free of the mammary tumor virus. Three outgrowth lines of preneoplastic hyperplastic alveolar nodules which arose in old females subjected to hormonal hyperstimulation, and six tumors developing from these outgrowths, were tested. It was found that the transformed mammary tissues are immunogenic in isogenic hosts, despite absence from this host-parasite interaction of the viral agent usually associated with these transformations. Normal lactating mammary gland, and mixture of heart and kidney tissue fragments also elicited immunogenic effects manifested vis-à-vis challenge with the mammary carcinomas and preneoplastic tissues, and it is suggested that at least one of the immunogens detected here is an organ-specific antigen of wider distribution than mammary parenchyma only. Although heightened resistance was occasionally demonstrated in response to immunization, the more common effect was enhancement. Serum from the immunized mice could passively transfer to normal isogenic recipients either heightened resistance or enhanced susceptibility to challenge, depending on the time after termination of the immunizing experience at which the serum was derived. These findings are discussed in the light of the dynamic relationships between hosts and neoplastic cells in this and other models of neoplasia.

Recent communications from our laboratories have described the existence of strong surface antigens of spontaneous mammary carcinomas of mice infected with the mammary tumor virus (MTV) which are controlled by the presence or biological activities of the agent, and similar findings have been reported by other investigators (1–3). These immunogens are capable of eliciting significant degrees of heightened resistance against subsequent tumor implants in syngeneic hosts free of the virus, they are fully cross-reactive, and they are already expressed on MTV-infected preneoplastic and even normal mammary tissues.

---

* The experiments carried out by Yoram Segev are in partial fulfillment of the requirements for the M.D. degree.

187

It has also been observed that these tumors may in some instances act immunogenically in autochthonous and isogenic hosts which are infected with the MTV (2, 4–8), despite the presumed specific immunological tolerance of such animals (9, 10). In such infected isogenic mice, this antigenicity is cross-reactive in animals of some strains (5) but not in those of others (6). These observations point to the occurrence of a second category of mouse mammary tumor antigens, independent of the presence of the etiological virus. This impression has been confirmed recently by Heppner and Pierce, who, by means of the Hellström colony inhibition technique found evidence for two types of tumor associated antigens in mouse mammary carcinomas, one apparently distinct for each neoplasm and one, presumably virus-controlled, common to many (11). Further confirmation of an MTV-independent antigenicity comes from the observations of Morton et al. (12).

On the other hand, it is possible to interpret differently at least some of the experiments which have been considered as evidence for MTV-independent mammary tumor antigens. It is conceivable that immunization procedures can break a state of tolerance induced by neonatal exposure to the virus, and some immune responses against MTV antigens in such mice have indeed been demonstrated (13). The non-cross-reactivity of the immunogens of MTV (+) tumors in some MTV (+) hosts does argue for a virus-independent antigenicity, but it is not impossible that there exist in addition to the virus-controlled common antigen(s), antigenic determinants consequent to viral action but nonetheless specific for each neoplasm, or at least not frequently duplicated.

The question of the origins and biological nature of the antigenic configuration of cells is clearly of primary importance to the biologist and, in systems dealing with human host-foreign cell relationships or which serve as models of such relationships in man, to the clinician. The qualitative and quantitative manifestations of immunological reactivity depend not only on the chemical and physical nature of the antigens presented, but also on their relation to the structural specificities of the tissues of the reacting animal, and on the animal's present and preceding experiences with the same and with related chemical configurations. A clear understanding of the complement of antigenicities on the surface of target cells is thus requisite to an analysis of the multifaceted directions which the immune response against them may take. Such information is certainly vital to any attempt at manipulating immunological reactivity in a manner designed to affect in the most desirable way the host's stance vis-à-vis the alien cells—increased ability to destroy them where these are pathogenic, enhanced receptivity where they are beneficial, as in the case of restorative normal tissue transplants.

We have, therefore, continued our series of investigations into the nature of the immunogenicity of spontaneous mammary carcinomas of mice, a model of host-tumor interaction which, because of its very complexity, appears to us to be one of the most relevant examples of neoplasia in man. The present communication is concerned with experiments designed to demonstrate by direct means the existence of immunogens of these cancers entirely independent of the MTV. To this effect, we conducted transplantation experiments in the highly inbred BALB/cCrgl strain of mice, in which no etiologic viral agent for mammary neoplasia appears to be present.

MATERIALS AND METHODS

The techniques of continuous isogenicity testing throughout the course of the experiments; implantation and challenge with tumor fragments and viable tumor cell suspensions; mammary fat-pad clearing, implantation of outgrowths of preneoplastic hyperplastic alveolar nodules (HAN), and the gross and histological evaluation of their growth; and bleeding and serum preparation have all been detailed in the preceding series of reports on the immunology of mouse mammary tissues (4, 5, 9, 10, 14, 15).

The animals employed in the present experiments were mice of the BALB/cCrgl strain, bred and maintained in Jerusalem from a nucleus of breeding pairs generously made available by Dr. K. B. DeOme of the Cancer Research Genetics Laboratory (CRGL) of the University of California in Berkeley. The animals were used here during the first few generations of the establishment of the CRGL stock in Israel, and there was no indication of any changes in their isogenicity status with regard to the CRGL parent strain.

The mice were fed a diet of standard pellets and water ad lib., and were housed in groups of five to 10 in metal cages. They were ear-tagged for identification, and the investigator examining each mouse periodically for tumor development did not have before him the code identifying the different treatment groups.

Tumor volumes were calculated from the formula $V = 0.4 ab^2$, where a is the major and b the minor diameter bisecting the palpable tumor mass at right angles to each other, as described by Attia and Weiss (5).

The outgrowths of HAN (termed HOG) were all of the "D" series, and were obtained through the kindness of Dr. D. Medina of the CRGL; they were derived from primary nodules appearing in the mammary glands of aged BALB/c females which had been hormonally hyperstimulated for a prolonged period by means of daily injections of estradiol and simultaneous implantation of several pituitary isografts (16, 17). These outgrowths were maintained by serial passage in isogenic animals, and typical mammary adenocarcinomas appear within them with varying frequency. Several of these outgrowth lines themselves, and tumors appearing spontaneously from them, were studied in the present experiments.

As these tumors originated from HOG implants, and as the outgrowths themselves arose in animals subjected to extrinsic hormonal stimulation, the neoplasms could not be termed "spontaneous." However, in view of their large similarity to truly spontaneous mouse mammary carcinomas, including those which arise on infrequent occasions in MTV-free strains, and also in light of the fact that "natural" mammary carcinogenesis in the autochthonous animal is heavily influenced by similar, intrinsic hormonal factors, these cancers could be considered a reasonable

model of spontaneous mouse mammary neoplasia.

Results are described as significant only when $P < 0.05$, as by the appropriate parametric analyses detailed in the preceding communications.

RESULTS

Immunization studies with MTV-free BALB/c mammary carcinomas

To date, six tumors have been examined for immunogenic properties in isogenic hosts, and the experience with each will be summarized separately.

Tumor 1 (designated D1T5S): Young adult BALB/c females in groups of 20 each were given s.c. immunizing implants of 1 mm³ fragments of living tumor or living normal lactating mammary tissue, the latter derived from an isogenic nursing female. The tumor was here in the fourth transplant generation. A third group was given normal tail skin grafts, taken from the tumor donors. When the tumors reached an approximate size of 5 × 5 mm in a majority of the tumor-immunized group, after approximately four weeks, the growths were removed surgically from all the animals. At the same time, the fragments of lactating mammary gland (LMG) were removed from all animals of the second group in which the tissues could be found upon skin incision. The skin grafts from the control group were also excised at the same time. Ten days later the mice were bled, and their sera pooled by groups. Four days thereafter, they were challenged by s.c. injection into the left inguinal region of a freshly prepared suspension of 10^5 viable tumor cells, as indicated by the usual trypan-blue exclusion test. This challenge dose had been found in a preceding titration experiment to lead to progressive tumor development in approximately 50% of normal animals (TD_{50}). (In all subsequent experiments as well, in which challenge was with tumor cell suspensions, the number of cells was about 1 TD_{50} as determined by previous titration, unless stated otherwise.)

As is seen from Fig. 1, there was a pronounc-

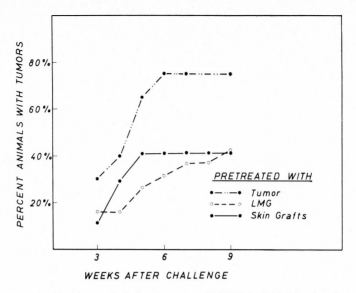

FIG. 1. Incidence of challenge tumors (D1T5S) in BALB/c females immunized prior to challenge with the tumor, isogenic LMG or isogenic normal skin grafts.

ed increase in the incidence of progressive tumors as a function of time after challenge in the tumor-immunized group.

This experiment was repeated, but with the tumor now in the ninth transplant generation, and with a challenge inoculum somewhat larger than 1 TD_{50}, 2×10^5 living cells. Under these conditions, there were no significant differences in tumor incidence between the differently pretreated groups, between 50 and 75% of the mice developing cancers. However, the growth rate of the cancers in the tumor and LMG immunized groups was moderately enhanced.

The pooled sera derived from the three groups 10 days after removal of the immunizing tissues were injected i.p. in 0.1 ml quantities to normal recipients (10 animals per group), 6 hr before these were challenged sc with 8.5×10^4 living tumor cells. Tumors appeared somewhat later and with a slightly lower incidence, in the mice given serum from the tumor bearers; the differences were not significant, however.

Tumor 2 (designated D2T3S): Groups of young adult BALB/c females were given s.c. immunizing implants (1 mm³) of the tumor, here in the eighth to ninth transplant generations, or of LMG, as in the preceding experiment. A third group was given 1 mm³ living implants of a mixture of heart and kidney fragments derived from the tumor donor, intended as a nonmammary tissue negative control, and a fourth group was injected with saline only. Fifteen to 34 animals were included in each group. One month after implantation, the tumors from all the animals were removed, as were the other immunizing tissues which could be detected. Nine days later, the mice were bled and their sera pooled, and eight days thereafter, they were challenged s.c. with tumor fragments of about 0.1 mm³ volume.

No differences were seen in the incidence rates of neoplasms which developed from the challenge inocula in the differently pretreated groups, more than half the animals in each giving rise to tumors. However, tumor devel-

190

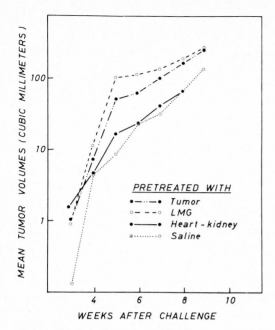

FIG. 2. Development of challenge tumors (D2T3S) in BALB/c females immunized prior to challenge with the tumor, isogenic LMG or isogenic heart-kidney fragments, or given saline only.

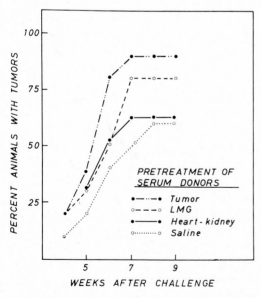

FIG. 3. Incidence of challenge tumors (D2T3S) in BALB/c females injected before challenge with sera from isogenic donors treated with the tumor, isogenic LMG, isogenic heart-kidney fragments or with saline only.

opment was enhanced in the animals pretreated with either the normal or neoplastic mammary tissue, as shown in Fig. 2.

In a passive transfer test with the sera, normal recipient females (10 mice per group) were given an intraperitoneal injection of 0.1 ml serum 6 hr before challenge, s.c., with 2.3×10^5 viable tumor cells. As shown in Fig. 3, the sera from the tumor and LMG groups appeared to increase the incidence of developing neoplasms.

In a similar passive transfer experiment, but employing 0.1 mm^3 tumor fragments instead of a cell suspension for challenge, no differences were observed in tumor incidence rates in the mice given the various sera, but the tumor-group serum again elicited an enhanced tumor growth rate as compared with serum from the saline control group. Serum from the heart-kidney group in this experiment also, surprisingly, acted as a growth enhancer, whereas serum from the LMG pretreated mice elicited no effect.

In a repeat active-immunization experiment with the same carcinoma, tumor-immunized mice developed tumors significantly sooner after challenge with 8×10^4 living cells than did the animals in the other two groups, pretreated, respectively, with LMG and heart-kidney fragments.

Tumor 3 (designated D7T4S): Groups of 18 to 32 young adult BALB/c females each were given immunizing implants (in this instance, of 0.1 mm^3 volume) of the tumor, LMG, or heart-kidney fragments or saline only. [Smaller immunizing implants were used in this and in several other experiments in view of observations that the development of enhancing immune factors may be favored by sensitization with neoplastic mammary tissue containing appreciable quantities of nonliving cells (Vaage, personal communication). It seemed appropriate, therefore, to determine whether reduction in the size of the immunizing stimulus would reduce the

191

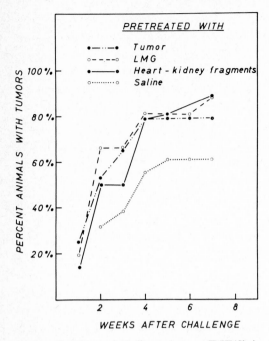

FIG. 4. Incidence of challenge tumors (D7T4S) in BALB/c females immunized prior to challenge with the tumor, isogenic LMG, or isogenic heart-kidney fragments, or given saline only.

likelihood of a resultant enhancement.] The tumor was in the second and third transplant generations. The immunizing tissues were removed 3.5 months later (this tumor grew very slowly in the first transplant generations), and the animals were bled four, 12, and 30 days thereafter. One week after the last bleeding, all the animals were challenged with 0.1 mm³ tumor fragments.

Pretreatment with tumor, as well as with LMG and heart-kidney fragments, resulted in an increased incidence of cancers arising from the challenge inocula within the observation period (Fig. 4).

Passive transfer experiments were then conducted, as described for the preceding experiments, with pooled sera taken at the three intervals after removal of the immunizing tissues. Each group of normal recipients consisted of 10 animals; the number of viable cells used for challenge was 1.4×10^6.

None of the sera obtained four days after excision of the immunizing tissues elicited a marked effect; there was a slight retardation in tumor development in the mice given serum from the heart-kidney pretreated donors. The second-bleeding sera behaved similarly: Those from the tumor and LMG treated animals exerted no effect, but serum from the heart-kidney group again exhibited some resistance-conferring properties, and now to a more pronounced extent. With the sera obtained at the third bleeding, a month after termination of the immunization experience, the picture was different (Fig. 5). The heart-kidney group serum was ineffective, whereas sera from both the tumor and LMG pretreated mice brought about an earlier appearance of the challenge growths.

The early humoral antibody response to

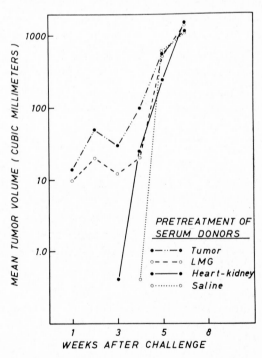

FIG. 5. Development of challenge tumors (D7T4S) in BALB/c females injected before challenge with sera from isogenic donors treated with the tumor, isogenic LMG, isogenic heart-kidney fragments or with saline only.

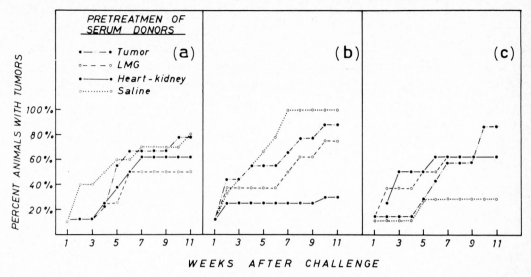

FIG. 6. Incidence of challenge tumors (D2aT2S) in BALB/c females injected before challenge with sera from isogenic donors treated with the tumor, isogenic LMG, isogenic heart-kidney fragments or with saline only. a) Sera derived from donors four days after termination of the immunizing experience; b) sera derived from donors 12 days after termination of the immunizing experience; c) sera derived from donors 28 days after termination of the immunizing experience.

most antigens is predominantly IgM, and IgG antibodies appear in quantities only after an interval of some days to weeks. Antigens presented as constituents of intact cells may be especially likely to favor and prolong the macroglobulin response, and 7S antibodies may indeed not appear in large numbers until removal of the immunizing tissue, which can also act to depress specific responsiveness. Enhancing activity is associated exclusively, or largely, with IgG antibodies, and the present observation of enhancement elicited only with the late serum is thus compatible with the likely dynamics of the production of resistance and enhancement factors towards the same cellular antigen.

The bimodality of serum effects, depending on the time elapsed between excision of the immunizing tissues and obtaining of the serum, is further demonstrated in the following experiment.

Tumor 4 (designated D2aT2S): Groups of young adult BALB/c males, 22 to 32 each, were immunized with 0.1 mm³ fragments of the tumor, LMG, heart-kidney or saline only. The tumor was here in the seventh and eighth transplant generations. The immunizing tissues were removed after two months, and the animals bled four, 12 and 28 days later. The sera from each group were pooled. Five days after the last bleeding, the animals were challenged with 0.1 mm³ tumor fragments.

There were no significant differences between the groups in the incidence of developing tumors appearing at different times after challenge, and only a slight indication of enhanced tumor growth rate in the tumor-immunized mice.

The passive transfer trials were performed with normal female recipients, eight to 10 per group, as described in the previous experiments. Challenge was with 10^6 viable cells.

No significant effect on tumor incidence rate was elicited by any of the sera obtained in the first bleeding after termination of immunization (Fig. 6a), but the sera from all

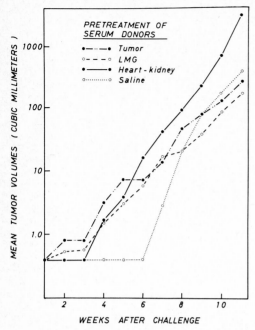

FIG. 7. Development of challenge tumors (D2aT2S) in BALB/c females injected before challenge with sera derived from isogenic donors 28 days after termination of their immunizing experience with the tumor, isogenic LMG, isogenic heart-kidney fragments or with saline only.

three tissue-pretreated groups slightly retarded tumor appearance; the heart-kidney group serum bestowed significant resistance at the second bleeding (Fig. 6b); and third-bleeding sera from all three groups—tumor, LMG, and heart-kidney—appeared to transfer enhancement (here, fewer viable cells were apparently contained in the challenge inoculum, as evident from the low incidence of tumors in the mice injected with serum from the saline control group). The data on tumor growth rates were very similar. The first-bleeding tumor-group serum exhibited a slight resistance effect; all the tissue-group sera showed some resistance properties at the second bleeding; and all three sera elicited enhancement (i.e., earlier appearance of palpable growths), at the last bleeding (Fig. 7).

It appears from the above experiments that the immune response to these MTV (–) mammary carcinomas is more usually manifested by enhancement. That this is not always the case, and that the nature of the response may be affected importantly by changes in the immunization experience, is indicated by the following experiments.

Tumor 5 (designated D2T8S): Groups of 24 to 30 young adult BALB/c females each were immunized by implantation of 0.1 mm³ fragments of the tumor, LMG, heart-kidney or saline only. The tumor was here in its first transplant generation. The immunizing tissues were removed after four months (this tumor also grew very slowly in the first transplant generations). One month later, the animals were challenged with 0.1 mm³ living tumor pieces. (In the interval between the removal of the immunizing tissues and challenge, the mice were bled several times, but data are not yet available on passive transfer studies with these sera.)

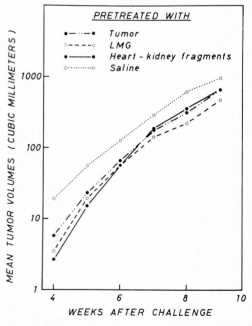

FIG. 8. Development of challenge tumors (D2T8S) in BALB/c females immunized prior to challenge with the tumor, isogenic LMG or isogenic heart-kidney fragments, or given saline only.

TABLE 1. *Incidence of challenge tumors (D8T3S) in BALB/c males and females immunized prior to challenge with the tumor, isogenic LMG, or isogenic heart-kidney fragments*

| Immunizing tissue | Tumor incidence at following weeks after challenge (%) | | | | | | | | | | | |
| | 3 | | | | 4 | | | | 5 | | | |
	Male	P	Female	P	Male	P	Female	P	Male	P	Female	P
Tumor (D8T3S)	62	NS	73	< 0.01	66	NS	73	< 0.05	66	NS	85	0.005
LMG	47	NS	60	NS	68	NS	60	NS	68	NS	65	< 0.1
Heart-kidney	64	—	35	—	71	—	35	—	78	—	35	—

NS = Not significant

Pretreatment with LMG, but not with tumor or heart-kidney, reduced slightly the incidence of developing tumors; treatment with all three of the tissues effected a slight degree of retardation of tumor development (Fig. 8).

Tumor 6 (designated D8T3S): Groups of 10 to 25 young adult male and female BALB/c mice each were immunized with 1 mm³ fragments of the tumor, LMG or heart-kidney. The tumor was here in the ninth and tenth transplant generations. One month later, the immunizing tissues were excised, and three weeks afterwards all the animals were challenged with 1 mm³ pieces of living tumor tissue.

As appears from Table 1, immunization with tumor resulted in a significant degree of enhancement in the females, as indicated by the larger proportion of animals developing neoplasms after challenge than in the heart-kidney pretreated group; no effect was evident in the male animals.

In another experiment with the same tumor, here in the fifth and sixth transplant generations, groups of 13 to 18 young adult males were given an immunizing implant of the tumor or of LMG, or a graft of tail skin from either the tumor bearer or from normal isogenic males (no differences were detected between these two skin graft groups, and they were therefore considered as one for purposes

of analysis). Two weeks later, the animals were challenged with about 10⁵ living tumor cells. This inoculum failed to give rise to progressively growing neoplasms in the great majority of the animals, and, accordingly, the mice were challenged a month later with tumor fragments (1 mm³). Thus, the first, abortive challenge constituted a second immunizing experience, with living tumor tissue, of the animals in all three groups.

As seen from Table 2, there was a significantly lower incidence of challenge tumors (the few animals which did give rise to tumors from the first challenge are excluded from the calculations) in the group pretreated with LMG plus tumor cells, and a nearly significant decrease in tumor incidence among the

TABLE 2. *Incidence of challenge tumors (D8T3S) in BALB/c males immunized prior to challenge with the tumor, isogenic LMG or isogenic skin grafts*

Immunizing tissue	Tumor incidence 2 months after challenge (%)	P
Tumor (D8T3S) + tumor cells	31	< 0.1
LMG + tumor cells	11	< 0.005
Skin grafts + tumor cells	64	—

All three groups of animals were challenged a first time with a suspension of 10⁵ tumor cells, which failed to give rise to tumors in most of the mice; the animals were therefore challenged a second time, one month later, with tumor fragments.

195

mice which had experienced tumor plus tumor. It thus appears that a second immunizing stimulus, with tumor, superimposed on a primary one of tumor or LMG, can elicit resistance against a mammary carcinoma under conditions where a single immunizing stimulus alone provoked no discernible response, or one manifested by enhancement.

Immunization studies with MTV-free outgrowths of preneoplastic hyperplastic alveolar nodules

The following experimental scheme was followed: The no. 4 mammary fat pads of 21-day-old female BALB/c mice were cleared. When the animals reached six to 10 weeks of age, 0.1 to 0.5 mm³ fragments of tissue were implanted in one of the cleared pads. One experiment was conducted with each of the HOG D1, D2 and D7, and in each experiment, LMG and heart-kidney immunization groups were included.

In order to heighten the immunizing stimulus [the mammary gland of mice represents an immunologically privileged site (18)], tissue fragments were simultaneously also placed s.c. in the inguinal region. Six weeks later, the fat pads containing the immunizing tissues were excised, and at the same time the s.c. placed fragments were removed, where these could be found. Two weeks later, the animals were bled (data on serum activity will be presented elsewhere), and one week thereafter the mice were challenged. Challenge was by implantation into the contralateral cleared fat pad of either the same or one of the other HOG. Each challenge group consisted of 10 to 20 animals. After 6 weeks, the fat pads containing the challenge HOG were excised, stained and preserved. The extent of occupancy of the pads by the challenge HOG was determined visually, by use of a dissecting microscope, and observations on the gross morphology of the tissues were recorded. Estimation of the percent occupancy of the

TABLE 3. *Development o outgrowths of hyperplastic alveolar nodules (HOG) in BALB/c females immunized prior to outgrowth challenge with HOG tissue, isogenic LMG or isogenic heart-kidney fragments*

Immunizing tissue	% of fat-pad filled with HAN-HOG challenge tissue		
	Median	Mean	P
Experiment A: HOG D2			
HOG-D1	30	35	NS
LMG	50	55	0.02
Heart-kidney	40	42	—
Experiment B: HOG D2			
HOG-D7	47	45	NS
LMG	30	39	< 0.05
Heart-kidney	60	52	—
Experiment C: HOG D1			
HOG-D2	20	27	< 0.02
LMG	30	42	NS
Heart kidney	60	50	—

NS = not significant.

pads was confirmed by at least two workers, who did not know the origin of the pads under examination.

This is obviously a very gross means of estimating the occurrence of an immune response against the challenging HOG tissues, and especially in view of the unfortunate fact that this tissue can be implanted only into the mammary fat pad, an immunologically privileged or at least partially privileged locality. Low degrees of responsiveness are therefore very likely to be obscured. Nonetheless, immunization with one of the HOG tested (D2) and with LMG resulted in a significant effect against at least two of the three corresponding HOG challenges (Table 3).

It is seen from Experiments A and B in Table 3 that LMG in one instance induced a slight but significant degree of enhanced growth of the challenge HOG-D2 tissue, and in a second elicited the opposite effect. These experiments were conducted at different times, and undoubtedly unappreciated variables affected the host-tumor interactions. It would appear, nonetheless, that experimental parameters other than those usually taken into consideration, or intrinsic changes in the host and tumor cell populations, can result in opposite manifestations of reactivity vis-à-vis the same target.

In both of these experiments, the immunizing HOG tissues D1 and D7 failed to evoke a significant effect. In contrast, immunization with HOG-D2 bestowed a significant degree of resistance against challenge with HOG-D1 (Experiment C), although in the same experiment this immunizing tissue failed to elicit an effect against the corresponding challenge (not shown in Table 3). It is also to be noted that immunization with HOG-D1 was ineffective not only against HOG-D2 (Experiment A), but also against challenge with the other HOG (not shown in Table 3).

In these experiments, immunization with heart-kidney fragments was considered as representing the base-line control, the above described tumor immunization studies being still in progress when analysis of HOG immunogenicity was begun. The findings from the tumor experiments indicate that heart-kidney immunization may not, in effect, constitute a negative control treatment, and the HOG work must therefore be repeated with saline, or perhaps normal skin graft, control groups to provide a more correct basis for comparison.

That experience with LMG and with at least some of the HOG tissues constitutes an immunizing stimulus directed towards HOG challenge is nonetheless indicated by the present observations, and also by the morphological appearance of the HOG tissues in the pretreated animals. In normal BALB/c hosts of the same age, the D2 HOG appeared as a rather typical lobular-alveolar tissue, thickly occupying the mammary fat pad. In contrast, HOG-D2 growing in the pads of animals previously exposed to any of the HOG was grossly abnormal in most, though not in all,

hosts: The fat pads were filled with a poorly organized, heterogenous growth in which ductile elements and grossly swollen, bloated and cystic areas could be seen prominently. Foci of inflammation were prominent within the area of growth. [A ductile tendency of hyperplastic alveolar outgrowths of nodules induced by the MTV or by carcinogens has been associated by several investigators with the occurrence of an active immune response (10 and G. Slemmer, personal communication).] The HOG-D2 challenge tissue growing in mice pretreated with LMG or heart-kidney showed similar abnormalities, but less frequently so, and to a lesser extent.

A tendency towards ductile development was also seen in HOG-D1 growing in hosts pretreated with LMG or heart-kidney, but not in the animals pretreated with any of the HOG, in whom the appearance of the D1 outgrowth was as normally lobular-alveolar as it was in untreated normal mice. As was seen in Table 3 (Experiment C), immunization with HOG-D2 bestowed a significant degree of resistance against challenge with HOG-D1, and it may be, therefore, that reduced growth and abnormal growth are alternative manifestations of the consequences of HOG immunization against HOG-D1 challenge, or that different antigens are responsible for the different effects.

Some of the challenge tissue fat pads of the animals tested with HOG-D7 still await examination, but it seems that in this case, too, pretreatment with HOG-D1 or with heart-kidney resulted in considerable abnormalcy in the morphology of this outgrowth as compared with its characteristics in untreated mice.

The details of these morphological observations, including the results of histological examination, will be presented at a later date. Even this brief description suffices, however, to indicate the prominent presence of structural manifestations of the responsiveness to a first experience with these preneoplastic tissues.

Further work is necessary to prove the immunological nature of this responsiveness, but the assumption that this is the case would appear to be reasonable. In this event, the present findings would point to the existence of a surface antigen(s) on cells of HOG-D2 which are also expressed on cells of HOG-D1 and on normal LMG cells, and thus would appear to fall within the category of organ-associated antigens; this antigen(s) may not, however, be truly organ-specific in that it may be expressed as well in other tissues, such as heart and kidney. HOG-D1 would then appear to possess this antigen in a less actively immunogenic form (Table 3, Experiment A) than HOG-D2.

DISCUSSION AND SPECULATION

A number of transplantation experiments were conducted with MTV-free mammary carcinomas and HAN outgrowth tissues of uninfected BALB/c mice, with the aim of determining whether the preneoplastic and neoplastic transformations of mammary parenchyma of mice are accompanied by antigenic changes even in the absence of the virus. The underlying assumption of these studies was that heightened resistance or enhancement towards challenge tissues, as demonstrated in active immunization and serum passive transfer experiments, could be correctly ascribed to immunological reactions; a large portion of all recent studies in transplantation immunology indeed proceed from this assumption. It should be remarked at the outset, however, that it is not inconceivable that changes in the host's stance towards implanted tissues can also arise from a variety of physiological, nonimmunological alterations induced by a primary experience with such tissues. This possibility seems the less remote when immunization and challenge is with cells very reactive hormonally, as in the present case. Although these findings are discussed in an immunological frame of reference, it must be remembered, therefore, that more rigorous proof than here presented is necessary to show beyond a doubt that immunological reactions are exclusively, or primarily, responsible.

The three salient points which emerge from the present observations are the following: Neoplastic and preneoplastic mammary tissues not infected with the viral agent usually associated with these transformations are nonetheless immunogenic in isogenic hosts. Second, at least one of these MTV-independent antigens is strongly expressed in normal lactating mammary gland, and is expressed apparently also in at least some other organs (heart and kidney were tested here, always in a mixture of tissue fragments). Third, the immune responses elicited by a primary exposure to the transformed and normal mammary tissue and, frequently, to heart-kidney cells as well, are much more usually manifested by enhancement than by heightened resistance. This was true even when immunization was with relatively small quantities of freshly obtained living tissue, suggesting that induction of enhancement was an intrinsic property of these cells and could not be ascribed to a sensitizing stimulus of large amounts of dead tissue.

It would appear, therefore, that an organ-associated antigen of wider distribution than mammary parenchyma only is strongly expressed on mammary tumor and HAN-HOG cells not infected with MTV. A similar observation has been reported by Müller (19), who found that enhancing antibodies elicited in mice by immunization with spontaneous, MTV(+) mammary carcinomas could be absorbed with cells from a variety of tissues, including kidney.

The alternative interpretation, that heart-kidney, and perhaps LMG also, elicit entirely nonspecific effects, seems unlikely: Both enhancement and resistance could be transferred passively with serum, depending on when it was derived in relation to the immunizing experience; and, an implantation procedure as such does not affect the growth of subsequent mammary challenge tissues, as evident from the failure of skin transplants in these and many of the earlier experiments to induce such changes.

Mammary neoplasia in mice is very much more frequent in animals infected pre- or neonatally with the MTV or one of its variants than in those uninfected, and the present system may thus be in a sense artificial. The question arises whether the organ-associated, and perhaps other, antigen(s) here detected are at all expressed on the "natural," MTV-infected mammary neoplasms, and if so, whether they are identical with the seemingly MTV-independent antigens of infected mammary cancers previously reported (6, 7). Müller's observations indicate an affirmative answer to the second question, but further work is necessary to clarify these antigenic relationships.

A more fundamental question presented by these observations pertains to the possibly causal connection between the presence of organ-specific or organ-associated immunogens on the surface of a cell, and a particular predilection by such cells to induce a specific immune response manifested by enhancement. Do such antigens perhaps have a uniquely marked capacity for stimulating, in autochthonous and isogenic animals, reactions leading to enhancement? The evolution on the surface of auto-antigenic cells of special configurations which can modulate immunological recognition in the direction of enhancement would obviously have major import in facilitating the peaceful integrity of organisms consisting of multiple, potentially self-sensitizing tissues. The dominant appearance of such antigenic determinants on the surface of autochthonous neoplastic cells

would have clear survival value for them, and would constitute a classic instance of preemption by a population of parasites of a mechanism normally contributory to the existence of the host, but now accruing to the benefit of the former and detriment of the latter.

In allogeneic and xenogeneic animals, these postulated special configurations may be relatively too insignificant to alter the immune manifestations which tend, when evoked by alien living tissue, to be predominantly in the direction of resistance. This discussion is, of course, still purely speculative, but it has the virtue of being susceptible to experimental approaches.

If the category of antigen(s) here detected is at least potentially capable of being expressed on the surface of MTV-infected cells as well, the possibility of competition for phenotypic appearance of different groups of antigens becomes very real. Here, again, the neoplastic variant would obviously gain by any ability to modulate such competition in the direction of those antigens which stimulate immune responses not destructive to the cell. The occurrence of such competition could well explain why only a fraction of MTV(+) mammary tumors of some strains appear to possess MTV-independent antigens (2, 6), and why in others (5) this is a much more common phenomenon.

A more practical consideration posed by the present data is whether a pronounced tendency to the induction of enhancement can be overcome by treating the host with those nonspecific immunological stimulators, such as the methanol extraction residue fraction of attenuated tubercle bacilli (2, 20, 21), which seem to channel subsequent immune responses strongly towards 19S antibody (22–24) and cellular reactivity (Kuperman and Weiss, in preparation). Experiments in this direction are in progress, in collaboration with E. Robinson and T. Mekori of Rambam Hospital in Haifa.

The observation that serum from tissue-immunized donors could elicit either enhancement or resistance in normal recipients, depending on when after primary sensitization it was obtained, is consistent with related findings by other investigators (19), and underlines the complexity of the consequences of the immune reaction to antigenic cells.

The seemingly lesser immunogenicity of the preneoplastic than of the neoplastic tissues here studied could have resulted from the unfavorable technical circumstances for demonstrating immune reactions to the HAN-HOG. On the other hand, it is possible that there may be a progressive increase in the expression of the responsible MTV-independent antigens from normal mammary parenchyma to fully malignant variants. It could be imagined that the latter, growing beyond the confines of the immunologically privileged mammary glands, would be the most dependent on a covering of enhancement-inducing antigenic markers. Might it indeed be conceivable that realization of the degree of neoplastic potential is to some extent a function of the quantitative expression of such immunogens?

The immunogenicity displayed by MTV-free mammary carcinomas and HOG in MTV(–) isogenic hosts appeared to be weak in relation to that of MTV-containing transformed mammary tissues in uninfected test animals. This observation, too, is consistent with a predominance of organ-associated antigens among these surface immunogens, organ-specific determinants being generally weak immunologic stimuli in the autochthonous and isogenic host. Nonetheless, the present results show that the MTV is not a necessary factor in the demonstrable immunogenicity of neoplastic and preneoplastic mammary tissues of the mouse.

The senior author expresses his gratitude to his mentor and former colleague, Professor K. B. DeOme, for his continued interest and stimulating suggestions and counsel. The authors state their appreciation to Dr. Margaret Kripke for her constructive advice throughout the course of these studies.

Supported by grants from Concern Foundation of Los Angeles; the Leukemia Research Foundation, Inc.; the Damon Runyon Memorial Fund, Inc.; the Medical Division of the American Friends of Hebrew University in Los Angeles; and the Samuel Lautenberg and Celia Sievitz Fellowships.

REFERENCES

1. DEZFULIAN, M., LAVRIN, D. H., SHEN, A., BLAIR, P. B. and WEISS, D. W. Immunology of spontaneous mammary carcinomas in mice. Studies on the nature of the protective antigens, in: "Carcinogenesis: A broad critique." Baltimore, Williams and Wilkins, 1967, p. 365.
2. WEISS, D. W. Immunological parameters of the host-parasite relationship in neoplasia. Ann. N. Y. Acad. Sci. 164: 431, 1969.
3. WEISS, D. W. Immunological parameters of host-tumor relationships: Spontaneous mammary neoplasia of the inbred mouse as a model. Cancer Res. 29: 2368, 1969.
4. WEISS, D. W., FAULKIN, L. J., JR. and DEOME, K. B. Acquisition of heightened resistance and susceptibility to spontaneous mouse mammary carcinomas in the original host. Cancer Res. 24: 732, 1964.
5. ATTIA, M. A. M. and WEISS, D. W. Immunology of spontaneous mammary carcinomas in mice. V. Acquired tumor resistance and enhancement in strain A mice infected with mammary tumor virus. Cancer Res. 26: 1787, 1966.
6. VAAGE, J. Non-virus-associated antigens in virus-induced mouse mammary tumors. Cancer Res. 28: 2477, 1968.
7. VAAGE, J., KALINOVSKY, T. and OLSON, R. Antigenic differences among virus-induced mouse mammary tumors arising spontaneously in the same C3H/Crgl host. Cancer Res. 29: 1452, 1969.
8. VAAGE, J. and WEISS, D. W. Immunization against spontaneous and autografted mouse mammary carcinomas in the autochthonous C3H/Crgl mouse. Cancer Res. 29: 1920, 1969.
9. LAVRIN, D. H., BLAIR, P. B. and WEISS, D. W. Immunology of spontaneous mammary carcinomas in mice. III. Immunogenicity of C3H preneoplastic hyperplastic alveolar nodules in C3Hf hosts. Cancer Res. 26: 293, 1966.
10. LAVRIN, D. H., BLAIR, P. B. and WEISS, D. W. Immunology of spontaneous mammary carcinomas in mice. IV. Association of the mammary tumor virus with the immunogenicity of C3H nodules and tumors. Cancer Res. 26: 929, 1966.
11. HEPPNER, G. and PIERCE, G. In vitro demonstration of tumor-specific antigens in spontaneous mammary tumors of mice. Int. J. Cancer 4: 212, 1969.
12. MORTON, D. L., MILLER, G. F. and WOOD, D. A. Demonstration of tumor specific immunity against antigens unrelated to the mammary tumor virus in spontaneous mammary adenocarcinomas. J. nat. Cancer Inst. 42: 289, 1969.

13. BLAIR, P. B., LAVRIN, D. H. DEZFULIAN, M. and WEISS, D. W. Immunology of the mouse mammary tumor virus (MTV): Identification *in vitro* of mouse antibodies against MTV. *Cancer Res.* **26**: 647, 1966.

14. ATTIA, M. A., DEOME, K. B. and WEISS, D. W. Immunology of spontaneous mammary carcinomas in mice. II. Resistance to a rapidly and a slowly developing tumor. *Cancer Res.* **25**: 451, 1965.

15. DEZFULIAN, M., ZEE, T., DEOME, K. B., BLAIR, P. B. and WEISS, D. W. Role of the mammary tumor virus in the immunogenicity of spontaneous mammary carcinomas of BALB/c mice and in the responsiveness of the hosts. *Cancer Res.* **28**: 1759, 1968.

16. MEDINA, D. and DEOME, K. B. Influence of mammary tumor virus on the tumor-producing capabilities of nodule outgrowths free of mammary tumor virus. *J. nat. Cancer Inst.* **40**: 1303, 1968.

17. MEDINA, D. and DEOME, K. B. Carcinogen-induced mammary tumors from preneoplastic nodule outgrowths in BALB/c mice. *Cancer Res.* **30**: 1055, 1970.

18. BLAIR, P. B. and MORETTI, R. L. The mammary fat pad as a privileged transplantation site. *Transplantation* **5**: 542, 1967.

19. MÜLLER, M. Immunologic interactions between isologous or F_1 hybrid hosts and spontaneous mammary tumors in CBA/Bln mice. *Cancer Res.* **27**: 2272, 1967.

20. WEISS, D. W., BONHAG, R. and LESLIE, P. Studies on the heterologous immunogenicity of a methanol-insoluble fraction of attenuated tubercle bacilli (BCG). II. Protection against tumor isografts. *J. exp. Med.* **124**: 1039, 1966.

21. WEISS, D. W. Immunology of spontaneous tumors, in: Lecam, L. and Neyman, J. (Eds.), "Proceedings of the Fifth Berkeley Symposium on Mathematical Statistics and Probability." Berkeley, University of California Press, 1967, p. 657.

22. STEINKULLER, C. G., KRIGBAUM, L. G. and WEISS, D. W. Studies on the mode of action of the heterologous immunogenicity of a methanol-insoluble fraction of attenuated tubercle bacilli (BCG). *Immunology* **16**: 255, 1969.

23. YASHPHE, D. and WEISS, D. W. Modulation of the immune response by a methanol-insoluble fraction of attenuated tubercle bacilli (BCG). Primary and secondary responses to sheep red blood cells and T2 phage. *Clin. exp. Immunol.* **7**: 269, 1970.

24. YASHPHE, D., STEINKULLER, C. and WEISS, D. W. Modulation of immunological responsiveness by pretreatment with a methanol-insoluble fraction of killed tubercle bacilli. *Israel J. med. Sci.* **5**: 259, 1969.

PROLIFERATION OF MACROPHAGE AND GRANULOCYTE PRECURSORS IN RESPONSE TO PRIMARY AND TRANSPLANTED TUMORS

A. D. HIBBERD and D. METCALF

Cancer Research Unit, Walter and Eliza Hall Institute, Melbourne, Australia

ABSTRACT

The *in vitro* agar culture system for growing hemopoietic colonies has been used to determine levels of macrophage and granulocyte precursors in the bone marrow and spleen of mice with primary and transplanted tumors. The tumor-bearing state generally resulted in an increased number of precursors in the bone marrow, and particularly in the spleen. Consistent rises were also observed in blood monocytes and granulocytes and in the serum level of the factor stimulating bone marrow colony growth *in vitro*. The proliferation of these precursor cells in response to tumors may represent an important component of the immune response to tumor cells.

INTRODUCTION

There is clear evidence that host animals can respond immunologically to antigenically-distinct tumor cells, particularly those induced by viruses and chemical carcinogens. Such responses are primarily mediated by specific lymphoid and plasma cells. Granulocytes and macrophages are not normally considered as components of a specific immune response, yet their presence at sites of immunological reaction suggests that these cells are also involved (even if nonspecifically) in the mediation of immune responses.

The precursor cells of granulocytes and macrophages in the bone marrow and spleen can proliferate in semi-solid agar cultures forming colonies of granulocytes, macrophages or mixtures of both cell types (1–3). These precursor cells are referred to as *in vitro* colony-forming cells (CFC). Colony formation *in vitro* requires the constant presence of a factor known as the colony stimulating factor (CSF) (4, 5) and the number of colonies developing is related to the concentration of CSF (6). The agar culture system thus allows the precise enumeration of precursors of granulocytes and macrophages in a tissue, or alternatively, allows the titration of CSF levels in various biological fluids.

CSF is detectable in the serum and urine of normal mice (4, 7) and humans (8, 9 and S. H. Chan, unpublished data), and may function as a normal regulator of granulocyte and monocyte production (10). CSF levels have been shown to be elevated in the serum of mice (4, 7) and humans (11) with various types of leukemia and acute infections.

It has been shown that *in vitro* CFC proliferate in the spleen and bone marrow following stimulation by a variety of antigens, e.g. pertussis (10), polymerized flagellin and sheep red cells (12) and in GVH reactions (A. D. Hibberd, unpublished data). The present study was undertaken to determine the response of *in vitro* CFC in mice to primary or transplanted syngeneic tumors and to determine the effect of tumor growth on CSF levels.

MATERIALS AND METHODS

The mice used were of the inbred strains AKR, BALB/c, C3H, CBA, C57BL 129/J and the F_1 hybrids (NZB $\times$ C57BL)F_1 and (BALB/c $\times$ C57BL)F_1. The transplantable tumors were kindly supplied by Dr. N. Warner of the Immunogenetics Laboratory. Dispersed suspensions of tumor cells in Eisen's solution were prepared by passing the tumor tissue through a stainless steel sieve.

The agar culture technique for mouse bone marrow cells and spleen cells and the composition of the agar-Eagle's medium have been described elsewhere (4, 7). Dispersed cell suspensions of bone marrow or spleen being assayed for CFC content were cultured in replicate 35 mm plastic Petri dishes (Falcon Plastics, Los Angeles) using 50,000 bone marrow and 100,000 spleen cells in 1 ml cultures. For stimulation of colony formation, the CSF used was 0.15 ml per culture of a human urine concentrate prepared according to the techniques described elsewhere (9). This was mixed with the agar-medium containing the cell suspension before gelling occurred. Cultures were incubated for seven days in a humidified atmosphere of 10% CO_2 in air, and the colonies were scored at $\times$ 25 magnifications using a dissecting microscope. In each assay run, control cultures of pooled three-month-old normal C57BL bone marrow cells were included. Colony counts on these control cultures were related to a standard value of $100/10^5$ C57BL bone marrow cells to determine the standardization ratio for individual assay runs. The CFC estimates from experimental animals assayed on different days were standardized by using this ratio. For cytological examination, colonies were removed using a fine pipette and stained with 0.6% orcein in 60% acetic acid, classifying colony cells according to the criteria described elsewhere (3).

All sera were ether-extracted to remove lipoidal inhibitory material (13) before assay for colony stimulating activity. Sera were assayed in duplicate cultures of 75,000 C57BL bone marrow cells at two dose levels, 0.1 and 0.05 ml and the colony stimulating activity expresses the mean number of colonies stimulated by 0.1 or 0.05 ml of serum, after standardization of colony counts against a standard pool of C57BL serum used in each assay run.

RESULTS

Response of in vitro *CFC and serum CSF in mice with primary lymphoid leukemia.* A survey was made of AKR mice with spontaneous lymphoid leukemia, measuring blood white cell levels, the femur content of *in vitro* CFC, and serum levels of CSF. The results (Table 1) indicated that almost all of the AKR mice with lymphoid leukemia exhibited elevated granulocyte and monocyte levels. In individual animals, there was no correlation between either total tumor mass or levels of leukemic cells in the blood and the degree of elevation of granulocyte and monocyte levels.

In parallel studies, an analysis was made of labeling patterns in the white cells of normal and leukemic AKR mice following pulse labeling with tritiated thymidine. The data (Table 2) indicated that the rise in the percentage of labeled polymorphs in the blood equalled or exceeded that in normal mice, and similar data were obtained for blood monocytes. These results indicate that the high blood levels of granulocytes and monocytes are likely to be due to an increased production, rather than to a prolonged intravascular life span of these cells.

The femur content of *in vitro* CFC was highly variable in the leukemic mice. Although the mean levels were approximately the same as in normal AKR mice, five of the 27 leukemic mice examined had elevated levels, and, in contrast, 14 of the 27 had levels below the lower limit in normal mice. The cellular composition in the marrow of leukemic animals may vary significantly from one bone marrow sample to another in the same animal, since

203

TABLE 1. *Effect of lymphoid leukemia development on white cell levels, bone marrow CFC and serum colony stimulating activity*

| Type | No. of animals | Mean tumor mass (mg) | Mean white cells/mm³ | | | | | | Total femur cell count × 10⁶ | Total CFC per femur | Serum colony stimulating activity[b] |
			Total[a]	Lymphocytes	Polymorphs	Eosinophils	Monocytes	Leukemic cells			
Normal	11	—	12,800 (6,700 to 20,600)	9,600 (4,800 to 13,500)	2,600 (1,400 to 5,100)	150 (0 to 600)	500 (0 to 1,200)	—	16.4 (12.3 to 32.0)	19.2 (8.7 to 37.4)	15 (2 to 71)
Lymphoid leukemia	27	2,180 (400 to 4,663)	35,100 (5,400 to 103,500)	7,200 (1,100 to 38,000)	16,300 (2,200 to 49,000)	200 (0 to 1,000)	1,600 (300 to 3,900)	9,800 (0 to 59,500)	17.1 (9.6 to 24.3)	16.6 (0 to 99.0)	37 (2 to 182)

a Arithmetic mean plus range of values.
b Mean number of colonies stimulated to develop from 75,000 C57BL bone marrow cells by 0.10 ml of serum.

three of the animals in this group had no detectable *in vitro* CFC in the marrow sampled, yet exhibited blood granulocyte levels as high as 10,000/mm³. The bone marrow showed varying degrees of infiltration by leukemic cells, but no correlation was observed in individual mice between the degree of infiltration and the level of *in vitro* CFC. Previous studies have shown that the presence of leukemic cells in the cultures does not inhibit colony formation by normal bone marrow cells, and in fact potentiates the growth of such colonies (14).

Serum CSF levels were elevated in most leukemic mice, but in individual animals there was no correlation between serum CSF levels and either bone marrow content of CFC or blood white cell levels.

Response in mice with transplanted tumors. A survey of mice bearing a variety of s.c. transplanted syngeneic tumors at a stage when the tumor mass approximated 10 to 20% of body weight indicated that the incidence of *in vitro* CFC was consistently elevated in the spleen, compared with levels in control mice (Table 3). In the bone marrow of tumor-bearing mice, the incidence of *in vitro* CFC per 10⁵ cells was generally also elevated, but in many of these animals there was a reduction in total cellularity, so that the total number of CFC in the bone marrow was often no higher than normal. Levels of CSF in the sera of tumor-bearing animals were uniformly elevated. The peripheral white cell levels were elevated moderately in most tumor-bearing animals, and in all cases there was an elevation in polymorph levels.

Two tumors were chosen for more detailed study of the host responses following s.c. transplantation: HPC-28, a Bence Jones protein-secreting plasma cell tumor of BALB/c mice which, when transplanted s.c., infiltrated the bone marrow and spleen as well as producing a local s.c. tumor; WEHI-10, a breast tumor of C3H mice producing moderate sple-

TABLE 2. *Rise in percent labeling of polymorphs in the peripheral blood of leukemic AKR mice following pulse labeling with tritiated thymidine*

Type of mouse	Percent labeled polymorphs at various hours after labeling[a]							
	0	2	6	12	18	24	48	72
Normal AKR	0	0	0	0	0	0	30.6	69.3
	0	0	0	0	2.0	0	20.5	57.1
	0	0	0		1.0	2.3		
	0	0	0				17.9	60.6
	0							85.8
Leukemic AKR	0	0	0	0	0	0.7	57.5	86.0
	0	0	0	0	13.4	2.7	55.2	69.0
	0	0	0		1.3		14.0	67.2
	0	0	0.8				68.6	80.3
	0							56.2
	0							

[a] Each value represents the percent labeled polymorphs in a different mouse at stated time intervals after i.v. injection of 5 µc/g tritiated thymidine. Data from 500 consecutive white cells.

TABLE 3. *Response of* in vitro *CFC, serum CSF and white cell levels to transplanted tumors*

Tumor number	Tumor type	Strain	CFC/ 10^5 bone marrow cells	CFC/ femur $\times 10^3$	CFC/ total spleen	Serum colony stimulating activity[a]	Blood white cell levels
HPC-11	PCT	(NZB × C57BL)F$_1$	100	22.2	1,300	66	26,000
HPC-2	PCT	(NZB × C57BL)F$_1$	304	63.8	22,300	56	15,600
Control	—	(NZB × C57BL)F$_1$	100	25.0	200	15	7,500
Control	—	(NZB × C57BL)F$_1$	96	25.0	200	21	9,700
HPC-42	PCT	BALB/c	300	57.0	4,700	35	10,200
WEHI-11	Sarcoma	BALB/c	186	38.7	4,000	25	23,100
WEHI-16	LL	BALB/c	140	28.0	4,400	42	24,800
WEHI-22	LL	BALB/c	112	28.9	2,100	33	10,000
Control	—	BALB/c	100	20.0	300	10	11,800
Control	—	BALB/c	100	29.5	200	3	6,100
Control	—	BALB/c	76	19.4	300	13	25,700
Control	—	BALB/c	100	29.5	300	21	9,000
HPC-13	PCT	(BALB/c × NZB)F$_1$	188	29.1	9,300	51	20,000
Control	—	(BALB/c × NZB)F$_1$	96	29.3	300	22	9,500
BT-1	BT	C3H	276	72.5	800	14	13,400
BT-2	BT	C3H	226	32.8	1,100	89	3,700
Control	—	C3H	100	26.0	100	7	4,600
Control	—	C3H	100	27.0	200	10	7,500

[a] Mean number of colonies stimulated to develop from 75,000 C57BL bone marrow cells by 0.05 ml of serum. PCT = plasma cell tumor; LL = lymphoid leukemia; BT = breast tumor.

nomegaly but with no evidence of tumor cell metastasis, either to the bone marrow or spleen.

Groups of BALB/c and C3H mice were transplanted s.c. with 2 × 10^6 cells of HPC-28 or WEHI-10. Six mice were examined at each time point and serial observations were made until the animals were moribund. The response of *in vitro* CFC in the bone marrow is shown in Fig. 1. In mice bearing HPC-28 there was an early rise in the total number of CFC reaching maximum levels eight to 12 days after transplantation, followed by a fall in total numbers after day 16. This subsequent fall

205

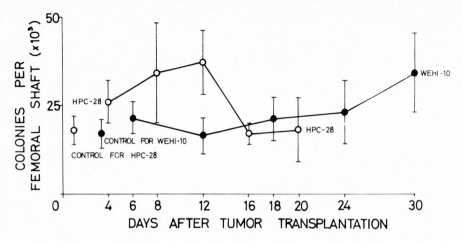

FIG. 1. Response of *in vitro* colony-forming cells in the bone marrow of mice transplanted with a plasma cell tumor (HPC-28) or a breast tumor (WEHI-10). Vertical bars ± two SE of mean.

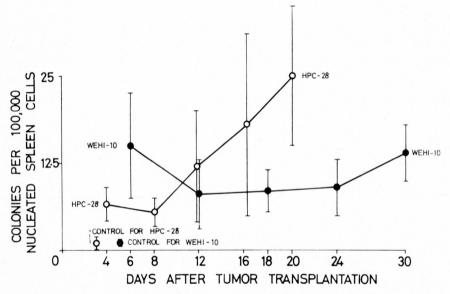

FIG. 2. Response of *in vitro* colony-forming cells in the spleen of mice transplanted with a plasma cell tumor (HPC-28) or a breast tumor (WEHI-10). Vertical bars ± two SE of mean.

in bone marrow CFC was associated with a reduction in the total cellularity of the bone marrow from mean levels of 24.0×10^6 to 14.0×10^6 per shaft, the percentage of CFC per 10^5 bone marrow cells remaining higher than normal throughout. In individual bone marrows, no correlation was observed between the percentage of infiltrating tumor cells and the incidence of *in vitro* CFC.

The response of bone marrow CFC to WEHI-10 was less complex. No changes occurred in total bone marrow cellularity with tumor growth and there was a progressive rise in the total numbers of CFC which paralleled the increase in tumor mass.

Fig. 2 shows that in both types of tumor-bearing animal, the percent incidence of *in vitro* CFC in the spleen was greatly elevated

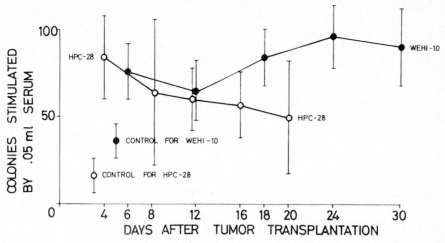

FIG. 3. Serum colony stimulating activity in mice transplanted with a plasma cell tumor (HPC-28) or a breast tumor (WEHI-10). Vertical bars ± two SE of mean.

above normal. As the total spleen weight was also elevated in both types of animal, the total spleen content of CFC was even higher when compared with spleens of control animals. Thus in the advanced stages of tumor growth there was a 50- to 100-fold increase in total *in vitro* CFC in the spleen (day 20, HPC-28: 18,000 ± 10,200 per spleen; control: 120 ± 40 per spleen; day 30, WEHI-10: 3,310 ± 220 per spleen; control: 76 ± 36 per spleen).

Occasional CFC were observed in some tumor masses, and this was accompanied by the occasional presence of granulocytic cells in these tumors.

Serum levels of CSF were uniformly elevated at all time points examined after transplantation of both types of tumor (Fig. 3). The colonies stimulated by sera from tumor-bearing animals were typical of those stimulated by normal serum CSF, being initially granulocytic in nature and later transforming to colonies of macrophages.

Response of mice to allogeneic tumor grafts. The response of mice to the injection of allogeneic tumor cells was investigated using the BALB/c tumor HPC-28 (H-2b). Five million tumor cells were injected into 129/J (H-2d),

CBA (H-2k) and B10D2 (H-2b) mice, the latter mice being co-isogenic with BALB/c mice for the major histocompatibility locus. No detectable tumor growth occurred in any of the three types of recipient, and the inoculated cells could be regarded as possibly being equivalent to an injection of nonviable antigenic material. As is shown in Table 4, there was a rise in *in vitro* CFC in all three types of animal, the responses being least marked in B10D2 mice which were the closest related to the BALB/c tumor strain.

Tumor cell content of CSF. Tumor cells are known to contain and produce material capable of stimulating colony formation *in vitro* (15, 16) and assays were performed on HPC-28 and WEHI-10 for their content of CSF using the extraction procedure described elsewhere (10). As control tissue, normal C57BL spleens were extracted in parallel with the tumor tissue. The results (Table 5) indicated that both tumors contained low levels of CSF, and that the content of CSF did not change significantly with progressive enlargement of the tumors.

DISCUSSION

The results indicated that the presence of a

TABLE 4. *Response of allogeneic mice to HPC-28 (H-2b)*

Mouse strain	Total spleen content of CFC[a]				Serum colony stimulating activity[a,b]			
	Days after transplantation				Days after transplantation			
	5	10	15	Control	5	10	15	Control
129/J (H-2d)	9,900 ± 2,400	2,400 ± 480	3,100 ± 2,280	160 ± 50	70 ± 17	142 ± 14	112 ± 17	57 ± 17
CBA (H-2k)	1,400 ± 1,300	3,100 ± 2,200	2,400 ± 1,000	70 ± 40	76 ± 26	151 ± 26	89 ± 17	48 ± 6
B10 D2 (H-2b)	250 ± 70	1,300 ± 1,200	820 ± 190	160 ± 50	82 ± 5	115 ± 11	101 ± 12	45 ± 8

[a] Mean ± two SE; six animals examined in each group at each time point.
[b] Mean number of colonies stimulated to develop from 75,000 C57BL bone marrow cells by 0.05 ml sera.

TABLE 5. *Colony stimulating activity of extracts of HPC-28 and WEHI-10*

Tissue	Days after transplantation	Mean tumor mass (g)	Total tumor colony stimulating activity[a]
HPC-28	12	2.0 ± 0.9	300 ± 470
	14	4.6 ± 0.7	250 ± 190
	18	4.3 ± 0.2	840 ± 810
WEHI-10	18	0.8 ± 0.8	270 ± 260
	24	3.4 ± 0.4	120 ± 40
	30	3.6 ± 2.0	240 ± 240
Normal C57BL spleen[b]	—	—	57; 47; 44; 53; 57; 44

[a] Calculated number of colonies stimulated to develop from 75,000 C57BL bone marrow cells by extract from whole tumor ± 2 SE; five tumors pooled at each time point.
[b] Calculated total number of colonies stimulated per 0.1 g of extracts of spleen from six different adult C57BL mice.

spontaneous or transplanted tumor induces a fairly uniform rise in serum CSF levels and a rise of 10- to 100-fold in granulocyte and macrophage precursors (*in vitro* CFC) in the spleen. The changes in the bone marrow were quantitatively less marked and were more variable. When the bone marrow was invaded by tumor cells, there was often depletion in bone marrow cellularity, accompanied by a variable depletion in the numbers of granulocyte and macrophage precursors. With the exception of the latter instance, the overall response to the presence of a growing tumor was an increase in both spleen and bone marrow levels of granulocyte and macrophage precursors. Since these are the only two organs containing these cells, and since there was an associated increase in blood levels of their progeny—granulocytes and macrophages— it is likely that the observed increases in CFC were due to an increased production or generation of these cells, rather than to an accumulation of these cells through failure to form progeny cells.

A number of possible explanations can be

advanced to account for the proliferation of CFC in tumor-bearing animals, but none entirely fit the known facts. The proliferation may simply be a response to the presence of dying tumor cells which require digestion and phagocytosis. This seems unlikely since the sequential study showed the response to occur early following tumor transplantation, at a time when few dying cells would be expected to be present. Alternatively, the responses may be due to the secondary infections in tumor-bearing animals since infections have been shown to elevate serum CSF levels (11, 17) and levels of *in vitro* CFC (D. Metcalf, unpublished data). However, previous studies have shown that granulocyte and serum CSF levels are equally as high in germ-free mice with lymphoid leukemia as in conventional leukemic mice (18), implying that secondary bacterial or protozoal infections are not necessarily involved in producing this response. Finally, the changes may be induced by the direct metabolic activity of the tumor cells themselves. Tumor cells contain and release CSF (15, 16), and CSF has been shown *in vivo* to stimulate a rise in blood granulocyte levels and in bone marrow and spleen CFC (10). However, this mechanism would be very unlikely to explain the results obtained with tumor transplants to allogeneic mice, in which few tumor cells could have survived, and in none of the experiments was there a good correlation in individual mice between serum CSF levels and *in vitro* CFC levels.

Could the rise in serum CSF levels and the proliferation of CFC be responses initiated by antigenic stimulation—in particular by tumor-specific antigens? Lymphoid leukemic cells in AKR mice exhibit tumor-specific antigens (19) as do breast tumor cells in C3H mice (20). Preliminary evidence suggests that plasma cell tumors also elicit tumor-specific antibody and homograft rejection responses in syngeneic hosts (21 and N. Warner, unpublished data). The injection of various anti-gens, e.g. pertussis, flagellin, sheep red cells and Freund's complete adjuvant induces both an acute rise in serum CSF levels and rises in the bone marrow, spleen and blood content of *in vitro* CFC (10, 12 and D. Metcalf, unpublished data). These antigen-induced rises in CFC are more marked in the spleen than in the bone marrow, as was the case in the present experiments. These considerations raise the possibility that the observed rises in serum CSF levels and the proliferation of granulocyte and macrophage precursors in the bone marrow and spleen could be para-immunological responses initiated by antigens specific to the tumor cells.

The exact mechanisms producing the observed responses in granulocyte and monocyte precursors require further investigation, but the increased production of differentiated progeny by these cells may constitute an important component of host resistance to a developing antigenic tumor. This applies particularly to the macrophages which are known to collaborate with lymphoid and anti-body-forming cells in some immune responses and which, in the presence of antibody directed against tumor cells, may represent an important system for the destruction of antigenic neoplastic cells.

Supported by the Carden Fellowship Fund of the Anti-Cancer Council of Victoria.

REFERENCES

1. PLUZNIK, D. and SACHS, L. The cloning of normal "mast" cells in tissue culture. *J. cell comp. Physiol.* **66**: 319, 1965.
2. BRADLEY, T. R. and METCALF, D. The growth of mouse bone marrow cells *in vitro*. *Aust. J. exp. Biol. med. Sci.* **44**: 287, 1966.
3. METCALF, D., BRADLEY, T. R. and ROBINSON, W. Analysis of colonies developing *in vitro* from mouse bone marrow cells stimulated by kidney feeder layers or leukemic serum. *J. cell. Physiol.* **69**: 93, 1967.
4. ROBINSON, W., METCALF, D. and BRADLEY, T. R. Stimulation by normal and leukemic mouse sera of colony formation *in vitro* by mouse bone marrow cells. *J. cell. Physiol.* **69**: 83, 1967.
5. METCALF, D. and FOSTER, R. Behavior on trans-

fer of serum stimulated bone marrow colonies. *Proc. Soc. exp. Biol. (N.Y.)* **126**: 758, 1967.

6. METCALF, D. Studies on colony formation *in vitro* by mouse bone marrow cells. II. Action of colony stimulating factor. *J. cell. Physiol.* (in press).

7. METCALF, D. and FOSTER, R. Bone marrow colony stimulating activity of serum from mice with viral-induced leukemia. *J. nat. Cancer Inst.* **39**: 1235, 1967.

8. METCALF, D. and STANLEY, E. R. Quantitative studies on the stimulation of mouse bone marrow colony growth *in vitro* by normal human urine. *Aust. J. exp. Biol. med. Sci.* **47**: 453, 1969.

9. STANLEY, E. R. and METCALF, D. Partial purification and some properties of the factor in normal and leukaemic human urine stimulating mouse bone marrow colony growth *in vitro*. *Aust. J. exp. Biol. med. Sci.* **47**: 467, 1969.

10. BRADLEY, T. R., METCALF, D., SUMNER, M. and STANLEY, E. R. Characteristics of *in vitro* colony formation by cells from haemopoietic tissues, in Farnes, P. (Ed.); "Hemic cells *in vitro*." Baltimore, Williams and Wilkins, 1969, v. 4, p. 22.

11. FOSTER, R., METCALF, D., ROBINSON, W. A. and BRADLEY, T. R. Bone marrow colony stimulating activity in human sera. Results of two independent surveys in Buffalo and Melbourne. *Brit. J. Haemat.* **15**: 147, 1968.

12. McNEILL, T. A. Antigenic stimulation of bone marrow colony forming cells. III. Effect *in vivo*. *Immunology* (in press).

13. STANLEY, E. R., ROBINSON, W. A. and ADA, G. L. Properties of the colony stimulating factor in leukaemic and normal mouse serum. *Aust. J. exp. Biol. med. Sci.* **46**: 715, 1968.

14. METCALF, D. Potentiation of bone marrow colony growth *in vitro* by the addition of lymphoid or bone marrow cells. *J. cell. Physiol.* **72**: 9, 1968.

15. PARAN, A., ICHIKAWA, Y. and SACHS, L. Production of the inducer for macrophage and granulocyte colonies by leukaemic cells. *J. cell. Physiol.* **72**: 251, 1968.

16. METCALF, D., MOORE, M. A. S. and WARNER, N. L. Colony formation *in vitro* by myelomonocytic leukemic cells. *J. nat. Cancer Inst.* **43**: 983, 1969.

17. FOSTER, R., METCALF, D. and KIRCHMYER, R. Induction of bone marrow colony stimulating activity by a filterable agent in leukemic and normal mouse serum. *J. exp. Med.* **127**: 853, 1968.

18. METCALF, D., FOSTER, R. and POLLARD, M. Colony stimulating activity of serum from germfree normal and leukemic mice. *J. cell. Physiol.* **70**: 131, 1967.

19. OLD, L. J., BOYSE, E. A. and STOCKERT, E. The G (Gross) leukemia antigen. *Cancer Res.* **25**: 813, 1965.

20. WEISS, D. W., LAVRIN, D. H., DEZFULIAN, M., VAAGE, J. and BLAIR, P. B. Studies on the immunology of spontaneous mammary carcinomas of mice, in: Harris, R. J. C. (Ed.), "Specific tumour antigens." Copenhagen, Munksgaard, 1967, p. 210.

21. LESPINATS, G. Induction d'une immunité vis-à-vis de la graffe de plasmocytosarcomes chez la souris BALB/c. *Europ. J. Cancer* **5**: 421, 1969.

TUMOR-DISTINCTIVE CELLULAR IMMUNITY
TO HUMAN SARCOMA AND CARCINOMA

FARKAS VÁNKY and JAN STJERNSWÄRD*

Radiumhemmet and Department of Orthopaedic Surgery, Karolinska Sjukhuset, and Department of Tumor
Biology, Karolinska Institutet, Stockholm, Sweden

ABSTRACT

The possible existence of tumor-distinctive cellular immune reactions in cancer
patients was studied *in vitro*. In a mixed-lymphocyte-target-interaction test, peripheral lymphocytes and draining lymph node cells of the cancer patient were
cultured *in vitro* with autochthonous malignant or nonmalignant, or with allogeneic target, cells in which DNA synthesis had been blocked. In 11 out of 20
patients with active disease at the time of testing, peripheral lymphocytes were
stimulated to increased DNA synthesis by autochthonous tumor cells but not
by autochthonous lymphocytes. Allogeneic lymphocytes were stimulated more
strongly by lymphocytes than by tumor cells from the patient. Tumor cells stimulated the patient's own lymphocytes more frequently than they stimulated allogeneic
lymphocytes. Autochthonous frozen tumor cells stimulated peripheral lymphocytes to the same degree. Lymphoid cells from a lymph node adjacent to the tumor
stimulated autochthonous lymphocytes. The converse, the stimulation of local lymph
node cells by peripheral autochthonous lymphocytes, was not observed. In four of
four patients, the lymph node cells draining the tumor stimulated autochthonous
peripheral lymphocytes at least to the same degree as did autochthonous tumor
cells. In two patients, local lymph node cells were not stimulated by autochthonous
tumor cells, although they were stimulated by allogeneic lymphocytes; autochthonous peripheral lymphocytes were, however, stimulated by the same tumor
cells, as well as by the autochthonous local lymph node cells. This may indicate the
existence of a tumor-distinctive immunological anergy in the local lymph node
draining the tumor.

These results thus point to the existence of tumor-distinctive cellular immune
reactions *in vitro* against autochthonous cancer, and they indicate that tumor
specific immunological nonreactivity in the lymph nodes draining the tumor
may occur.

INTRODUCTION

Existing clinical evidence indicates that autochthonous cancer may be hampered in its

growth by some host mechanisms (1), and *in
vitro* studies indeed indicate that human tumor
cells may differ in antigenicity from the host's
normal cells. Burkitt's lymphoma cells (2–6),
anaplastic carcinoma of the postnasal space

---

* Reprint requests to Dr. J. Stjernswärd.

211

(7, 8), malignant melanoma (9–11), neuro-blastoma (12), colon carcinoma (13), lipoid sarcoma (14), osteogenic sarcoma (15), bron-cogenic carcinoma (16), renal carcinoma (17), cancer of the testis (18) and leukemic cells (19) may evoke immunological reactions which are tumor-distinctive, as detected by humoral antibody formation or by cellular immune responses. Admixture of the patient's own lymphocytes with his reinjected tumor has been found to inhibit the take of the trans-plant (20). The cellular immune response of the patient, most probably of the delayed hypersensitivity type, is the main vector of an immunological surveillance mechanism, in-hibiting tumor growth (21). Regression of primary human skin tumor or different types of metastases to the skin by experimentally induced delayed hypersensitivity reactions around the tumor nodules supports this hypo-thesis (22).

When leukocytes from immunogenetically disparate donors are mixed in culture they undergo blastoid transformations, DNA syn-thesis and mitosis (23–26). This mixed lym-phocyte interaction represents an immuno-logically specific response by lymphocytes in culture to allogeneic cellular transplantation antigens (26).

We have presented evidence suggesting that the patients' own lymphocytes can be stimu-lated to increased DNA synthesis by autoch-thonous tumor cells, but not by autochthonous nonmalignant cells (5). Further studies by a "mixed-lymphocyte-target-interaction test" (MLTIT), in which the peripheral lympho-cytes of the patient are cultured *in vitro* with autochthonous malignant or nonmalignant cells, indicate that the cancer patient's lym-phocytes may, in fact, be stimulated by autoch-thonous tumor cells. Lymphocytes from patients with Burkitt's lymphoma or naso-pharyngeal carcinoma (5, 6), renal carcinoma (17), carcinoma of the testis (18) or bronco-genic carcinoma (16) have been found to be stimulated to increased DNA synthesis by autochthonous tumor cells. The present study was undertaken to determine, in patients with various forms of sarcoma and carcinoma, whether the patient's own lymphocytes may be stimulated by autochthonous tumor cells.

MATERIAL AND METHODS

MLTIT. Lymphocytes were obtained from periph-eral venous blood. Fifty ml quantities were de-fibrinated by shaking with glass beads. White cells were isolated by sedimentation in the pre-sence of 3 % dextran (Dextran 250, mol wt 250,000, Pharmacia, Uppsala) at 37 C for 30 min.

Tumor tissue obtained at surgery was put imme-diately into cold Earle's basal tissue culture me-dium (BME) with 10 % heat inactivated fetal calf serum, 100 IU/ml of penicillin and 100 µg/ml of streptomycin added. The tumor was then minced and passed through a steel net.

Two $\times$ 10^6 living lymphocytes, designated as "effector" cells or stimulated cells, were mixed with 10^6 cells designated "target" cells or stimu-lating cells, in which DNA synthesis had been blocked. Viability of effector cells was determined by vital staining. DNA synthesis was inhibited in the target cells by adding mitomycin-C (Nutritional Biochemical Corp., Cleveland, Ohio, lot 8799), 25 µg to 10^7 cells in a volume of 3 ml of tissue culture medium (27).

The effector cells were cultured with the target cells in screw-cap vials containing 4 ml BME. Tests were run in triplicate whenever possible. Some vials contained only lymphocytes and phy-tohemagglutinin (PHA) (Wellcome Research Lab., Beckenham, England), in a final dilution of 1:100 in 4 ml BME. After five days' incubation at 37 C in a humidified 5 % CO_2 chamber, 4 µc tritium labeled thymidine (thymidine methyl-H^3, specific activity 5.0 c/mmole, batch 67, Radiochemical Centre, Amersham, England) were added to each vial. After 12 hr incubation, the DNA was iso-lated from each vial by precipitation with 10 % trichloroacetic acid. Subsequently, the H^3 activity was measured in a Packard liquid scintillation counter.

Frozen and thawed target cells. Ten $\times$ 10^6 cells in 15 % glycerine in BME, in a total volume of 1 ml, were kept at +5 C for at least 30 min. Thereafter they were slowly frozen, at the rate of 1 C per min, to –28 C, except for the interval –6 C to –12 C when the temperature was reduced 6 C in 1 min; thereafter, the temperature was reduced 10 C/min to –80 C. The tube was then rapidly thawed; it was brought from –80 C to +37 C by holding in a water-bath for 20 sec. After washing twice in BME, mitomycin-C was added.

Patients studied. All patients studied carried a tumor at the time their blood was collected. Peripheral blood was always collected preoperatively because it has been shown that the lymphocyte response to PHA decreases postoperatively (28). Each diagnosis was confirmed histopathologically.

RESULTS

Cellular immune reactions against autochthonous cancer. The details of an individual test to demonstrate tumor-distinctive cellbound immune reactions by the MLTIT are shown in Table 1. Stimulation of peripheral blood lymphocytes from the patient to increased DNA synthesis on exposure to mitomycin-C-treated autochthonous tumor cells, allogeneic lym-

phocytes, and PHA is shown. The patient's lymphocytes were stimulated to increased DNA synthesis by his own tumor cells, indicating that these cells were recognized as foreign.

In this and similar tests, allogeneic lymphocytes and PHA were always included as control stimulating targets, to make certain that any failure of the patient's lymphocytes to respond to autochthonous tumor cells could not be due to their nonviability. As expected, the response to these stimuli was considerable. Mitomycin-C-treated cells alone were included as negative controls, to assure that DNA synthesis had been blocked.

The responsiveness of peripheral lymphocytes from 20 patients after contact with mitomycin-C-treated autochthonous tumor cells, allogeneic lymphocytes or PHA is presented in Table 2. Eleven out of the 20 patients

TABLE 1. *Search for tumor-specific cellular immunity. DNA synthesis of the peripheral lymphocytes of a cancer patient and of a normal donor upon exposure to mitomycin-C-treated autochthonous sarcoma cells, autochthonous and allogeneic lymphocytes and PHA in vitro in the MLTIT*

Stimulated cells (effector cells)	Stimulating cells (target cells)-mitomycin-C-treated	Count/10 min	Reactivity index[a]
Lymphocytes of cancer patient[b]	Autochthonous lymphocytes	7,171 (3,971, 10,371)	1.0
	Autochthonous tumor cells	19,517 (12,692, 27,710, 18,150)	2.7
	Frozen and thawed autochthonous tumor cells	23,333 (16,630, 14,058, 39,312)	3.2
	Allogeneic lymphocytes	76,514 (38,677, 114,351)	10.7
	PHA only	268,265 (171,307, 365,224)	382.8
	None	4,906 (4,990, 4,823)	0.6
Lymphocytes of healthy donor	Lymphocytes of that donor	7,943 (8,976, 6,911)	1.0
	Lymphocytes of the cancer patient	62,209 (55,660, 68,759)	7.8
	Tumor cells of the cancer patient	9,347 (13,250, 5,663, 9,128)	1.1
	Frozen and thawed tumor cells of the cancer patient	9,878 (13,297, 8,323, 8,014)	1.0
	PHA only	841,267 (873,466, 809,069)	112.8
	None	7,728 (7,728)	0.9
No effector cells	Lymphocytes of the cancer patient	2,304 (1,793, 2,866)	0.3
	Tumor cells of the cancer patient	1,647 (1,450, 1,844)	0.2
	Frozen and thawed tumor cells of the cancer patient	2,083 (1,864, 2,300)	0.2
	Lymphocytes of healthy donor	2,034 (2,235, 1,834)	0.2
	PHA only	1,774 (1,998, 1,560)	0.2
	None	1,460 (1,460)	0.1

[a] Reactivity index is expressed as the ratio of count/10 min in the test system to count/10 min against mitomycin-C-treated autochthonous lymphocytes.
[b] 2×10^6 effector cells cultured with 10^6 target cells in 4 ml tissue culture media.

TABLE 2. Reactivity of peripheral lymphocytes from patients with various sarcomas and carcinomas against mitomycin-C-treated autochthonous tumor cells, allogeneic lymphocytes and PHA as compared with reactivity to autochthonous lymphocytes in the MLTIT

Stimulated cells: Autochthonous lymphocytes

Reactivity index when test was performed with tumor cells from patients with the following disease

Reactivity index	Disease	Stimulating cells (mitomycin-C-treated): Autochthonous lymphocytes	Autochthonous tumor cells	Allogeneic lymphocytes	PHA
< 1.5	Synovial sarcoma	1.0	0.2	0.8	500.0
< 1.5	Angio-sarcoma	1.0	0.8	10.5	33.1
< 1.5	Osteo-sarcoma	1.0	0.8	1.4	3.8
< 1.5	Osteo-sarcoma	1.0	1.2	2.0	65.0
< 1.5	Fibro-sarcoma	1.0	0.3	14.7	125.1
< 1.5	Fibro-sarcoma	1.0	1.4	13.8	49.6
< 1.5	Lipo-sarcoma	1.0	1.0	2.5	93.7
< 1.5	Giant cell sarcoma	1.0	1.2	39.0	200.0
< 1.5	Breast carcinoma	1.0	1.1	1.4	43.6
1.5 to 2.0	Osteo-sarcoma	1.0	1.5	3.6	54.8
1.5 to 2.0	Osteo-sarcoma	1.0	1.9	7.7	63.7
2.0 to 5.0	Chordoma	1.0	2.2	5.3	248.8
2.0 to 5.0	Reticulum cell sarcoma	1.0	2.7	17.7	382.8
2.0 to 5.0	Rhabdomyo-sarcoma	1.0	3.3	3.6	176.6
2.0 to 5.0	Glioma	1.0	2.1	3.0	351.1
2.0 to 5.0	Renal carcinoma	1.0	2.3	5.5	10.0
2.0 to 5.0	Breast carcinoma	1.0	2.2	2.5	62.5
2.0 to 5.0	Seminoma	1.0	2.7	4.5	94.1
> 5.0	Myxo-sarcoma	1.0	6.6	10.3	NT
> 5.0	Thyroid carcinoma	1.0	5.3	NT	76.5

[a] See footnote to Table 1.

TABLE 3. Comparison between the ability of malignant and nonmalignant cells from the same donor to stimulate allogeneic peripheral lymphocytes from healthy donors to increased DNA-synthesis in the MLTIT

Stimulated cells: Peripheral lymphocytes of healthy donors

Diagnosis	Stimulating cells (mitomycin-C-treated): Autochthonous lymphocytes	Lymphocytes of the patient	Tumor cells of the patient	PHA
Osteo-sarcoma	1.0	1.3	0.4	10.4
Osteo-sarcoma	1.0	13.4	0.7	37.6
Reticulum cell sarcoma	1.0	7.8	1.1	112.8
Lipo-sarcoma	1.0	6.0	0.7	571.4
Giant cell sarcoma	1.0	2.1	1.0	50.4
Angio-sarcoma	1.0	1.3	0.4	17.4
Fibro-sarcoma	1.0	4.6	0.6	315.7
Breast carcinoma	1.0	1.0	0.5	15.8
Seminoma	1.0	1.1	1.5	190.2
Chordoma	1.0	NT	3.6	185.6
Renal carcinoma	1.0	1.6	2.2	9.4
Breast carcinoma	1.0	9.2	3.3	61.5

reacted against autochthonous tumor cells with an index above 1.5. The lymphocytes from all patients which were stimulated by autochthonous tumor cells were stimulated by allogeneic cells, with a reactivity of between 2.5 and 10.3. In a number of instances, the reactivity index towards autochthonous tumor was of the same order as towards allogeneic cells. The results indicate that the strength of the tumor-distinctive immunological stimulus may at times be as strong as that of the allogeneic cell's histocompatibility antigens. No correlation between the extents of autochthonous cell and PHA stimulation was evident. The lymphocytes from three of the eleven patients who were not stimulated by autochthonous tumor cells were not stimulated by allogeneic lymphocytes either, and in one of these instances, the lymphoid cells also failed to respond well to PHA. This patient's lymphocytes may thus have been nonspecifically nonreactive, and negative results obtained against autochthonous tumor cells in such cases should be discounted.

The data also seem to indicate that lymphocytes from patients with carcinoma are more likely to be stimulated by the autochthonous neoplastic cells (four out of five) than are lymphocytes from patients with sarcoma (seven of 15).

Comparison between the ability of malignant and nonmalignant cells to stimulate allogeneic lymphocytes in the MLTIT. If the malignant and nonmalignant cells from the same patient possess the same isoantigens, quantitatively and qualitatively, allogeneic effector lymphocytes from a healthy donor should be stimulated to increased DNA synthesis to the same degree by the two types of target cell. This was tested with target cells from 12 of the patients and Table 3 summarizes the results. Tumor cells and lymphocytes from the same cancer patient did not appear to stimulate allogeneic lymphocytes to the same extent. The allogeneic tumor cells were effective in four of 12 patients tested (mean index = 2.6), as compared with the allogeneic normal cells which effected transformation in seven of 12 patients (mean index = 6.4).

The ability of autochthonous and allogeneic lymphocytes to be stimulated by the same tumor cells. The reactivity indexes in the 12 instances where autochthonous and allogeneic lymphocytes were incubated with cells from the same tumor are summarize din Table 4. The autochthonous lymphocytes were stimulated more frequently (seven of 12) by the tumor cells than were the allogeneic lymphocytes (four of 12). This finding may support the tumor-distinctiveness of the reactions observed in

TABLE 4. *Comparison between the ability of the same tumor cells to stimulate autochthonous and allogeneic lymphocytes*

Stimulated cells	Stimulating cells (mitomycin-C-treated)	Diagnosis of target cell donor											
		Chordoma	*Renal carcinoma*	*Breast carcinoma*	*Seminoma*	*Osteo-sarcoma*	*Osteo-sarcoma*	*Reticulum cell sarcoma*	*Fibro-sarcoma*	*Lipo-sarcoma*	*Giant cell sarcoma*	*Angio-sarcoma*	*Breast carcinoma*
Auto-chthonous lymphocytes	Tumor cells	2.2	2.3	2.2	2.7	1.9	1.5	2.7	1.4	1.0	1.2	0.8	1.1
Allogeneic lymphocytes[a]	Tumor cells	3.6	2.2	3.3	1.5	0.7	0.4	1.1	0.6	0.7	1.0	0.4	0.5

[a] From healthy donors

TABLE 5. *Correlation between the ability of the same tumor cells from various tumors to stimulate autochthonous and allogeneic lymphocytes*

Reactivity of		
Autochthonous lymphocytes from tumor patients	Allogeneic lymphocytes from healthy donors	Observed frequencies
+	+	4
+	−	3
−	+	0
−	−	5

+ = lymphocytes stimulated to increased DNA-synthesis by the patient's tumor cells.
− = not stimulated.

the MLTIT in autochthonous combinations.

The variation of the observed frequencies of reactivity are summarized in Table 5. In none of the experiments were only allogeneic lymphocytes stimulated. Either both types of lymphocytes were stimulated (four of 12) or neither (five of 12) or only autochthonous lymphocytes (three of 12) but never allogeneic ones alone.

Sarcoma cells stimulated allogeneic lymphocytes less frequently (none of seven) than did carcinoma cells (four of five) (Table 4).

The ability of lymphoid cells from nodes draining the tumor area to stimulate and be stimulated. In five of the patients, the immune reactivity of lymphoid cells from lymph nodes adjacent to and draining the tumor-area was tested. The reactivity of both local lymph node cells and peripheral blood lymphocytes to autochthonous tumor and lymphoid cells was compared. The results are presented in Table 6. Mitomycin-C-treated lymph node cells from four of four patients stimulated autoch-

TABLE 6. *Reactivity of lymphocytes from local lymph nodes and from the peripheral circulation to tumor and lymphoid target cells*

Stimulated cells	Stimulating cells (mitomycin-C-treated)	Reactivity index when test was performed with tumor cells from patient with the following diseases				
		Osteo-sarcoma	Osteo-sarcoma	Osteo-sarcoma	Fibro-sarcoma	Breast carcinoma
Autochthonous peripheral lymphocytes	Autochthonous peripheral lymphocytes	1.0	1.0	1.0	1.0	1.0
	Autochthonous tumor	1.5	0.8	1.9	1.4	2.2
	Autochthonous local lymph node cells	1.5	NT	3.5	1.7	2.4
	Allogeneic peripheral lymphocytes	3.6	1.4	7.7	13.8	2.5
Autochthonous local lymph node cells	Autochthonous local lymph node cells	1.0	1.0	1.0	1.0	1.0
	Autochthonous peripheral lymphocytes	NT	NT	1.2	1.4	0.3
	Autochthonous tumor	0.2	1.0	0.6	0.5	0.3
	Allogeneic peripheral lymphocytes	1.1	1.0	6.2	5.9	1.0

NT = not tested

thonous peripheral lymphocytes, with a reactivity index about the same as that towards autochthonous tumor cells. As the target lymphoid cells came from a node draining the tumor, the reactivity towards these cells could be explained by localization of tumor antigens or tumor cells in the lymph node; local lymph node cells were not stimulated by autochthonous peripheral blood lymphocytes.

Significantly, local lymph node cells were not stimulated by the autochthonous tumor targets. In two of five patients, this nonreactivity may be considered as conclusive and not due to any nonviability, as evidenced by their good reactivity to allogeneic cells. In contrast, the peripheral lymphocytes of several patients were stimulated by the autochthonous tumor cells. These results thus point to the existence in some patients of a tumor-distinctive immunological anergy in the lymph node cells draining the tumor.

Frozen target cells. So as to be able to follow the possible tumor-distinctive immune reactivity of the same patient during different clinical stages, it is necessary to have available the same tumor cells as targets.

Tumor cells were frozen. Their ability to stimulate autochthonous or allogeneic cells in the MLTI-test was tested and compared with that of fresh tumor biopsy cells. The results depicted in Table 7 show the reactivity index in seven experiments, and they show that frozen tumor cells may also be effective in the test system.

DISCUSSION

The autochthonous peripheral blood lymphocytes of 11 of 20 patients with a tumor burden at the time of testing were stimulated to increased DNA synthesis when incubated with mitomycin-C- treated cancer cells. Similarly treated peripheral lymphocytes or, as reported elsewhere (17), nonmalignant tissue of the same origin as the tumor, did not stimulate autochthonous lymphocytes to in-

TABLE 7. *Ability of frozen and thawed as compared to fresh tumor biopsy cells to stimulate autochthonous and allogeneic lymphocytes*

Stimulated cells	Stimulating cells (mitomycin-C-treated)	Reactivity index when test was performed with tumor cells from patients with following disease						
		Reticulum cell sarcoma	*Osteo-sarcoma*	*Osteo-sarcoma*	*Giant cell sarcoma*	*Fibro-sarcoma*	*Breast carcinoma*	*Seminoma*
Autochthonous lymphocytes	Autochthonous lymphocytes	1.0	1.0	1.0	1.0	1.0	1.0	1.0
	Autochthonous tumor cells	2.7	1.5	1.9	1.2	1.4	2.2	2.7
	Autochthonous tumor cells, frozen[a]	3.2	1.9	2.6	1.8	2.2	1.2	1.6
Allogeneic lymphocytes	Lymphocytes from the patient	7.8	1.3	13.4	2.1	4.6	9.2	1.1
	Tumor cells from the patient	1.1	0.4	0.7	1.0	0.6	3.3	1.5
	Tumor cells from the patient frozen	1.2	0.5	0.8	1.9	14.9	1.7	0.9

[a] Cells frozen to –80 C in sterile glycerine (15% with tissue culture media), stored at –90 and rapidly (20 sec) thawed in waterbath at 37 C.

creased DNA synthesis to the same extent as did the malignant cells. This supports the presence of tumor-distinctive cellular immune reactions *in vitro*. The tumor-distinctiveness of this reaction is supported by the finding that autochthonous peripheral lymphocytes appeared to be stimulated more frequently by the cancer cells than were allogeneic lymphocytes: the more frequent reactivity of autochthonous lymphocytes may indicate that the patient is sensitized against his own tumor cells.

The decreased ability of sarcoma cells to stimulate allogeneic lymphocytes may reflect losses of normal isoantigen on malignant cells. However, it is noted that differences in HL-A antigens have not been observed between malignant and nonmalignant cells derived from the same tissue in at least some instances: HL-A antigens were found to be the same on leukoblasts and lymphocytes from the same patient (29, 30). Another explanation for the failure of sarcoma cells to stimulate the effector cells may be a "crowding-out" of normal isoantigens by new tumor antigens, to which allogeneic lymphocytes are not reactive before immunization. Still other plausible explanations present themselves. The stimulating antigens may be covered by antibodies. A toxic effect, brought about by lysosomes (31) or by mitosis-inhibiting polypeptides from the malignant cells (32), may also contribute to the low reactivity towards allogeneic tumor cells. It is also quite possible that connective tissue cells in themselves have expressed fewer isoantigenic determinants than do lymphocytes or epithelial cells.

In the lymphocyte transformation test with lymphoid cells derived from donors with different histocompatibility antigens, increased DNA synthesis is observed (23–26) and the reaction occurs without any known prior immunization of the cell donors. Lymphocytes from donors presensitized against certain nontissue antigens such as tuberculin (33),

also react *in vitro* against the antigen, but only if the donor is presensitized. The immunocompetent cells might, a priori, have different thresholds for reaction against various antigens (34). During the evolution of multicellular organisms, an identification code may have developed, expressed by the isoantigens on the cell surface. The immune systems may have an existing immunity against different isoantigens, and thus be able to react against them anamnestically on bona fide first contact. The most important function of normal isoantigens might then be to act as detector systems for genetic abberations occuring in somatic cells (35, 36).

Lymph node cells from a gland draining a tumor area stimulated autochthonous peripheral lymphocytes to increased DNA synthesis. Local lymph node cells were not, however, stimulated by autochthonous peripheral lymphocytes. One explanation may be that antigen(s) or tumor cells have been trapped in the local lymph node cells draining the tumor area. The lymph node which drains the injection site of an antigen has been demonstrated to trap a relatively constant proportion of antigen, which thereafter is retained for a variable period of time (37, 38). Indeed, certain antigens when associated with macrophages are much more immunogenic than in their native form, the difference in immunogenicity being greater the smaller the quantities compared (39). Microscopic examination of the lymph node cells in suspension showed no intact tumor cells, but tumor fragments or products may well have been present. Another explanation may come from the finding that antigen-activated human lymphocytes generate, in addition to a migration inhibiting factor (40) and "lymphotoxin" (41), a soluble "mitogenic" factor (42); if the local lymph node cells contain tumor cell components they may be antigen-activated and generate such mitogenic factor(s) which could then stimulate the DNA metabolism of autochthonous peripheral blood lymphocytes. This possibility is subject to experimental tests.

Local lymph node cells of two patients were not stimulated by the autochthonous tumor targets, although they were stimulated by allogeneic cells. Autochthonous peripheral lymphocytes were, however, stimulated by the same tumor cells, as well as by the local lymph node cells. These results may be interpreted as reflecting a specific tolerance or paralysis of the local lymph node cells to tumor antigens. In fact, the mixed lymphocyte reaction test has been demonstrated to serve as an *in vitro* test for tolerance (43–45). Our findings may thus be analogous to the results of others who showed that local lymph node cells which were tolerant to the histocompatibility antigens of an allogeneic strain did not transform when exposed in a mixed leukocyte culture to cells from that strain. This nonreactivity was considered to be immunologically specific, since the lymphocytes were able to transform after exposure to other antigens (43–45). A correlation between lymphocyte transformation and classical humoral and cellular immune responses has been found (46).

We wish to express our sincere gratitude to Dr. Anna-Marta Vanky and Miss Susanne Stenbrink for valuable technical assistance.

Supported by grants from the King Gustav V:s Jubilee Fund, the Cancer Society in Stockholm, the Swedish Cancer Society, the Gösta Milton Fund, and the Brummer Fund.

REFERENCES

1. EVERSON, T. C. and COLE, W. H. "Spontaneous regression of cancer." Philadelphia, W. B. Saunders Co., 1966.
2. HENLE, G. and HENLE, W. Immunofluorescence in cells derived from Burkitt's lymphoma. *J. Bact.* **91**: 1248, 1966.
3. KLEIN, G., CLIFFORD, P., KLEIN, E. and STJERNSWÄRD, J. Search for tumor-specific immune reactions in Burkitt's lymphoma patients by the membrane immunofluorescence reaction. *Proc. nat. Acad. Sci. (Wash.)* **55**: 1528, 1966.
4. OLD, L. J., BOYSE, E. A., OETTGEN, H. F., DE HARVEN, E., GEERING, C., WILLIAMSON, D. and CLIFFORD, P. Precipitating antibody in human serum to an antigen present in cultured Burkitt's lymphoma cells. *Proc. nat. Acad. Sci. (Wash.)* **56**: 1699, 1966.
5. STJERNSWÄRD, J., CLIFFORD, P., SINGH, S. and SVEDMYR, E. Indication of cellular immunological reactions against autochthonous tumor in cancer patients studied in vitro. *E. Afr. med. J.* **7**: 484, 1968.
6. STJERNSWÄRD, K., CLIFFORD, P. and SVEDMYR, E. General and tumor-distinctive cellular immunological reactivity, in: Burkitt, D. and Wright, D. (Eds.), "Burkitt's lymphoma." Edinburgh, E. & S. Livingstone, 1970.
7. CHU, E. H. V., STJERNSWÄRD, J., CLIFFORD, P. and KLEIN, G. Reactivity of human lymphon cytes against autochthonous and allogeneic normal and tumor cells in vitro. *J. nat. Cancer Inst.* **39**: 595, 1967.
8. HENLE, W., HENLE, G., BURTIN, P., CACHIN, Y., CLIFFORD, P., DE SCHRYVER, A., DE THE, G., DIEHL, V., HO, H. C. and KLEIN, G. Antibodies to EB virus in nasopharyngeal carcinoma of the head and neck, other neoplasms and control groups. *J. nat. Cancer Inst.* **44**: 225, 1970.
9. MORTON, D. L., MALMGREN, R. A., HOLMES, E. L. and KETCHAM, A. S. Demonstration of antibodies against human malignant melanoma by immunofluorescence. *Surgery* **64**: 233, 1968.
10. LEWIS, M. G., IKONOPISOV, R. L., NAIRN, R. C., PHILIPS, T. M., HAMILTON-FAIRLEY, G., BODENHAM, D. C. and ALEXANDER, P. Tumor-specific antibodies in human malignant melanoma and their relationship to the extent of the disease. *Brit. Med. J.* **3**: 547, 1969.
11. MUNA, N. M., MARCUS, S. and SMART, C. Detection by immunofluorescence of antibodies specific for human malignant melanoma cells. *Cancer (Phila.)* **23**: 88, 1969.
12. HELLSTRÖM, I., HELLSTRÖM, K.-E., PIERCE, G. and BILL, H. A. Demonstration of cellbound and humoral immunity against neuroblastoma cells. *Proc. nat. Acad. Sci. (Wash.)* **60**: 1231, 1968.
13. HELLSTRÖM, K-E. and HELLSTRÖM, I. Cellular immunity against tumor antigens. *Advanc. Cancer Res.* **12**: 167, 1969.
14. MORTON, D. L., HALL, W. T. and MALMGREN, R. A. Human liposarcomas: Tissue culture containing foci of transformed cells with viral particles. *Science* **165**: 813, 1969.
15. MORTON, D. L., MALMGREN, R. A., HALL, W. T. and SCHIDLOVSKY, G. Immunologic and virus studies with human sarcomas. *Surgery* **66**: 152, 1969.
16. STJERNSWÄRD, J., JOHANSSON, B., SVEDMYR, E. and SUNDBLAD, R. Indication of tumor-specific cellbound immunological reactivity and depressed general reactivity in a pair of twins. *Clin. exp. Immunol.* **6**: 429, 1970.
17. STJERNSWÄRD, J., ALMGARD, L.-E., FRANZEN, S., VON SCHREEB, T. and WADSTRÖM, L. B. Tumor-distinctive immunological reactions in patients with renal carcinomas. *Clin. exp. Immunol.* **6**: 963, 1970.
18. STJERNSWÄRD, J. and CLIFFORD, P. Tumor-distinctive cellular immune reactions against autochthonous cancer, in: Severi, L. (Ed.),

"Immunity and tolerance in oncogenesis." *Fourth Perugia Quadr. Int. Conf. on Cancer, Perugia 1969.* 1970, p. 749.

19. Fridman, W. H. and Kourilsky, F. M. Stimulation of lymphocytes by autologous leukemic cells in acute leukemia. *Nature (Lond.)* **224**: 277, 1969.

20. Southam, C. M., Brunschwig, A., Levin, A. G. and Dizon, Q. S. Effect of leukocytes on transplantability of human cancer. *Cancer (Phila.)* **19**: 1743, 1966.

21. Burnet, M. F. "Cellular immunology." Melbourne, Melbourne University Press, 1969.

22a. Klein, E. Immunotherapy of cutaneous and mucosal neoplasms. *N.Y. St. J. Med.* 900, 1968.

22b. Stjerswärd, J. and Levin, A. Delayed hypersensitivity induced regression of human neoplasms. *Cancer (Phila.)* (in press).

23. Bach, F. H. and Hirschhorn, K. Lymphocyte interaction. A potential histocompatibility test in vitro. *Science* **143**: 813, 1964.

24. Bain, B., Vas, M. R. and Lowenstein, L. The development of large immature mononuclear cells in mixed leucocyte cultures. *Blood* **23**: 108, 1964.

25. Dutton, R. W. Further studies of the stimulation of DNA-synthesis in cultures of spleen cell suspensions by homologous cells in inbred strains of mice and rats. *J. exp. Med.* **122**: 759, 1965.

26. Wilson, B. B. and Billingham, W. Lymphocytes and transplantation immunity. *Advanc. Immunol.* **6**: 189, 1967.

27. Bach, F. H. and Voynow, M. K. One-way stimulation in mixed leukocyte culture. *Science* **153**: 545, 1966.

28. Riddle, P. R. and Berenbaum, M. C. Postoperative depression of the lymphocyte response to phytohaemagglutinin. *Lancet* **i**: 746, 1967.

29. Kourilsky, F. M., Dausset, J. and Bernard, J. Normal leukocyte antigens of human leukemic leukoblasts—a qualitative study. *Cancer Res.* **28**: 372, 1968.

30. Kourilsky, F. M., Dausset, J., Feingold, N., Dupuy, J. M. and Bernard, J. Leukocyte groups and acute leukemia. *J. nat. Cancer Inst.* **41**: 81, 1968.

31. Allison, A. C. and Mallucci, L. Uptake of hydrocarbon carcinogens by lysosomes. *Nature (Lond.)* **203**: 1024, 1964.

32. Holmberg, B. Studies on a polypeptide inhibiting cell growth obtained from human ascites tumor fluid. Ph.D. thesis, Stockholm 1968.

33. Pearmain, G., Lycette, R. R. and Fitzgerald, P. H. Tuberculin-induced mitosis in peripheral blood leucocytes. *Lancet* **i**: 637, 1963.

34. Lengerova, A. and Viklicky, V. Relative "strength" of histocompatibility barriers as compared on the basis of different criteria. *Folia Biol. (Praha)* **15**: 333, 1969.

35. Klein, G. Tumor antigens. *Ann. Rev. Microbiol.* 20, 1966.

36. Haughton, G. Isoantigenic complexity: a speculative essay. *Folia Biol. (Praha)* **15**: 239, 1969.

37. Ada, G. L., Nossal, G. J. V. and Pye, J. Antigens in immunity. III. Distribution of iodinated antigens following injections into rats via the hind footpads. *Aust. J. exp. Biol. med. Sci.* **42**: 295, 1964.

38. Nossal, G. J. V., Ada, G. L. and Austin, L. M. Antigens in immunity IV. Cellular localization of ^{125}I-labelled flagella in lymph nodes. *Aust. J. exp. Biol. med. Sci.* **42**: 311, 1964.

39. Humphrey, J. H. The fate of antigens and its relationship to the immune response. *Antibiot. et Chemotherap.* **15**: 7, 1969.

40. Bennett, B. and Bloom, B. R. Reactions in vivo and in vitro produced by soluble substances associated with delayed type hypersensitivity. *Proc. nat. Acad. Sci. (Wash.)* **59**: 756, 1968.

41. Kolb, W. P. and Granger, G. A. Lymphocyte in vitro cytotoxicity: characterization of human lymphotoxin. *Proc. nat. Acad. Sci. (Wash.)* **61**: 1250, 1968.

42. Maini, R. N., Bryceson, A. D. M., Wolstencroft, R. H. and Dumonde, D. C. Lymphocyte mitogenic factor in man. *Nature (Lond.)* **224**: 43, 1969.

43. Wilson, D. B., Silvers, W. K. and Nowell, P. C. Quantitative studies on the mixed lymphocyte interaction in rats. II. Relationship of the proliferative response to the immunologic status of the donors. *J. exp. Med.* **126**: 655, 1967.

44. Schwarz, M. R. The mixed lymphocyte reaction: an in vitro test for tolerance. *J. exp. Med.* **127**: 879, 1968.

45. Dutton, R. W. The effect of antigen on the proliferation of spleen cell suspensions from tolerant rabbits. *J. Immunol.* **93**: 814, 1964.

46. Benezra, D., Gery, I. and Davies, A. M. The relationship between lymphocyte transformation and immune responses. II. Correlation between transformation and humoral and cellular immune responses. *Clin. exp. Immunol.* **5**: 155, 1969.

ANTILYMPHOCYTE SERUM AND ENHANCEMENT

M. TAKASUGI* and W. H. HILDEMANN

Department of Medical Microbiology and Immunology, University of California, Los Angeles, California, USA

ABSTRACT

By selective absorptions of rabbit antiserum against A/Sn mouse spleen cells, it was found that antibodies, especially of the 7S or IgG class, directed toward both graft and host cell antigens prolonged the survival of an allogeneic tumor graft in congenic A.BY hosts. At least two sites of action appear to account for the immunosuppression observed following xenogeneic antilymphocyte serum treatment. Thus, antibodies cytotoxic for host lymphocytes and enhancing antibodies specific for donor cell antigens were both demonstrated to be immunosuppressive in the present experiments. Depending on the test system involved, xenogeneic antisera directed against lymphoid cells may be expected to contain antibodies effective against species-specific antigens, alloantigens and tissue-specific antigens.

INTRODUCTION

Following the key discovery by Kaliss (1) of the role of mouse antibodies in immunological enhancement, rabbit antibodies directed against mouse tumors were tried and also found to be effective in promoting tumor growth in incompatible hosts (2). Feldman and Globerson (3) pursued this line of research by conducting a series of experiments on enhancement using rabbit antiserum to induce unresponsiveness. Interest in immunosuppression following administration of xenogeneic serum reached new heights when Woodruff and Anderson (4) demonstrated the effectiveness of rabbit antiserum directed toward lymphocytes in repressing rejection of skin and organ grafts. The perplexing problem of how antilymphocyte serum (ALS) achieves immunosuppression was raised by this observation. One possibility was that enhancement and the ALS effect might have a similar basis. In the present studies, designed to explore this possibility, antiserum was similarly produced in rabbits by immunization against tumor or spleen and lymph node cells from the tumor strain.

As the name antilymphocyte serum implies, the effects of the rabbit antiserum are assumed to be directed against a major component of the machinery of immunity, the mouse lymphocyte in the model considered here. When a series of injections of antilymphocyte serum is administered, a depression of the peripheral lymphocyte count has been observed, and

* Supported by Public Health Service training grant 5T01 AI 0249 from the National Institute of Allergy and Infectious Diseases. Present address: Department of Surgery, University of California, Los Angeles.

221

this, according to Monaco and co-workers (5, 6), is primarily responsible for the inhibition of graft rejection. Alternate explanations for the ALS effect have been suggested, and reviewed by Levey and Medawar (7, 8). They include "blindfolding" of the effector system, immunological thymectomy by the antilymphocyte serum, sterile activation of lymphocytes, and classical enhancement. Other mechanisms, such as increased opsonization, have also been proposed (9). Most of these possibilities were rejected by the reviewers as insufficient to explain ALS effects. However, the arguments cited to date are not compelling in eliminating enhancement as an important mechanism.

Enhancement by serum antibodies alone cannot fully explain the prolongation of mouse skin allografts achieved with rabbit antiserum, since allogeneic antiserum is so ineffective in this regard (10). However, enhancement could well augment the weakened immunity associated with the lymphopenia which regularly follows ALS administration. To the extent that the rabbit antibodies are directed against mouse species-specific antigens, both host cells and allograft cells would of course react with the antibodies. As ALS is composed of a heterogeneous family of antibodies, more than one mechanism of immunosuppression may well be involved. The difficulty of correlating a single assay with ALS effectivity (11) in the prevention of graft rejection argues for multiple sites of action for ALS. Obviously some effects are stronger than others. Moreover, rejection of test-skin allografts may lack the sensitivity to detect weaker effects. Allogeneic test systems such as tumor growth or orthotopic kidney grafts which commonly allow prolonged graft survival may, on the other hand, possess the desired sensitivity to reveal more subtle reactions.

The antisera used in the early enhancement studies and in the later antilymphocyte experiments were similar and possibly identical. A clearer definition of each effect was now sought by attempting to isolate the differently directed activities of the serum. Enhancement usually involves allogeneic antiserum, thereby limiting the antibody effect to antigens of donor target tissue absent in the host. Xenogeneic ALS, on the other hand, possesses a predominance of antibodies directed against species-specific antigens. The most important distinction is that enhancement thus involves antibodies directed against the graft whereas ALS effects are directed against the host. That allogeneic graft and host share many antigens clearly complicates interpretation of ALS effects. However, by absorption of the sera with various cells of graft and host origin, a clearer distinction between the two effects becomes possible.

MATERIALS AND METHODS

Production of serum and serum fractions. Two female New Zealand rabbits weighing approximately 3 kg were injected intradermally three times a week with 10^8 A/Sn spleen cells or 2.5×10^8 sarcoma I (Sa I) cells, for two weeks. Seven days after the last injection, the rabbits were bled, the blood was defibrinated, and the serum was harvested. One experiment was performed with rabbit anti-Sa I, to demonstrate antibody activity against this tumor. Thereafter, antiserum produced against A/Sn spleen cells was used in experiments calling for whole or absorbed serum, because of its higher activity. The rabbits were given booster injections of 10^8 A/Sn spleen cells every other day for one week and then bled for hyperimmune antiserum five days later. This serum was fractionated by gel filtration on a Sephadex G-200 column, as described previously (12). The first peak from several chromatographic runs was combined, concentrated and designated as rabbit 19S (IgM) antibody. The second peak was also pooled, concentrated and designated as rabbit 7S (IgG) antibody. Both fractions were stored without additives at –90 C in a Revco freezer.

Tumor-host system. Sarcoma I, an A strain tumor with H-2a antigens was assayed for growth in congenic A.BY hosts carrying H-2b antigens. Tumor volume was estimated by measuring the two diameters at right angles to each other and applying the formula V = .4(ab²), where 'a' stands for the major and 'b' for the minor diameter (13). The tumor was injected mid-dorsally and measured every three to five days for at least 20 days.

Antibody activity. A) Hemagglutination: Titration of hemagglutinating activity was carried out in Microtiter "V" plates. To each well 0.025 ml saline was added, and the same amount of antiserum was serially diluted across each row with Microtiter dilutors. To each well 0.025 ml of a 2% mouse red blood cell suspension in saline was added. The plates were tapped to mix the cell suspension, and then allowed to settle for 4 hr before reading by the following criteria:

A sharp circle at the point in the well   –
Blurring around the edges of the circle   1+
Cells covering part of the floor of the well 2+
Cells covering complete floor of the well   3+
Hemagglutination titers were designated as the highest dilution giving a positive reading.

B) Cytotoxicity: Cytotoxic tests were also carried out in Microtiter "V" plates using Medium 199 as the diluent. Serial dilutions of 0.025 ml antibody were made and 10^5 lymph node cells in 0.01 ml diluent were added to each well. Following addition of 0.025 ml of a 1:3 dilution of guinea pig complement, the plates were incubated at room temperature for 4 hr before the test was scored for the percentage of cells killed as shown by trypan blue exclusion under phase contrast microscopy. Fifty percent cell-death end points were chosen to designate cytotoxic titers.

Absorption. Two ml of antiserum or antiserum fractions were allowed to react with 1.0 ml packed red blood cells or spleen cells in an ice bath for 1 hr. The suspension was mixed at intervals with a Pasteur pipette to resuspend the cells. After four such absorptions, the removal of xenogeneic antibodies appeared to be complete, based on negative reactions with new test-cells.

Peripheral lymphocyte count. Total leukocyte counts were made on retroorbital sinus blood taken into a Unopette blood diluting pipette, and counted in a hemocytometer. Differential counts were done on cover slips after staining with Wright's blood stain. The lymphocyte count was obtained by multiplying the percentage of lymphocytes by the total leukocyte count.

RESULTS

The effect of rabbit antisera on the growth of sarcoma I in A.BY mice. Antiserum produced in rabbits against the A strain tumor Sa I had a titer of only 1:16 in hemagglutinating activity against A/Sn red blood cells. When the same immunization schedule was followed using A/Sn spleen cells, the titer was 1:64. Both antisera were capable of prolonging the survival of Sa I cells when 0.2 ml of the anti-Sa I or 0.1 ml of the anti-A/Sn spleen cells sera were injected into A.BY hosts inoculated with the tumor (Fig. 1). The failure of Sa I cells to invoke higher antibody activity in rabbits was attributed to low concentrations of antigens on the tumor cell surface membranes.

The effect of rabbit antiserum fractions on the growth of Sarcoma I in A.BY mice. Since some loss of antibody activity always accompanies column chromatography, only rabbit anti-A/Sn spleen cells were used in the fractionation of antiserum. When both 19S and 7S fractions were reconcentrated and tested by hemagglutination, near equal titers, of 1:128 against A/Sn red blood cells and 1:64 against A.BY erythrocytes, were found for

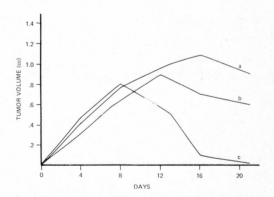

FIG. 1. Prolonged survival of tumor Sa I following treatment of male A.BY mice with rabbit antiserum. The curves represent mean tumor volumes at intervals after inoculation of 5×10^5 tumor cells in the following groups of animals: a) three of five mice given 0.2 ml rabbit anti-Sa I (two of the five which showed no prolonged survival of the tumor are not included); b) five of five mice given 0.1 ml rabbit anti-A/Sn spleen cells; c) five control mice given 0.2 ml normal serum. Serum was administered i.p. immediately after a s.c. injection of the tumor cells.

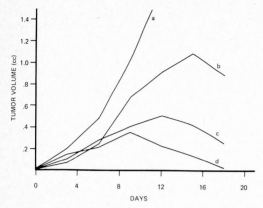

FIG. 2. Prolonged survival of tumor Sa I following treatment of female mice with rabbit antiserum fractions. The curves represent mean tumor volumes at intervals after inoculation 10⁶ tumor cells in the following groups: a) three normal A/Sn mice; b) three A.BY mice given 0.2 ml 7S antibody; c) three A.BY mice given 0.2 ml 19S antibody; d) three untreated A.BY mice. The rabbit anti-mouse lymphocyte fractions were administered i.p. immediately after a s.c. injection of the tumor.

phocyte counts in these controls remained well within the normal range of two to six million lymphocytes/ml.

In ALS treated mice challenged with Sa I, only a slight decrease in lymphocyte count was observed on the day following treatment, and recovery had taken place by the next count taken on the fourth day. In contrast, mice treated with ALS but without exposure to Sa I exhibited a marked lymphopenia of several days. It appears, therefore, that two opposing effects are occurring simultaneously in ALS-treated mice with growing tumors. While the antiserum depresses the lymphocyte level, the immune mechanism is not completely destroyed and responds to the antigenic stimulation of the tumor by cell proliferation. The result is an attenuation of the lymphopenia and a later lymphocytosis. The tumor grew larger and for a longer duration than in untreated hosts under these conditions.

both fractions. When 0.2 ml of either fraction was given to female A.BY hosts inoculated with 10⁶ Sa I cells, 7S antibody was found to possess greater immunosuppressive activity, although a slight delay in regression was observed in mice treated with rabbit IgM (Fig. 2). It is noted that others have found that virtually all of the activity of antilymphocyte serum resides in the 7S fraction (14).

The effect of rabbit antiserum and antiserum fractions on the peripheral lymphocyte count in A.BY hosts. To evaluate the effect of the lymphopenia following ALS injections, the peripheral lymphocyte count was followed in ALS-treated hosts during growth and rejection of Sa I and in mice given only ALS (Fig. 3). Lymphocytosis was observed accompanying the rejection of the tumor in untreated control mice. The absence of increased lymphocyte levels for the same period in animals without tumors eliminated possible infections during retroorbital bleeding as the cause of lymphocytosis. The peripheral lym-

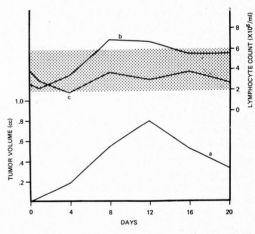

FIG. 3. The peripheral blood lymphocyte levels in Sa I tumor-bearing mice treated with ALS. a) The mean growth curve of Sa I in three male A.BY mice given 5 × 10⁵ tumor cells s.c. followed by 0.1 ml rabbit antilymphocyte serum i.p.; b) the mean lymphocyte count for the same mice during the period of observation; c) the mean lymphocyte count in three male A.BY mice not carrying the tumor following administration of 0.1 ml rabbit ALS. The shaded area represents the normal range of lymphocytes in the peripheral blood of untreated A.BY mice.

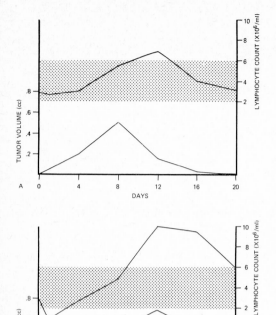

FIG. 4. The peripheral blood lymphocyte levels in Sa I tumor-bearing mice treated with rabbit anti-mouse lymphocyte fractions. A) The graph shows the peripheral blood lymphocyte response (above) and the mean growth curve of Sa I (below) in three female A.BY mice given a s.c. injection of 10⁶ tumor cells followed immediately by 0.1 ml rabbit 19S antibody. B) The conditions for this test were identical to those represented in Graph A above, except that 0.1 ml 7S antibody was given i.p.

The shaded areas represent the normal range of peripheral blood lymphocyte levels in untreated A.BY mice.

The peripheral lymphocyte count was also followed in A.BY mice treated with rabbit 19S or 7S antibodies rather than with whole ALS (Fig. 4A, B). Little or no lymphopenia was observed after 19S injection and a strong lymphocyte response accompanied the normal rejection pattern of the tumor. On the other hand, a sudden depression of the peripheral lymphocyte count was detected after

7S treatment, and the lymphocyte numbers did not return to the original level until the fifth day. Although complete rejection of the tumor did not occur, a delayed but strong lymphocytosis developed, reaching an average level of 10×10^6 lymphocytes/ml on the 12th day. Meanwhile, the tumor volume showed a slight decline between the 12th and 16th day, suggesting that immunity had developed but was inadequate to destroy the tumor. After this decline, the tumor grew progressively. The growth pattern and lymphocyte response taken together suggest that immunity to the graft was delayed by the early lymphopenia, allowing the tumor to grow beyond effective immunological control.

Direction of activity by rabbit antimouse lymphocyte serum (RAMLS). Immunologic reactions across xenogeneic barriers may be assumed to differ substantially from the corresponding responses across less formidable allogeneic barriers. In the present context, mouse antigens recognized by rabbits may be classified into three groups. These are 1) antigens specific to the cell type used in immunization (organ- or tissue-specific antigens), 2) histocompatibility antigens (strain-specific antigens) and 3) antigens peculiar to the mouse (species-specific antigens). Theoretically, the first two classes should be more important in ALS effects, since most species-specific antibodies would be quickly absorbed by other tissue upon i.p. injection before reaching the circulating lymphocytes or a distant allograft.

Antibodies against lymphocyte-specific antigens are probably responsible for the lymphopenia and consequent prolongation of tumor survival. The effectiveness of rabbit antibodies formed against A/Sn lymphocytes in depressing lymphocyte levels in A.BY hosts is consistent with the congenic relationship of these strains.

Antibodies against histocompatibility antigens present on the tumor graft would be ex-

225

pected to cause enhancement, as evidenced by the delayed regression following antiserum treatment. If rabbits can discern antigens of the H-2 system, antibodies should be present in the antiserum elicited by A/Sn spleen cells. Alloantigens other than those of the H-2 system could not play a role in these studies, because of the congenic nature of the tumor donor and recipient mouse strain.

To specify the target of RAMLS activity, absorption studies were carried out with the red blood cells and spleen cells from the graft and host strain. Completeness of absorption and activities of each serum were tested by hemagglutination of red cells and cytotoxic tests against lymph node cells from each strain.

Table 1 shows the design of a series of absorption experiments intended to distinguish the possible antibody effects. The original rabbit antiserum was produced against A/Sn spleen cells and could be assumed to possess antibodies directed against H-2a, lymphocyte-specific, and mouse-specific antigens. The hemagglutinating and cytotoxic titers of the original serum against both A/Sn and A.BY cells were 1:64.

The results of absorption and the effect of absorbed antisera on the growth of sarcoma I in male and female A.BY hosts are shown in Table 2. The presence of antibodies with

TABLE 1. *Design of experiments*

Serum	Absorption	Antibodies removed	Target of absorbed antiserum	Interpretation if tumor survival is prolonged
1	A/Sn RBC	Anti-H-2a Antimouse	Lymphocyte	Antilymphocyte effect
2	A. BY RBC	Antimouse	1) Lymphocyte 2) Tumor cells	1) Antilymphocyte effect 2) Enhancement
3	A/Sn spleen	Antilymphocyte Anti-H-2a Antimouse	——	Nonspecific effects
4	A. BY spleen	Antilymphocyte Antimouse	Tumor cells	Enhancement

TABLE 2. *Enhancement and antilymphocyte effect of rabbit anti-A/Sn spleen serum*

Serum no.	Absorption[a]	Hemagglutination titer A/Sn RBC	Hemagglutination titer A.BY RBC	Cytotoxicity titer A/Sn LNC[g]	Cytotoxicity titer A.BY LNC	Females[b] Delayed regression[d]	Females[b] Progressive growth[e]	Males[c] Delayed regression[d]	Males[c] Progressive growth[e]
1	A/Sn RBC	0	0	16	32	5/5	0/5	1/5	4/5
2	A.BY RBC	2	0	32	32	4/5	1/5	3/5	2/5
3	A/Sn SC[f]	0	0	0	0	1/5	0/5	1/5	0/5
4	A.BY SC	2	0	16	0	3/5	1/5	2/5	0/5
5		64	64	64	32	2/5	3/5	4/5	0/5
NRS[h]		8	8	—[i]	—[i]	1/5	0/5	0/5	0/5

[a] Antiserum was absorbed four times with half the volume of packed cells. Each animal was given 0.2 ml of this serum i.p.
[b] Females received 10^6 Sa I cells s.c. on the back.
[c] Males received 5×10^5 Sa I cells s.c. on the back.
[d] Tumor volume greater than 0.20 ml on day 15, less than 0.20 ml on day 20.
[e] Tumor volume greater than 0.20 ml on day 20.
[f] SC = spleen cells
[g] LNC = lymph node cells
[h] NRS = normal rabbit serum
[i] — = not done

H-2a specificities which could cause enhancement is demonstrated by the retention of hemagglutinating activity against A/Sn red blood cells after absorption with A.BY erythrocytes and spleen cells. Similarly, A/Sn cytotoxic antibodies remained after complete absorption of all A.BY activity with A.BY spleen cells. Also, the presence of antilymphocyte antibodies was confirmed by the retention of A/Sn lymphocytotoxic activity in the rabbit antiserum after exhaustive absorption with A/Sn red blood cells. This result could conceivably be explained by the difference in sensitivity between the two tests. For example, serum #4 possessing only specificities against H-2a antigens exhibited a hemagglutination titer of 1:2 and a cytotoxic titer of 1:16. However, the activity of serum #1 against A.BY lymph node cells reveals antibodies directed against lymphocyte-specific antigens. If antibodies against H-2a were incompletely absorbed by A/Sn red cells, activity should have been greater against A/Sn than A.BY lymph node cells. Thus, antibodies specific for H-2a antigens present only on the tumor, and antilymphocyte antibodies directed against the host immune mechanism could be separated by absorption and tested for ALS and enhancement activity.

When the effect of absorbed antisera on tumor growth was followed in A.BY mice, the only cell suspension which removed all immunosuppressive activity was A/Sn spleen cells. Tumor survival was clearly prolonged in mice treated with the other three antisera. This demonstrates the coexistence of enhancing antibodies and antilymphocyte antibodies in the original serum.

Since IgG antibody was earlier shown to be more immunosuppressive than IgM, the experiment was repeated with 7S antibody reconcentrated to hemagglutination and cytotoxic titers of 1:128 and 1:256. Similar results were obtained and are shown in Table 3. Since enhancement was a definite possibility in these experiments, lymphocyte counts were followed in A.BY mice treated with absorbed 7S antibody. The results in most cases, including those of serum #4 which included putative enhancing antibody, did not show progressive growth but only a delay in regression which was accompanied by lymphocytosis, as would be expected. Since antibodies directed toward the tumor graft were capable of prolonging its survival, the observed enhancement was attributable to the administered 7S or IgG antibodies.

DISCUSSION

Since xenogeneic antibodies are not limited to the unidirectional activity found in allogeneic graft-host combinations, the site of

TABLE 3. *Enhancement and antilymphocyte effect of rabbit anti-A/Sn spleen IgG[a]*

| | | Hemagglutination titer | | Cytotoxicity titer | | Tumor challenge | | | |
| | | | | | | Females | | Males | |
Serum fraction no.	Ab- sorp- tion	A/Sn RBC	A.BY RBC	A/Sn LNC	A.BY LNC	Delayed regression	Progressive growth	Delayed regression	Progressive growth
1	A/Sn RBC	0	0	32	16	0/3	3/3	2/3	1/3
2	A.BY RBC	0	0	16	8	0/3	1/3	1/3	1/3
3	A/Sn SC	0	0	0	0	0/2	0/2	0/2	0/2
4	A.BY SC	0	0	0	0	1/2	1/2	2/3	0/3
5		128	128	256	256	0/3	3/3	3/3	0/3
NRS		8	8	0	0	0/2	0/2	0/3	0/3

[a] Same conditions as in Table 2.

227

activity of such antibodies and their influence on tumor allograft survival in congenic mice was investigated. In the usual experiment utilizing antilymphocyte serum for immunosuppression, a series of ALS injections is administered to the recipient before and after introduction of the graft. A severe loss of lymphocytes is reflected in peripheral lymphopenia and in the competency of the host to reject the graft. The depression of lymphocyte levels by continuing ALS treatment appears to destroy the central mechanism of rejection, and thereby obscures any other graft-promoting effect of the xenogeneic serum. To detect such effects, a single injection of rabbit antiserum was administered concurrently with the tumor inoculum. The injection of the antiserum at the strength used depressed the peripheral lymphocyte level briefly, but did not prevent mice from responding and rejecting the allogeneic tumor. By avoiding an obliteration of the immune response, effects other than antilymphocyte activity could be observed.

The results of the present studies indicate that at least two effects dependent on ALS treatment were responsible for inhibiting the immune response to sarcoma I. The most obvious was the destructive activity of antibodies to host lymphocytes. The present results once again confirmed that cytotoxic action against lymphocytes is a major cause of the decline in peripheral lymphocyte levels after ALS treatment; surely, a severe lymphopenia cripples the hosts' capacity to reject foreign grafts. The ability of rabbit antiserum absorbed with A/Sn red blood cells to prolong graft survival provided strong support for antilymphocyte activity in the present experiments. A/Sn red cells should remove most antibodies with H-2a specificities, including those shared with H-2b mice. Since species-specific antibodies would not be expected to react preferentially with lymphocytes, the majority should be removed by absorption *in vivo*

with host cells in general before they react with circulating lymphocytes. This leaves a specific antilymphocyte effect.

When the peripheral lymphocyte response was quantitated after ALS treatment, a lymphopenia was succeeded by lymphocytosis despite progressive growth of the tumor. Although other factors such as peripheral inhibition may have participated, the ultimate failure to reject the tumor graft appeared to depend, at least partially, on the lateness in the mobilization of the immune response as represented by the lymphocytosis.

The ability of rabbit antiserum produced against A/Sn spleen cells and absorbed with A.BY spleen cells to delay rejection suggested enhancement as a participating factor. A.BY spleen cells should remove antibodies directed against lymphocyte antigens and also against species-specific antigens present in the immunizing inoculum, thereby leaving antibodies against H-2a specificities characteristic of A/Sn mice. The effectiveness of this absorbed serum with antibodies directed only against antigens of the tumor cells was interpreted as specific enhancement. Complete inhibition of the lymphocytosis associated with graft rejection, as reported in an allogeneic system (15), was not found here: and, only a prolongation of tumor survival, reflecting weak enhancement, was achieved.

Cerilli and Treat (16) also studied the effect of ALS on the transplantation of tumors and concluded that enhancement did not play a significant role since tumor cells were much less effective in absorbing the immunosuppressive effect of rabbit ALS than were lymphocytes. However, the lack of reduction in leukoagglutinating activity following absorption with tumor cells in their studies attests to the incompleteness of absorption, and their regimen of 0.025 ml administered every third day beginning six days prior to the test favors strong lymphocytotoxicity which could well mask the involvement of any enhancement.

It is well known that lymphocytes may possess a higher concentration of normal antigens on their surface than many tumor cells. In the present studies with Sa I, the tumor proved to be a weak agent in immunization and in absorption. That enhancement is secondary to the lymphocytotoxic effect in our studies too is suggested by the greater incidence of progressive growths and delayed rejections which were observed following treatment with serum absorbed with red cells than with A.BY spleen cells.

Enhancement in the allogeneic system employed in the present experiments requires antibodies directed specifically against antigens on sarcoma I. This means that antibodies must interfere with the rejection response engendered in A.BY hosts against H-2a antigens on the tumor. That rabbits can recognize H-2a antigens among many presented in a xenogeneic combination has been described by Brent et al. (17) and Shorter and Elveback (18). Our results confirm those observations, since serum from rabbits immunized with A/Sn spleen cells and absorbed with A.BY cells showed greater activity against A/Sn than A.BY cells. Prolongation of tumor survival by these absorbed sera with activity directed toward the tumor graft implies that enhancement can participate in the immunosuppression following xenogeneic ALS treatment.

We wish to thank Dr. Paul I. Terasaki for stimulating discussions and for his interest during the development of this study.

Supported by Pubic Health Service Research Grant AI 07970 from the National Institute of Allergy and Infectious Diseases.

REFERENCES

1. KALISS, N. and MOLOMUT, N. The effect of prior injections of tissue antiserums on the survival of cancer homoiografts in mice. *Cancer Res.* **12**: 110, 1952.
2. KALISS, N. Immunological enhancement of tumor homografts in mice. A review. *Cancer Res.* **18**: 992, 1958.
3. FELDMAN, M. and GLOBERSON, A. Studies on the mechanism of immunological enhancement of tumo rgrafts. *J. nat. Cancer Inst.* **25**: 631, 1960.
4. WOODRUFF, M. F. A. and ANDERSON, N. F. Effect of lymphocyte depletion by thoracic duct fistula and administration of anti-lymphocyte serum on the survival of skin homografts in rats. *Nature (Lond.)* **200**: 702, 1963.
5. MONACO, A. P., WOOD, M. L., GRAY, J. G. and RUSSELL, P. S. Studies on heterologous anti-lymphocyte serum in mice. II. Effect on the immune response. *J. Immunol.* **96**: 229, 1966.
6. GRAY, J. G., MONACO, A. P., WOOD, M. L. and RUSSELL, P. S. Studies on heterologous anti-lymphocyte serum in mice. I. In vitro and in vivo properties. *J. Immunol.* **96**: 217, 1966.
7. LEVEY, R. H. and MEDAWAR, P. B. The mode of action of anti-lymphocytic serum, in: Wolstenholme, G. E. W. and O'Connor, M. (Eds.), "Antilymphocytic serum." Ciba Foundation Symposium. Boston, Little, Brown and Co., 1967, p. 72.
8. LEVEY, R. H. and MEDAWAR, P. B. Nature and mode of action of antilymphocyte serum. *Proc. nat. Acad. Sci. (Wash.)* **56**: 1130, 1966.
9. GREAVES, M. F., TURSI, A., PLAYFAIR, J. H. L., TORRIGIANI, G., ZAMIR, R. and ROITT, I. M. Immunosuppressive potency and in vitro activity of antilymphocyte globulin. *Lancet* **i**: 68, 1969.
10. BRENT, L. and MEDAWAR, P. B. Quantitative studies on tissue transplantation immunity. V. The role of antiserum in enhancement and desensitization. *Proc. roy. Soc. B* **155**: 392, 1961.
11. JEEJEEBOY, H. F. Studies on the mode of action of heterologous antilymphocyte plasma. I. A comparison of the immunosuppressive properties of dog and rabbit anti-rat lymphocyte plasma. *Transplantation* **5**: 273, 1967.
12. TAKASUGI, M. and HILDEMANN, W. H. Regulation of immunity toward allogeneic tumors in mice. I. Effect of antiserum fractions on tumor growth. *J. nat Cancer Inst.* **43**: 843, 1969.
13. ATTIA, M. A., DeOME, K. B. and WEISS, D. W. Immunology of spontaneous mammary carcinomas in mice. II. Resistance to a rapidly and a slowly developing tumor. *Cancer Res.* **25**: 451, 1965.
14. JAMES, K. and MEDAWAR, P. B. Characterization of antilymphocyte antibody. *Nature (Lond.)* **214**: 1052, 1967.
15. TAKASUGI, M. and HILDEMANN, W. H. Regulation of immunity toward allogeneic tumors in mice. II. Effect of antiserum and antiserum fractions on cellular and humoral response. *J. nat. Cancer Inst.* **43**: 857, 1969.
16. CERILLI, G. J. and TREAT, R. C. The effect of antilymphocyte serum on the induction and growth of tumor in the adult mouse. *Transplantation* **8**: 774, 1969.
17. BRENT, L., COURTENAY, T. and GOWLAND, G. Immunological reactivity of lymphoid cells after treatment with antilymphocytic serum. *Nature (Lond.)* **215**: 1461, 1967.
18. SHORTER, R. G. and ELVEBACK, L. R. Evaluation of strain-specific effects in the immunosuppressive action of heterologous antithymus sera in mice. *Transplantation* **9**: 253, 1970.

TUMOR-ASSOCIATED IMMUNOGLOBULINS

ISAAC P. WITZ

Department of Microbiology, Tel Aviv University, Tel Aviv, Israel

There are several possible mechanisms, not mutually exclusive, to account for the successful outgrowth of antigenic tumors in the primary host. Antibody mediated self- (or auto-) enhancement has been suggested as one of them (1–4). Enhancing antibodies present in the autochthonous host may interfere with tumor rejection either by affecting the immune mechanism of the host, rendering it completely or partially inactive, or by blocking antigenic determinants on the tumor cell surface. Such a blocking may interfere with the afferent limb of the immune response (5) by rendering tumor cells nonimmunogenic or less so, or may prevent immune lymphocytes from destroying the target tumor cells (efferent inhibition), or both (5).

An efferent enhancement mechanism implies that intrinsically potent effector lymphocytes from immunized donors are blocked from attacking and destroying antibody-coated target cells, while the antibodies themselves are apparently harmless to the cells which they coat. The existence of efferent enhancement of tumor allografts has been suggested by G. Möller's *in vivo* experiments (6, 7) and has been strongly supported by the *in vitro* studies of E. Möller (8) and Brunner and co-workers (9). In these experiments, tumor cells could be protected *in vitro* from destruction by allogeneic lymphocytes from immunized donors by blocking the target cells with alloantibodies directed against the same target cells.

An efferent type of enhancement can also be postulated for autochthonous systems, and could explain the successful growth of autochthonous tumors despite the fact that autochthonous hosts react (or can be induced to react) against tumor-specific transplantation antigens. This host reactivity may be characterized by antitumor immunity at the level of the whole animal or by the ability of isolated autochthonous lymphoid cells to kill or to prevent the growth of the tumor cells (10–16). Using the sensitive method of colony inhibition (17), it has been shown by the Hellströms and their collaborators (18) that lymph node cells from animals whose primary tumors regressed or were removed can destroy, or at least inhibit, the multiplication of the autochthonous tumor cells *in vitro*. Blood lymphocytes from cancer patients had a similar capacity (19, 20). The same authors (21–23) and Heppner (24) further demonstrated that serum from animals and humans with actively growing tumors can abrogate this lymphocyte-mediated destruction of the tumor cells. It became clear that the serum affected the tumor target cells and not the effector lymphocytes, presumably by blocking receptor sites on the former. The removal of this protective effect of the serum following its incubation with an antiserum directed against immunoglobulin led to the conclusion that the active serum factor was an immunoglobulin.

From these results it was postulated that antibodies present in the serum of tumor-bearing humans and animals may interfere with lymphocyte-mediated destruction of autochthonous tumor cells, in a manner similar to the alloantibody-mediated prevention of tumor cell destruction by allogeneic immune lymphocytes. The question whether such a mechanism does, in fact, also operate *in vivo* is of extreme importance.

Accessibility of tumor antigens to circulating antibodies. In order for an efferent enhancement mechanism to be operative *in vivo*, the requirement that antigenic determinants on tumor cells be accessible to circulating antibodies must be met. *In vivo* localization studies of radioiodine labeled alloantibodies in mice (25–28) have shown that this question can be approached experimentally. It was found that allografts of mouse marrow cells could be traced in the recipients by injecting the carrier animals with radiolabeled alloantibodies directed at alloantigens of the donor. These antibodies did not cross-localize in ungrafted recipients, and they were fixed in the graft hosts to the implanted cells (29). Using the same experimental approach, attempts were made to discover whether tumor-specific antigens are accessible to circulating antibodies. Radioiodine-labeled antibodies derived from syngeneic mice immunized with irradiated Moloney lymphoma cells were injected into Moloney lymphoma-bearing mice and into corresponding normal animals. The results (30) showed that there was a significant increase in specific localization of the antibodies in the spleens of the lymphoma-bearing, as compared to the normal mice; however, only little or no localization in the tumors could be observed. One way to interpret the results was that the tumor cells lodging in the spleen of the lymphoma-bearing mice are better accessible to the circulation than those within the tumor mass, because of the better blood circulation through the spleen. Additional experiments (Witz, Shany and Klein, unpublished results) have revealed that anti-Moloney lymphoma antibodies can sometimes localize on ascitic Moloney tumor cells.

It would appear, accordingly, that antitumor antibodies with localizing properties can find their way to the tumor if the conditions of the circulation permit it, and the functional conditions for an efferent type of enhancement do thus exist.

Coating of tumor cells by immunoglobulin. A demonstration that tumor cells are covered *in situ* by antibodies would strongly support the hypothesis that an efferent enhancement mechanism operates in the autochthonous tumor-bearing host. There are several reports which indicate such *in vivo* coating of tumor cells by immunoglobulin.

Indirect evidence for coating of tumor cells by immunoglobulin is indeed quite convincing. Pilch and Riggins (31) demonstrated that humoral antibodies directed at cell surface antigens of methylcholanthrene-induced tumors appear in the serum of mice soon after surgical removal of the neoplasms. Use of a fluorescent reagent directed against mouse immunoglobulin did not, however, establish the presence of an immunoglobulin coat on the cells. Gold (32) reported essentially similar results: 70% of patients with nonmetastatic malignancies of the digestive system were reported to have antibodies directed against carcinoembryonic antigens, in contrast to patients with metastatic tumors who as a rule did not have these antibodies. In the same study it was reported that in four patients who did not have such antibodies, humoral antibodies directed against the carcinoembryonic antigens of the digestive system appeared soon after surgical removal of their tumors. The interpretation of these results has been that large masses of tumors absorb all of the antibodies from the circulation. Methycholanthrene-induced autochthonous sarcomas were found by Yoshida (11) to contain components of complement, thus indicating, indirectly, the presence of complement-fixing immunoglobulin attached to the neoplastic cells.

Direct evidence for the *in vivo* coating of tumor cells by antibodies was obtained by Klein et al. (33, 34), and by Tachibana who showed that Burkitt's lymphoma cells are coated with IgG. Witz et al. (35) demonstrated that membranous elements from autochthonous acetaminofluorene-induced rat hepatomas are associated with IgG. Similar results were obtained with benzo(a)pyrene-induced tumors in C3H and C57BL mice (36, 37). The immunoglobulins could be eluted from the tissue preparation with a low pH glycine buffer. Coating of Moloney lymphoma cells with

immunoglobulin was demonstrated by the following experiments: Moloney lymphoma ascites cells were removed from strain A mice nine to 11 days following implantation. The cells were washed twice with pH 7.2 phosphate buffer containing 10% inactivated calf serum. To various amounts of cells, a mixture containing I^{131} labeled globulin from a rabbit antimouse globulin antiserum and I^{125} labeled normal rabbit globulin was added. The mixture was incubated with the cells for 60 min at 37 C, and the cells were washed twice with buffer. The cells were then counted for the presence of I^{131} and I^{125} in a double channel analyzer, and the uptake by the tumor cells of antibodies directed against mouse globulin was calculated. Fig. 1 shows the results of such an experiment. It can be seen clearly that increasing numbers of Moloney lymphoma cells absorb increasing proportions of the anti-immunoglobulin antibodies, indicating that globulin is present on these tumor cells. The uptake of the labeled antimouse globulin antibodies could be inhibited by addition to the incubation mixture of excess unlabeled globulin isolated from the same rabbit antimouse globulin antiserum. It should be noted that not all lymphoma cells studied fixed the antimouse globulin antibodies, and in contrast to other tumors no immunoglobulin could be detected in acid eluates of ascites Moloney lymphoma cells; the amount of elutable immunoglobulin (if any was eluted) may have been too small to be detected.

Elution of immunoglobulin from tumor cells and from subcellular fractions, and the identification of the eluted immunoglobulins. With the aim of elucidating the biological activity of the immunoglobulins found in association with tumors, we* initiated experiments designed to determine the subcellular fraction

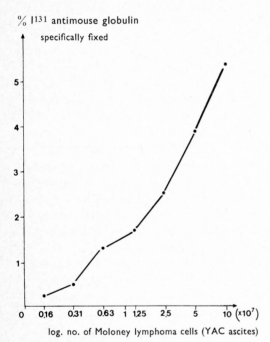

% I^{131} antimouse globulin

specifically fixed

log. no. of Moloney lymphoma cells (YAC ascites)

FIG. 1. *In vitro* fixation of I^{131} labeled globulin from a rabbit antimouse globulin antiserum onto Moloney lymphoma cells. I^{131} antimouse globulin specifically fixed is the fixation (% of added dose) of I^{131} labeled globulin from a rabbit antimouse globulin antiserum, minus the fixation (% of added dose) of I^{125} labeled globulin from an unimmunized rabbit.

*   These experiments are part of a Ph.D. thesis of M. Ran, to be submitted to the Senate of the Tel Aviv University.

richest in elutable immunoglobulin (using a pH 2.5 glycine buffer) and to identify the immunoglobulins present in these eluates. Tissue of primary benzo(a)pyrene-induced sarcomas was homogenized in 0.25 M sucrose, after removal of necrotic and hemorrhagic portions. The homogenate was then fractionated according to Fig. 2. The various sediments were washed at least twice with a pH 8.0 borate buffered saline, and were then subjected to extraction with ice-cold pH 2.5 glycine buffer for 30 min in a shaking ice bath. The mixtures were centrifuged for 30 min at 12,000 to 30,000 $\times$ g in the cold, and the supernatant fluids neutralized with 1.0 N NaOH. The neutralized supernatant fluids

were then dialyzed against borate buffered saline at pH 8.0.

Most of the experiments were performed with the fraction which sedimented after centrifugation at 105,000 $\times$ g (membrane-rich fraction). Analyzing eluates of this subcellular fraction by immunoelectrophoresis with an antiserum directed against mouse serum, it was found that the eluates originating from tumor tissue contained IgG, which was apparently the only serum protein present. No IgG was detected in eluates from the corresponding fractions originating from normal muscle. A semiquantitative determination of IgG (Table 1) revealed that eluates originating from the membrane-rich fraction of the

TABLE 1. *Elutable IgG2 from cells and from tissue sediments obtained following centrifugation at 105,000 $\times$ g*

	No. of experiments	No. of mice[a]	No. of IgG2 units eluted/mg tissue protein[b]	IgG2 relative activity of eluate (%)[c]
Benzo(a)pyrene induced primary tumors, C3H				
Individual tumors[d]				
(105,000 $\times$ g sediment) (mean $\pm$ SD)	5	6	5.6 $\pm$ 0.9	9.0 $\pm$ 2.8
Tumor pools[e]				
(105,000 $\times$ g sediment) (mean $\pm$ SD)	5	14	3.9 $\pm$ 2.1	14.3 $\pm$ 8.2
Intact tumor cells	4	10	8.6 $\pm$ 2.9	4.7 $\pm$ 3.7
Transplanted C3H tumors (originating from a benzo(a)pyrene induced tumor 105.000 $\times$ g sediment				
Line 1 transplant generation 1	1	6	1.3	3.0
Line 2 ,, ,, 11	1	2	0.6	7.1
Line 2 ,, ,, 12	1	3	1.7	3.9
Line 2 ,, ,, 13	1	9	2.0	6.7
Spontaneous mammary carcinoma, C3H				
105,000 $\times$ g sediment (mean $\pm$ SD)	6	16	4.0 $\pm$ 2.3	10.8 $\pm$ 13.9[f]
Normal muscle, C3H				
105,000 $\times$ g sediment	3	30	< 0.5[g]	0.0

[a] Cumulative number of mice, used for all experiments with each material.
[b] IgG2 unit = the minimal volume of eluate required to give a precipitation line with a monospecific IgG2 reagent, under standard conditions.
[c] IgG2 relative activity = the minimal amount of eluate protein required to give a precipitation line with a monospecific IgG2 reagent per total protein eluted (%).
[d] The tumors in this group were harvested from a single group of mice, all having been injected with benzo(a)pyrene at the same time. Individual tumors were analyzed.
[e] Tumors were harvested and pooled from various groups of mice which had been injected with benzo(a)pyrene at different times.
[f] Note the variation among the tumors. The IgG2 relative activity of large tumors was much higher than that of small tumors.
[g] Even the most concentrated eluates of 105,000 $\times$ g sediments of normal muscle did not produce a precipitation line with the IgG2 reagent.

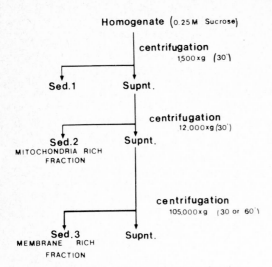

Homogenate (0.25 M Sucrose)

centrifugation
1,500 × g (30')

Sed. 1   Supnt.

centrifugation
12,000 × g (30')

Sed. 2   Supnt.
MITOCHONDRIA RICH
FRACTION

centrifugation
105,000 × g (30 or 60')

Sed. 3   Supnt.
MEMBRANE   RICH
FRACTION

FIG. 2.   Preparation of tissue subcellular fractions.

benzo(a)pyrene induced tumors contained at least 10 times more IgG (per tissue protein) than similar eluates of normal muscle. In general, it was observed that eluates from fast-growing tumors had a higher IgG2 relative activity than eluates from slowly growing ones. (IgG$_2$ relative activity is the minimal amount of eluate protein required to produce a precipitation line with a monospecific IgG$_2$ antiserum reagent, per total protein eluted.)

It was further found that the subcellular fractions in which membranes (both external and internal) are the major components (sediment III in Fig. 2) are the richest in elutable immunoglobulin. The amount of IgG eluted from the mitochondria rich fraction, for instance, was at least two to three times less than the amount eluted from the membrane-rich fraction. An indication that the eluted IgG was, in fact, associated with the surface of the tumor cells comes from the observation that immunoglobulin was found in acid eluates of intact washed tumor cells, separated mechanically from solid tumors.

Identification of the subclass to which the eluted IgG belonged was performed with mono-specific antiserum reagents against mouse IgG1 and IgG2 (Melpar, USA). In the eluates

of most tumors, only IgG2, and not IgG1, was detected; only a minority of the eluates contained IgG1 in addition to IgG2. Immnno-electrophoretic tests showed that the IgG2 from the eluates had a restricted mobility compared with IgG2 from serum (Fig. 3), indicating, perhaps, that only a selected population of IgG2 molecules is present in the eluates.

Subcellular fractions of other mouse tumors were also analyzed qualitatively and semi-quantitatively for the presence of elutable immunoglobulin. Some of the results are summarized in Table 1. IgG2 could be eluted from sediments (105,000 × g) of tumors transplanted from primary benzo(a)pyrene-induced sarcomas in C3H mice. Two different tumor lines were tested, line 1 in its first transplant generation and line 2 in its 11th to 13th transplant generations. The amounts of IgG2 eluted were substantially lower than those eluted from primary tumors. The variability in elutable IgG2 from membrane-rich sediments of spontaneous mammary carcinomas of C3H mice is of interest. It was observed that in most cases the eluates from large tumors contained relatively less non-IgG2 proteins than eluates from small ones. This was shown by a higher IgG2 relative activity of the former eluates compared to a lower IgG2 relative activity of eluates from small tumors.

Some biological activities of tumor eluates. IgG isolated from eluates of carcinogen-induced rat hepatomas had a 10- to 20-fold higher affinity for the microsomal fraction of tumors or of normal liver than IgG isolated from serum. This was measured *in vitro*, using the paired radioiodine label technique (35). IgG isolated from normal rat liver eluates also had a 10- to 20-fold higher affinity to the microsomal fractions than IgG isolated from serum. It was suggested that the eluted IgG represents a selected population of antitissue antibodies, fixed *in vivo* to their targets.

Preliminary experiments suggest that eluates

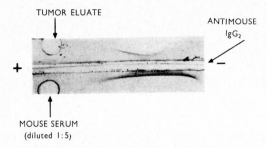

TUMOR ELUATE

ANTIMOUSE
IgG₂

+

MOUSE SERUM
(diluted 1:5)

FIG. 3. Immunoelectrophoretic analysis of mouse serum and a benzo(a)pyrene induced tumor eluate developed with a monospecific anti-IgG2 antiserum. Note the restricted mobility of the IgG2 from the eluate.

of benzo(a)pyrene-induced sarcomas have the capability of enhancing the growth of such transplanted tumors. This was shown by the finding that incubation of tumor cells with tumor eluates prior to their transfer to recipient mice enhanced growth. This enhancement was manifested by earlier appearance of tumors, a higher proportion of takes and the larger size of the tumors and, sometimes, a shorter survival time of the host mice. No data are yet available on the nature of the factors in the tumor eluates causing the enhancement, nor on its specificity. It can be assumed, however, that the enhancing capacity of the eluates can be attributed, at least in part, to an IgG of high binding affinity to the target cells.

Possible biological significance of the tumor-associated immunoglobulins. IgG found in association with tumors may originate either from immunoglobulin-producing cells within or around the tumor, or, alternatively, they may be produced distally and may then become absorbed onto the surface of the neoplastic cells. Phillips has recently shown (38) that some transplantable mouse tumors produce IgG and at least one component of complement. If the IgG2 is indeed produced by cells which are found in the close vicinity of the tumor itself, it would be of great interest to find out why mostly IgG2 producing cells migrate to the tumor.

At least two alternative mechanisms may function in the absorption of IgG molecules to tumor cells. One is "nonspecific" in nature, that is, the binding of IgG to cells without the agency of a specific antigen-binding site on the IgG molecule. The alternative specific mechanism implies that the tumor-associated IgG represents antibody directed against determinants on the cell membranes.

Nonspecific fixation of immunoglobulin molecules to various tissues is a well known phenomenon (for review, see Refs. 39, 40). Homocytotropic antibodies (41) may illustrate such a binding. Some antibody molecules directed against a variety of antigens have the capability of becoming firmly attached to tissues, the Fc fragment of the molecule apparently being responsible for this attachment (42–44). It is conceivable that immunoglobulin attached to cells by any means, specifically or even nonspecifically, may reduce their immunogenicity, and may protect them from various insults, including cell-mediated immunity. Both an afferent and an efferent enhancement of primary tumor-growth may thus occur as a result of such a nonspecific event. If host-tumor interactions are regarded in analogous terms to host-microbial parasite relations, one might reach the conclusion that it is of great selective advantage for a tumor to be able to "utilize," for its own protection, the characteristic of certain types of immunoglobulins to bind nonspecifically to tissues. An argument against the possibility that the tumor-associated immunoglobulin represents homocytotropic antibodies is the fact that in mice these antibodies usually belong to the fast-moving IgG1 immunoglobulin subclass (45, 46), whereas the immunoglobulins detected in association with the tumors were primarily of the IgG2 type. On the other hand, negatively charged tumor cells may nonspecifically attach to themselves, by electrostatic bonds, less negatively charged IgG2 molecules.

Alternatively, or in addition, the tumor-

235

associated IgG2 immunoglobulins may represent specific antibodies directed against determinants of tumor cells. This binding may also protect tumor cells from lymphocyte-mediated destruction, and thus constitute enhancement operating at the level of the target cell. This hypothesis is strengthened by the experimental evidence that IgG2 type antibodies indeed possess specific enhancing properties for tumor allografts (47–49).

If a specific fixation of IgG2 antibody to its antigen on the tumor cell surface indeed occurs, then an afferent enhancement would be somewhat more difficult to explain, due to the time factor involved. Humoral and cellular responses appear simultaneously, and in no case does the humoral response preceed the cellular response, a situation required for purely afferent enhancement mechanism to occru.

If our observations on the association between IgG2 and tumors represent, in fact, a phenomenon of efferent enhancement, a number of questions immediately present themselves. First, it is generally accepted that mouse IgG2 antibodies fix complement, and as such may be cytotoxic to cells to which they are bound. The fact that this did not appear to be the case here requires some consideration. The possibilities exist that complement was not activated, that there were insufficient amounts of complement, that the cells were resistant to the activity of complement, or that activated complement could not be fixed due to a deformation in the structure of the antibodies. The last point requires elaboration, and we examined the capability of subcellular fractions of tumors to induce alterations in the structure of immunoglobulins. Pilot experiments suggested that the lysosome rich subcellular fraction of tumors may, under certain experimental conditions, indeed induce changes in crude serum globulin preparations. These changes are manifested by an altered precipitation pattern of the treated immunoglobulins in gel-diffusion and in immunoelectrophoresis. No data are yet available as to which globulins were altered, what type of changes occurred, or what substance in the tumor fraction induced the observed alterations.

Another question concerns the nature of the antigen from which the IgG2 was eluted. As reported, the IgG2 was derived from membrane-rich subcellular fractions and from intact tumor cells, suggesting that the immunoglobulin was bound to external membranes. It would be of extreme importance to identify the antigenic determinant or the site of the tumor cell surface to which the immunoglobulin is bound, and to determine whether these determinants are specific for each tumor, in a manner similar to the tumor-specific transplantation antigens of such carcinogen-induced tumors, or whether the determinant is common to several tumors. The problem of avidity of the antibody to the tumor cells also requires further consideration. Hellström observed (22) that the enhancing antibodies in his system had extremely low avidity for the tumor cells; simple washing of the coated cells dissociated the cell-immunoglobulin complex. This finding is in agreement with the studies demonstrating that immunization with relatively high doses of antigen will result in low affinity (50) and low avidity (51) antibodies. A tumor-bearing animal is probably constantly sensitized with massive doses of antigen, resulting in antibodies of very low avidity to the immunogens. The IgG2 in the acid eluates may thus represent relatively high-avidity antibodies, the very low-avidity ones being removed in the process of washing; or alternatively, the eluted antibodies may represent molecules of a relatively low avidity for cell surface antigens as compared with antibodies which may not have been dissociated from the tissue with thelow pH buffer. Quantitative determinants of how much total immunoglobulin was bound to the tissue and what fraction was eluted would help in determining this point.

This investigation has been aided by a grant from The Jane Coffin Childs Memorial Fund for Medical Research.

The author wishes to thank Drs. N. Kaliss, G. Klein and D. Pressman for their valuable comments and criticisms of this paper.

REFERENCES

1. ATTIA, A. M. and WEISS, D. W. Immunology of spontaneous mammary carcinomas in mice. V. Acquired tumor resistance and enhancement in strain A mice infected with mammary tumor virus. *Cancer Res.* **26**: 1787, 1966.
2. DEZFULIAN, M., ZEE, T., DEOME, K. B., BLAIR, P. B. and WEISS, D. W. Role of the mammary tumor virus in the immunogenicity of spontaneous mammary carcinomas of BALB/c mice and in the responsiveness of the hosts. *Cancer Res.* **28**: 1759, 1968.
3. KALISS, N. Immunological enhancement. *Int. Rev. exp. Path.* **8**: 241, 1969.
4. KLEIN, G. Experimental studies in tumor immunology. *Fed. Proc.* **28**: 1739, 1969.
5. BILLINGHAM, R. E., BRENT, L. and MEDAWAR, P. B. Enhancement in normal homografts, with a note of its possible mechanism. *Transplant. Bull.* **3**: 84, 1956.
6. MÖLLER, G. Studies on the mechanism of immunological enhancement of tumor homografts. III. Interaction between humoral isoantibodies and immune lymphoid cells. *J. nat. Cancer Inst.* **30**: 1205, 1963.
7. MÖLLER, G. Antibody-induced depression of the immune response: A study of the mechanism in various immunological systems. *Transplantation* **2**: 405, 1964.
8. MÖLLER, E. Antagonistic effects of humoral isoantibodies on the in vitro cytotoxicity of immune lymphoid cells. *J. exp. Med.* **122**: 11, 1965.
9. BRUNNER, K. T., MAUEL, J., CEROTTINI, J. C. and CHAPUIS, B. Quantitative assay of the lytic action of immune lymphoid cells on ^{51}Cr-labelled allogeneic target cells in vitro; Inhibition by isoantibody and by drugs. *Immunology* **14**: 181, 1968.
10. KLEIN, G., SJÖGREN, H. O., KLEIN, E. and HELLSTRÖM, K. E. Demonstration of resistance against methylcholanthrene-induced sarcomas in the primary autochthonous host. *Cancer Res.* **20**: 1561, 1960.
11. YOSHIDA, T. O. Further evidence of immunologic reaction against methylcholanthrene-induced autochthonous tumors. *Jap. J. exp. Med.* **35**: 115, 1965.
12. MIKULSKA, Z. B., SMITH, C. and ALEXANDER, P. Evidence for an immunological reaction of the host directed against its own actively growing primary tumor. *J. nat. Cancer Inst.* **36**: 29, 1966.
13. SOUTHAM, C. M., BRUNSCHWIG, A., LEVIN, A. G. and DIZON, Q. S. Effect of Leukocytes on transplantability of human cancer. *Cancer (Phila.)* **19**: 1743, 1966.
14. TAKEDA, K., AIZAWA, M., KIKUCHI, Y., YAMAWAKI, S. and NAKAMURA, K. Tumor auto-immunity against methylcholanthrene-induced sarcomas of the rat. *Gann* **57**: 221, 1966
15. FEFER, A., McCOY, J. L., PERK, K. and GLYNN, J. P. Immunologic, virologic, and pathologic studies of regression of autochthonous Moloney sarcoma virus-induced tumors in mice. *Cancer Res.* **28**: 1577, 1968.
16. STJERNSWÄRD, J., CLIFFORD, P., SINGH, S. and SVEDMYR, E. Indication of cellular immunological reactions against autochthonous tumor in cancer patients studied in vitro. *E. Afr. med. J.* **45**: 1, 1968.
17. HELLSTRÖM, I. A colony inhibition (CI) technique for demonstration of tumor cell destruction by lymphoid cells in vitro. *Int. J. Cancer* **2**: 65, 1967.
18. HELLSTRÖM, I., HELLSTRÖM, K. E. and PIERCE, G. E. In vitro studies of immune reactions against autochthonous and syngeneic mouse tumors induced by methylcholanthrene and plastic discs. *Int. J. Cancer* **3**: 467, 1968.
19. HELLSTRÖM, I. E., HELLSTRÖM, K. E., PIERCE, G. E. and BILL, A. H. Demonstration of cell-bound and humoral immunity against neuroblastoma cells. *Proc. nat. Acad. Sci. (Wash.)* **60**: 1231, 1968.
20. HELLSTRÖM, I., HELLSTRÖM, K. E., PIERCE, G. E. and YANG, J. P. S. Cellular and humoral immunity to different types of human neoplasms. *Nature (Lond.)* **220**: 1352, 1968.
21. HELLSTRÖM, I., HELLSTRÖM, K. E., EVANS, C. A., HEPPNER, G. H., PIERCE, G. E. and YANG, J. P. S. Serum mediated protection of neoplastic cells from inhibition by lymphocytes immune to their tumor-specific antigens. *Proc. nat. Acad. Sci. (Wash.)* **62**: 362, 1969.
22. HELLSTRÖM, I. and HELLSTRÖM, K. E. Studies on cellular immunity and its serum-mediated inhibition in Moloney virus induced mouse sarcoma. *Int. J. Cancer* **4**: 587, 1969.
23. HELLSTRÖM, I., EVANS, C. A. and HELLSTRÖM, K. E. Cellular immunity and its serum mediated inhibition in shope-virus-induced rabbit papillomas. *Int. J. Cancer* **4**: 601, 1969.
24. HEPPNER, G. H. Studies on serum-mediated inhibition of cellular immunity to spontaneous mouse mammary tumors. *Int. J. Cancer* **4**: 608, 1969.
25. WITZ, I., YAGI, Y. and PRESSMAN, D. Availability of isoantigens to circulating antibodies. *J. Immunol.* **101**: 217, 1968.
26. WITZ, I., KALISS, N. and PRESSMAN, D. Isoantigens available to circulating antibodies. *J. Immunol.* **102**: 283, 1969.
27. WITZ, I., YAGI, Y. and PRESSMAN, D. Brain localizing activity of hetero and isoimmune sera directed against lymphocytic cells. *Proc. Soc. exp. Biol. (N.Y.)* **130**: 928, 1969.
28. WITZ, I., CUDKOWICZ, G. and PRESSMAN, D. Availability of transplantation alloantigens to circulating antibodies. Studies with alloantibodies of known specificity. *J. Immunol.* **102**: 1373, 1969.
29. WITZ, I., CUDKOWICZ, G. and PRESSMAN, D. Detection of hemopoietic allografts by localization of radiolabeled alloantibodies. *J. Immunol.* **104**: 19, 1970.

30. WITZ, I., KLEIN, G. and PRESSMAN, D. Moloney lymphoma antibodies from mice; localization in spleens of Moloney lymphoma bearing mice. *Proc. Soc. exp. Biol. (N.Y.)* **130**: 1102, 1969.

31. PILCH, Y. H. and RIGGINS, R. S. Antibodies to spontaneous and methylcholanthrene induced tumors in inbred mice. *Cancer Res.* **26**: 871, 1966.

32. GOLD, P. Circulating antibodies against carcino-embryonic antigens of the human digestive system. *Cancer (Phila.)* **20**: 1663, 1967.

33. KLEIN, G. and OETTGEN, H. F. Immunologic factors involved in the growth of primary tumors in human or animal hosts. *Cancer Res.* **29**: 1741, 1969.

34. KLEIN, G., CLIFFORD, P., HENLE, G., HENLE, W., GEERING, G. and OLD, L. J. EBV-associated serological patterns in a Burkitt lymphoma patient during regression and recurrence. *Int. J. Cancer* **4**: 416, 1969.

35. WITZ, I., YAGI, Y. and PRESSMAN, D. IgG associated with microsomes from autochthonous hepatomas and normal liver of rats. *Cancer Res.* **27**: 2295, 1967.

36. WITZ, I. and RAN, M. Studies on the association of immunoglobulins with tumors, in: L. Severi (Ed.) "Immunity and tolerance in oncogenesis." *Proc. IV Int. Quad. Conf. Cancer, 1969.* 1970, p. 345.

37. RAN, M. and WITZ, I.P. Tumor associated immunoglobulins. The elution of IgG_2 from mouse tumors. *Int. J. Cancer* **6**: 361, 1970.

38. PHILLIPS, M. E. Tumor antigens. I. Immunological studies of tissue and tumor antigens and serum protein production by a mouse rhabdomyosarcoma and mammary adenocarcinoma. *Int. Arch. Allergy* **37**: 54, 1970.

39. ISHIZAKA, K. Gamma globulin and molecular mechanisms in hypersensitivity reactions. *Progr. Allergy* **7**: 32, 1963.

40. BLOCH, K. J. The anaphylactic antibodies of mammals including man. *Progr. Allergy* **10**: 84, 1967.

41. BECKER, E. L. and AUSTIN, K. F. Mechanisms of immunologic injury of rat peritoneal mast cells. I. The effect of phosphonate inhibitors on the homocytotropic antibody mediated histamine release and the first component of rat complement. *J. exp. Med.* **124**: 379, 1966.

42. OVARY, Z. and KARUSH, F. Studies on the immunologic mechanism of anaphylaxis. II. Sensitizing and combining capacity in vivo of fractions separated from papain digest of antihapten antibody. *J. Immunol.* **86**: 146, 1961.

43. ISHIZAKA, K., ISHIZAKA, T. and SUGAHARA, T. Biological activity of soluble antigen-antibody complexes. VII. Role of an antibody fragment in the induction of biological activities. *J. Immunol.* **88**: 690, 1962.

44. PINTO, M. and MORE, R. Homologous skin-sensitizing activity of rabbit anti-hydrocortisone hemisuccinate antibodies. II. Inhibition and adsorption studies on "Early-antibody"—induced P-K type reaction. *Int. Arch. Allergy* **37**: 41, 1970.

45. MOTA, I., WONG, D. and SADUN, E. H. Separation of mouse homocytotropic antibodies by biological screening. *Immunology* **17**: 295, 1969.

46. MCVEIGH, T. A., Jr. and VOSS, E. W., Jr. Properties of purified mouse homocytotropic antibody. *J. Immunol.* **103**: 1349, 1969.

47. IRVIN, G. L., III., EUSTACE, J. C. and FAHEY, J. L. Enhancement activity of mouse immunoglobulin classes. *J. Immunol.* **99**: 1085, 1967.

48. TOKUDA, S. and MCENTEE, P. F. Immunologinic enhancement of sarcoma. I by mouse γ-globulin fractions. *Transplantation* **5**: 606, 1967.

49. TAKASUGI, M. and HILDEMANN, W. H. Regulation of immunity toward allogeneic tumors in mice. I. Effect of antiserum fractions on tumor growth. *J. nat. Cancer Inst.* **43**: 843, 1969.

50. GOIDL, E. A., PAUL, W. E., SISKIND, G. W. and BENACERRAF, B. The effect of antigen dose and time after immunization on the amount and affinity of anti-hapten antibody. *J. Immunol.* **100**: 371, 1968.

51. CELADA, F., SCHMIDT, D. and STROM, R. Determination of avidity of anti-albumin antibodies in the mouse. Influence of the number of cells transferred on the quality of the secondary adoptive response. *Immunology* **17**: 189, 1969.

THE USE OF
IRRADIATED IMMUNE LYMPHOID CELLS FOR
IMMUNOTHERAPY OF PRIMARY TUMORS IN RATS

PETER ALEXANDER and E. J. DELORME

Chester Beatty Research Institute Laboratories, Belmont, Sutton, Surrey, England

ABSTRACT

The growth of primary chemically induced sarcomas in rats can be slowed, and occasionally complete regressions induced, by injecting lymphoid cells from the thoracic duct lymph of rats immunized with a piece of the tumor to be treated. Irradiation of the immune lymphoid cells with 1,000 R of X-rays prior to injection does not diminish their antitumor activity. These experiments support the hypothesis that the cells responsible for the antitumor action are immunoblasts, and that they do not need to proliferate in the tumor-bearing host in order to exert their action. The use of irradiated lymphoid cells removes any possibility that this procedure may produce a dangerous graft-vs.-host disease in the tumor-bearing recipient.

INTRODUCTION

An effective method for exploiting the presence of tumor specific antigens of the transplantation type for the control of established tumors (either syngeneic transplants or primary) is the injection into the tumor-bearing animal of immune lymphoid cells (1). Since our research is aimed at finding immunotherapeutic procedures that might eventually be applicable to man, we concentrated on using allogeneic and xenogeneic lymphoid cells* obtained from donors immunized with a piece of the tumor to be treated. The tumor-bearing animals to which this therapy was applied have normal immunological reactivity, and consequently the foreign lymphocytes do not proliferate and cannot give rise to a graft-vs.-host reaction. It is important to distinguish this procedure from the injection of foreign lymphocytes into an immunologically suppressed animal (or into an F 1 hybrid), where a graft-vs.-host reaction occurs, in the course of which tumor cells are destroyed. The graft-vs.-host reaction is not, however, tumor specific, and normal cells are killed at the same time; treatment of immunologically suppressed animals with foreign lymphocytes is therefore associated with much toxicity.

The rationale for our procedure is that im-

---

* We found in a limited series of trials that immune syngeneic lymphoid cells were also effective against rat sarcoma, but since such cells can form a graft in the tumor-bearing host it is possible that their mode of action is different from that of foreign immune lymphocytes.

mune lymphoid cells have the capacity of destroying, as a result of direct cell-to-cell contact, specific target cells. If the lymphoid cells reach the tumor *in vivo*, they will cause tumor destruction by direct interaction. For this mechanism to apply, the injected cells need not grow or indeed survive for any length of time in the tumor-bearing animal. This procedure thus has some similarity to the administration of specific antibody, and we have referred to it as passive cellular immunity. We have studied this procedure in two experimental tumor systems: a) a variety of syngeneic ascites lymphomas in mice (2), and b) primary chemically induced sarcomas in rats (1). In both situations, antitumor effects were observed, but the nature of the effective lymphoid cells is, probably, different in the two systems (3). The present report is confined to the treatment of primary rat sarcomas* induced by a pellet of 3:4 benzpyrene.

The growth of more than 50% of these primary tumors was retarded, and occasionally complete regressions were obtained, by administering lymphoid cells taken from donor animals that had been immunized with a piece of the neoplasm to be treated. The donor animals were either allogeneic rats (1) or sheep or goats (5). To obtain the best antitumor effect, the procedure outlined below had to be followed:

1) The injected lymphoid cells had to be collected from the lymphatic circulation (i.e., from the thoracic duct in rats, or from efferent lymph of a stimulated node in the case of sheep and goats). Cells obtained from the spleen or lymph nodes of immunized animals had a better effect against the sarcomas than

against the lymphomas, although they showed some antitumor activity also against the latter (3, 6).

2) Only the cells present in the lymph between four and 10 days after immunization were effective.

3) The immune lymphoid cells were most effective if administered i.v. to the tumor-bearing animal.

4) Large numbers of cells (of the order of 10^8) have to be injected. This large number of foreign lymphoid cells did not cause any apparent ill effects. A graft-vs.-host reaction was seen only when the tumor-bearing animals were sick before treatment (e.g., with bronchiectasis) or had received whole-body irradiation.

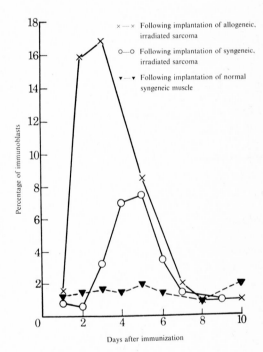

FIG. 1. Appearance in rat thoracic duct lymph of immunoblasts following stimulation with irradiated grafts of allogeneic sarcoma, syngeneic sarcoma and syngeneic muscle. The antigens were injected at multiple sites below the diaphragm. At each of the time points shown, three to five rats were cannulated and the lymph examined after a collection period of a few hours.

---

* The use of the carcinogen in relatively insoluble pellet form is important because in this way this cytotoxic agent remains localized, and does not damage lymphoid tissue. As a result, the animals are not in any way immunologically suppressed, unlike animals in which carcinogen has been applied in oil (4).

5) The tumor at the time of treatment must not exceed 2 cm in diameter.

The antitumor action of the immune lymphoid cells is confined to the particular tumor-which has been used for immunizing the donor animal. This indicates that the action of these cells is directed against the tumor specific antigens, which in the case of chemically induced neoplasms are unique to each tumor.

The cytotoxic action of the lymphoid cells obtained from the efferent lymph of a stimulated node against specific target cells was investigated in detail in an *in vitro* system (7). The cells that were responsible for killing the target cells by an immunologically specific reaction were not small lymphocytes but large, pyroninophilic blast cells which are released in large numbers into the afferent lymph of a stimulated node between 70 and 120 hr after application of the antigen (Fig. 1). These cells are referred to by us as immunoblasts, and a detailed description of their properties has been published (6). Once the immunoblast response has passed, the cells in the lymph are no longer cytotoxic.*

It must be emphasized that the appearance of immunoblasts in the lymph of draining nodes occurs in response to all types of antigenic stimulation, and that this reaction does not distinguish between cell-mediated and humoral antibody-mediated immune responses. Removal of draining lymph containing immunoblasts prevents the establishment of an immune state in the animal of both the humoral and cell-mediated type.

The cytotoxicity of the immunoblasts as assayed *in vitro* against target cells in tissue

culture was extremely radio-resistant and unaffected by doses of X-rays up to 5,000 R (8, 9). In view of this finding, we decided to investigate whether the antitumor action against primary rat sarcomas of the thoracic duct lymphocytes from immunized allogeneic donors was maintained if the lymphocytes were exposed to X-rays prior to injection into the tumor-bearing animals. The outcome of this experiment is not only of theoretical interest with regard to the mode of action of this form of immunotherapy, but may also be of practical value since by irradiating the lymphoid cells prior to injection, there is no longer any possibility of causing a hazardous graft-vs.-host reaction.

MATERIALS AND METHODS

The procedure used follows closely that previously described for the treatment of primary rat sarcomas (1, 5). Sarcomas were induced in outbred Wistar rats bred in our specific-pathogen free unit by a s.c. placed pellet of 3:4 benzpyrene. Only animals developing tumors between four and 10 months after implantation of the pellet were used; these tumors grow in an extremely uniform manner, and none has been observed to regress spontaneously. Tumors which arise after one year do not behave quite so predictably and are not used by us for this reason. When the tumors are between 1.5 and 2 cm in diameter, approximately one-half of the mass is removed surgically and the material obtained used to immunize three "donor rats" with multiple trocar implants placed s.c. in the lower half of the body.* These implants do not grow in the animals because they are not syngeneic with the rat in which the tumor arose.

Four days after immunization, the thoracic duct of the "donor" rats is cannulated and the lymph is drained for three days. Each day, collections of lymph are made and the cells are separated and washed free from the lymph plasma

---

* This finding is not in contradiction with the well established observation that cells taken from spleen and lymph nodes many weeks after immunization are still cytotoxic *in vitro*, because in these organs there are other types of cytotoxic cells which do not circulate in large numbers in lymph. These include macrophages and immunological memory cells (8).

---

* The efferent lymph coming from nodes situated below the level of the diaphragm drains directly into the thoracic duct, and all the cells coming from such nodes will therefore be collected when the duct is cannulated.

by centrifugation. The cells from the three donors are pooled and injected i.v. into the tumor-bearing rat. This is performed on three successive occasions; i.e., on the fifth, sixth and seventh day after partial removal of the tumor. The total number of cells injected was not identical for each tumor since the flow of lymph from the various donor rats could not be maintained constant. However, in each case the tumor-bearing animals received between 10^8 and 5×10^8 lymphocytes, of which approximately 10% were immunoblasts.

Irradiation was carried out with 220 kv X-rays at a dose rate of 800 R/min. During irradiation, the lymphocytes were suspended in cold tissue culture medium under conditions where oxygenation was adequate.

RESULTS

The effect of the treatment in the growth of the tumors was determined by measuring the average diameter of the tumor. The starting point is the diameter of the tumor on the day at which treatment was begun, that is five days after surgical removal of part of the tumor. The tumors at this time had actual diameters between 0.8 and 1.3 cm, but for convenience of representation, all tumor measurements have been converted so that the initial dimension shown in Fig. 2 is 1 cm. The actual numerical adjustment is small, since the actual starting dimensions were very

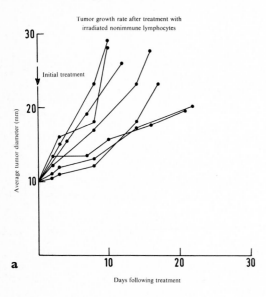

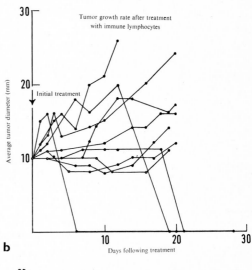

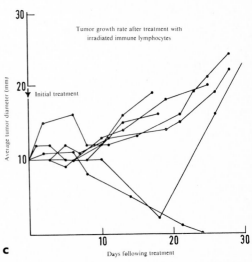

FIG. 2.   Growth rate of different primary sarcomata in rats following surgical removal of part of the tumor and treatment by i.v. injection of allogeneic lymphoid cells obtained from the thoracic duct lymph of donor animals. At the start of the experiment, the average diameter of the tumors ranged from 8 to 10 mm, but on the graphs, the dimensions were adjusted to the same starting point.
a) Control: Nonimmune thoracic duct cells.
b) Immune thoracic duct cells, unirradiated.
c) Immune thoracic duct cells irradiated with 1,000 R of X-rays prior to injection.

close to 1 cm. The animals were divided into four groups:

Group 1. Tumors treated with allogeneic thoracic duct cells from unimmunized rats.

Group 2. Unirradiated immune lymphoid cells; tumors treated with immune lymphoid cells from donors that had been immunized with the cancer to be treated (see Fig. 2b).

Group 3. Irradiated immune lymphoid cells; as Group 2, except that the lymphoid cells had been exposed to 1,000 R of X-rays (see Fig. 2c).

Group 4. Treatment with irradiated nonspecific lymphoid cells; in this group, irradiated lymphoid cells were injected that were directed against a different tumor. Each individual experiment involved the use of two tumor-bearing rats (rat A and rat B). Lymphocytes from donors immunized with tumors from rat A were injected into rat B, and vice versa. Three such experiments were performed, involving six tumor-bearing rats in all. The growth rate of these six tumors following injection was normal, and fell within the range shown for the controls shown in Fig. 2a.

The results of the experiments shown in Fig. 2a and 2b closely parallel our earlier findings (1, 5). We expressed the effect on tumor growth as the time required for the tumors to increase in diameter by a factor of 1.6. This we called the "fourfold increase time," because for a sphere, a diameter increase of 1.6 times is the same as an increase in volume of four times. In a large series (1, 10) of controls in which the tumor had only been biopsied, the "fourfold increase time" averaged 12 days, and in no case exceeded 18. Fig. 2a shows that the tumors in rats treated with nonimmune allogeneic lymphoid cells grew at the rate to be expected for animals that had received no treatment; in every one, the average diameter had increased by more than 1.6 times in less than 20 days.

The antitumor effect of the unirradiated immune lymphocytes closely reproduced the original experiment (1), in that four out of the seven tumors had a "fourfold increase time" of greater than 20 days, i.e., half the tumors grew significantly more slowly than any of the controls.

Fig. 2c shows that the growth inhibitory effect of the immune lymphoid cells is not abolished by irradiation. Indeed, the group of animals treated with irradiated lymphoid cells had a greater number of complete regressions that those treated with unirradiated immune lymphoid cells. While the number of animals treated was too small to be able to conclude that irradiated lymphoid cells are superior to unirradiated ones, it is clearly evident that irradiation has had no adverse effect.

Since all of the tumors in Group 4 grew at the normal rate, it is reasonable to conclude that the antitumor action of the irradiated lymphoid cells is immunologically specific, as had been found previously (1) for the unirradiated lymphoid cells, and presumably directed against the unique tumor-specific antigens of chemically induced sarcomas.

DISCUSSION

We had concluded earlier (5) that the cells responsible for slowing the growth of the primary sarcomas were immunoblasts, from the observation that only cells collected between four and 10 days after immunization were effective. The finding that irradiation with 1,000 R does not reduce the antitumor action of the lymphoid cells not only adds powerful support to the hypothesis that the cells responsible are immunoblasts, but provides direct proof of our original hypothesis that the injected cells do not have to proliferate in order to affect the tumor.

Our views on the mechanism by which the immunoblasts act *in vivo* have gone full circle. We began to question (11) our initial hypothesis that the injected cells homed to the tumor and there, by cell to cell interaction, killed tumor cells when we had found that xenogeneic lymphoid cells were as effective as lymphoid cells obtained from an animal of the same species. It seemed inconceivable at the time that heterologous lymphoid cells would persist for any length of time in the tumor-bearing host, and we believed that they were picked up immediately by the reticuloendothelial (RE) system. Many workers had earlier shown that heterologous lymphocytes were removed in this way, and certainly in our own experiments we failed to find heterologous lymphocytes in the circulation. However, evidence is accumulating that not all of the foreign immunoblasts are picked up by the RE system. By using scintillation counting, xenogeneic immunoblasts that have, in fact, been labeled *in vitro* have been detected in the tumors. The reason why such cells are not all removed by the RE system is that they extravasate rapidly. Immunoblasts have an extraordinary facility for passing through vascular barriers and penetrating to intercellular spaces (4, 6). The small lymphocytes do this at a much slower rate, and they are, in fact, picked up almost entirely by the RE system when injected i.v. into a foreign host. The immunoblasts which have extravasated persist for some days in extravascular tissue, and have been shown to synthesize immunoglobulin in a foreign host (i.e., sheep antibody is synthesized by these cells in mice) (6). We postulate that one of the functions of immunoblasts is to bring immunological reactivity to extravascular sites, and it is fortunate that even heterologous immunoblasts are able to do this for a time. This new knowledge about the physiology of immunoblasts eliminates the objections that had previously been believed to invalidate the "passive cellular immunity hypothesis" for the antitumor action of foreign lymphoid cells.

Before we knew that foreign immunoblasts can persist at extravascular sites, we explored the possibility that the antitumor action of xenogeneic and allogeneic immunoblasts depended on the transfer of an immunologically specific subcellular component from the immune lymphocytes to the tumor-bearing hosts. We found that the nucleic acids extracted from the immunoblasts exert a specific and presumably immunologically mediated antitumor action. The initial observations (12, 13) have been repeated and confirmed in a further series of experiments (6). Our hypothesis is that RNA from the immunoblasts produces a phenotypic transformation in some of the host cells, and causes these to acquire an immunologically specific antitumor activity. Whatever the mechanism, we were interested in the practical usefulness of cell-free extracts because there would be no possibility of inducing a graft-vs.-host reaction. However, the cell-free extracts are not as efficient as the cells themselves, and from the point of view of tumor immunotherapy, there now appears to be no advantage in using the nucleic acid extract rather than the cells since the hazard of a graft-vs.-host reaction can be avoided by using irradiated cells. A major obstacle to exploring the usefulness of irradiated immune lymphoid cells in the treatment of human malignant disease is that the number of cells that have to be injected to produce an antitumor effect is so very large. Based on the experiments with rats, more than 10^{12} cells would be needed in man. To produce this number of cells requires cannulation of something like eight nodes in sheep, and the availability of sufficient tumor to stimulate these eight nodes. Moreover, to attempt immunotherapy in advanced disease is a waste of time, and only patients with a small amount of residual disease could conceivably benefit from immunotherapy. Such patients do not have a hopeless prognosis, and a carefully conducted trial would be fneeded to establish whether the immunotherapy has been beneficial. We feel that before immunoblasts can be used in man, methods must be looked for to increase the proportion of the immunoblasts that reach the tumor.

Supported by grants from the Medical Research Council and the Cancer Research Campaign.

REFERENCES

1. DELORME, E. J. and ALEXANDER, P. Treatment of primary fibrosarcoma in the rat with immune lymphocytes. *Lancet* **ii**: 117, 1964.
2. ALEXANDER, P., CONNEL, D. I. and MIKULSKA, Z. B. Treatment of a murine leukaemia with spleen cells or sera from allogenic mice immunized against the tumor. *Cancer Res.* **26**: part 1. 1508, 1966.
3. ALEXANDER, P. Immunotherapy of leukaemia: The use of different classes of immune lymphocytes. *Cancer Res.* **27**: 2521, 1967.
4. ALEXANDER, P., BENSTED, J., DELORME, E. J., HALL, J. G. and HODGETT, J. The cellular immune response to primary sarcomata in rats. *Proc. roy. Soc. B.* **174**: 237, 1969.
5. ALEXANDER, P., DELORME, E. J. and HALL, J. G. The effect of lymphoid cells from the lymph of specifically immunized sheep on the growth of primary sarcomata in rats. *Lancet* **i**: 1186, 1966.
6. ALEXANDER, P. and HALL, J. G. The role of immunoblasts in host resistance and immunotherapy of primary sarcomata. *Advan. Cancer Res.* **13**: 1, 1970.
7. DENHAM, S., HALL, J. G., WOLF, A. and ALEXANDER, P. The nature of the cytotoxic cells in lymph following primary antigenic challenge. *Transplantation* **7**: 194, 1969.
8. DENHAM, S., GRANT, C., HALL, J. G. and ALEXANDER, P. The occurrence of two types of cytotoxic lymphoid cells in mice immunized with allogeneic tumor cells. *Transplantation* **9**: 366, 1970.
9. GRANT, C. K., DENHAM, S., HALL, J. G. and ALEXANDER, P. Antibody and complement-like factors in the cytotoxic action of immune lymphocytes. *Nature (Lond.)* **227**: 509, 1970.
10. HADDOW, A. and ALEXANDER, P. An immunological method of increasing the sensitivity of primary sarcomas to local irradiation with X-rays. *Lancet* **i**: 452, 1964.
11. ALEXANDER, P., BENSTED, J., DELORME, E. J., HALL, J. G., HAMILTON, L. D. G. and HODGETT, J. Treatment of primary sarcomas by enhancing host defense with immune lymphocytes or their RNA, in: "The proliferation and sium on Fundamental Cancer Research," University of Texas M.D. Anderson Hospital, spread of neoplastic cells." *21st Annual Symposium on Fundamental Cancer Research, University of Texas M.D. Anderson Hospital*. Baltimore, Williams and Wilkins Co., 1968, p. 693
12. ALEXANDER, P., DELORME, E. J., HAMILTON, L. D. G. and HALL, J. G. Effect of nucleic acids from immune lymphocytes on rat sarcomata. *Nature (Lond.)* **213**: 569, 1967.
13. ALEXANDER, P., DELORME, E. J., HAMILTON, L. D. G. and HALL, J. G. Stimulation of antitumor activity of the host with RNA from immune lymphocytes, in: Plesica, O. and Braun, W. (Eds.), "Nucleic acids in immunology." Berlin, Springer Verlag, 1969, p. 527.

TRANSFER OF TUMOR IMMUNITY WITH RNA

YOSEF H. PILCH, KENNETH P. RAMMING* and PETER J. DECKERS

Surgery Branch, National Cancer Institute, National Institutes of Health, Bethesda, Maryland, USA

ABSTRACT

RNA was extracted from the lymph nodes and spleens of guinea pigs previously immunized with a benzpyrene-induced C3Hf/HeN mouse sarcoma (BP-4). Normal C3H spleens cells were incubated with this RNA and injected into C3H mice which were then challenged with 10^4 viable BP-4 cells. Marked decrease in the incidence of tumor growth resulted. RNA from guinea pigs immunized with normal C3H tissues was ineffective. Treatment of the active RNA preparations with ribonuclease removed activity, while deoxyribonuclease or pronase treatment did not. Specificity of this response for the immunizing tumor was demonstrated.

In another system, RNA from the nodes and spleens of guinea pigs immunized with a Fisher 344 rat sarcoma (BP-1R) was mixed with dextran sulfate, a potent inhibitor of ribonuclease, and administered to normal Fisher rats which were then challenged with 10^4 BP-1R cells. Significant reduction in the incidence of tumor development was noted. Dextran sulfate alone or with nonspecific guinea pig RNA was ineffective.

In a syngeneic system designed to conclusively establish RNA mediation of immunity to tumor specific transplantation antigens, normal Fisher spleen cells were incubated with RNA from the spleens of Fisher rats immunized with BP-1R and given i.v. to Fisher rats which then received 3.5×10^4 BP-1R cells. Inhibition of tumor growth resulted. In another syngeneic system, *in vitro*, normal strain 2 guinea pig spleen cells were incubated with RNA extracted from the spleens of strain 2 guinea pigs immunized with a methylcholanthrene-induced strain 2 guinea pig sarcoma (MCA-A). Acellular areas of immune cytolysis of MCA-A cells were produced when aliquots of such RNA-incubated spleen cells were applied to MCA-A monolayers, but produced no cytolysis of normal strain 2 lung epithelial cells. Again, ribonuclease treatment abrogated the response, and specificity for the immunizing tumor was demonstrated.

INTRODUCTION

In recent years, a number of laboratories have studied the apparent conversion of normal, nonimmune lymphoid cells to specific immunoreactive status following incubation *in vitro* with RNA-rich extracts prepared from lymphoid tissues or macrophages exposed to specific antigens either *in vivo* or *in vitro* (1–6). Although considerable work in this area has suggested that a species of RNA of relatively

* Present address: Department of Surgery, Duke University School of Medicine, Durham, North Carolina, USA.

246

low molecular weight might be coding for antibody formation (2, 5, 7–9), much recent evidence suggests that persistent antigen, or antigenic determinant groups, possibly bound to a unique species of RNA may be involved in such reactions (9–14). Recently, Fishman and Adler have reported the identification of two types of immunologically active RNA from macrophages exposed to T2 phage *in vitro*. One was associated with phage antigen, induced IgG antibody formation, and may represent preformed informational macrophage RNA. The other was free of antigen, evoked IgM antibody formation, and may contain a type of immunoreactive RNA-antigen complex (15).

The transfer of immunity to cellular antigens has also been accomplished with "immune" RNA preparations. The transfer of transplantation immunity by incubation of autologous spleen cells *in vitro* with RNA extracted from regional lymph node cells of specifically immunized rabbits was demonstrated by Mannick and Egdahl in 1964 (16). Reinfusion of these RNA-incubated spleen cells caused the accelerated rejection of skin allografts taken from the same animal used to immunize the RNA donor. These findings have since been confirmed by Sabbadini and Sehon (17) and in our own laboratory (18). In addition, Wilson and Wecker (19) and Bondevik and Mannick (20) have shown that nonimmune lymphoid cells, incubated with RNA extracted from the lymphoid organs of animals immunized to histocompatibility antigens, cause specific immune cytolysis of target cells *in vitro*.

Since immunity to transplantation antigens could be mediated by immune RNA, it seemed likely that immunity to tumor specific transplantation antigens could also be transferred with RNA. Several authors working in a variety of systems have published reports of the inhibition or retardation of tumor growth mediated by preparations of "immune" RNA.

Alexander et al. reported growth retardation and occasional temporary regression of benzpyrene-induced sarcomas in rats treated by footpad injections of RNA extracted from lymph cells of sheep immunized with the particular rat tumor being treated (21, 22). Rigby has prolonged the survival of mice bearing Ehrlich ascites tumors by administering syngeneic spleen cells previously incubated with RNA from the spleens of mice immunized with this tumor (23). Londner et al. have reported a slowing of the growth of transplants of a spontaneously arising sarcoma in rats treated by the i.p. injection of RNA extracted from the spleens of rats immunized with the tumor being treated (24). Recently, Kennedy et al. have reported protection of C3H mice against transplants of a benzpyrene-induced sarcoma by footpad injections of RNA extracted from the lymph nodes and spleens of C57Bl mice immunized with this tumor (25).

The experiments which form the basis of this report were designed 1) to determine if immunity to tumor-specific transplantation antigens could be transferred by "immune" RNA extracted from the lymphoid organs of specifically immunized animals; 2) to investigate the possibility that such immunity could be mediated by heterologous immune RNA, that is, RNA extracted from the lymphoid organs of an animal species different from the tumor's host of origin; 3) to attempt the direct, systemic administration of antitumor "immune" RNA; 4) to develop in experimental animals models for the immunotherapy of human cancer.

MATERIALS AND METHODS

Mediation of immunity to tumor isografts in mice by xenogeneic RNA. Two benzpyrene-induced sarcomas, designated BP-4 and BP-1 induced and carried in female C3Hf/HeN mice, were used in their early transplant generations. Both these tumors were shown to contain distinct and different tumor-specific transplantation antigens, and no cross-reactivity between the antigens of these two tumors was demonstrated (Ramming and Pilch, in preparation).

Adult Hartley guinea pigs were immunized by injecting into each footpad a brei of 0.5 ml of a 40% w/v tumor cell suspension of either BP-1 or BP-4 sarcoma cells in Hank's balanced salt solution mixed with an equal volume of complete Freund's adjuvant. An i.p. injection of 1.0 ml of tumor cells without adjuvant was also given. One control group of guinea pigs received similar injections of C3H normal tissues—a mixture of lung, liver, kidney and spleen cells—instead of tumor cells. Another control group of guinea pigs received footpad injections of complete Freund's adjuvant only. After 10 to 14 days, the spleens, and axillary, popliteal and inguinal lymph nodes were excised and frozen in dry ice. RNA was extracted from these tissues as described previously (18). The RNA content of these preparations was determined by the orcinol reaction. This RNA was dissolved in Earle's balanced salt solution to a concentration of 400 to 1,000 µg/ml and made 0.7 M with respect to sucrose. In some experiments, the RNA was treated with ribonuclease, deoxyribonuclease or pronase prior to the addition of the sucrose, as previously described (26, Ramming and Pilch, in preparation).

Cell suspensions were prepared from the spleens of untreated C3H/HeN mice as previously described (26, 27), and were incubated in the RNA solutions at 37 C for 20 min at a concentration of 10^7 to 10^8 spleen cells/ml. The RNA-incubated spleen cells were washed once in Earle's balanced salt solution, counted, and the concentration adjusted to 5 to 10 × 10^7 cells/ml. In the course of these experiments, although not necessarily in every experiment, normal C3H spleen cells were incubated with the following experimental and control RNA preparations: 1) RNA from the lymphoid tissues of guinea pigs immunized with BP-4 mouse sarcoma (BP-4 RNA); 2) RNA from guinea pigs immunized with BP-1 sarcoma (BP-1 RNA); 3) RNA from pigs immunized with normal C3H tissues (normal C3H tissue RNA); 4) RNA from guinea pigs injected with Freund's adjuvant only (Freund's adjuvant RNA); 5) BP-4 RNA treated with ribonuclease (BP-4 RNA-ribonuclease), 6) BP-4 RNA treated with deoxyribonuclease (BP-4 RNA-deoxyribonuclease), and 7) BP-4 RNA treated with pronase (BP-4 RNA-pronase).

For each experiment, normal C3H mice were divided into groups of 20 to 30 animals. Mice in each group were given, on two successive days, i.p. injections of 0.5 ml containing 5 to 10 × 10^7 spleen cells which had been incubated in the RNA preparations designated for that group. Some control groups received normal C3H/HeN spleen cells which had not been incubated with RNA, and challenge control groups received no spleen cells at all. Mice in all groups received a s.c. inoculum of 10^4 BP-4 or 5 × 10^3 BP-1 tumor cells in the flank coincident with the first injection of spleen cells. All mice were then observed for subsequent tumor development.

Induction of immune cytolysis in vitro *with syngeneic RNA.* Two methylcholanthrene-induced sarcomas carried in inbred, female strain 2 guinea pigs and as monolayers in tissue culture were used. One was a liposarcoma designated MCA-A, the second an osteosarcoma designated MCA-25. Both tumors had been shown to contain tumor specific transplantation antigens by Holmes et al. (28), and no cross-reactivity between the two tumors had been observed.

Adult, female strain 2 guinea pigs were given a single intradermal injection of 10^6 viable MCA-A or MCA-25 tumor cells in the skin of the flank. When tumors became 2 to 3 cm in diameter, they were excised. After 10 to 14 days, intradermal injections of 5 × 10^6 viable cells of the same tumor were administered at two week intervals for a minimum of three months. At least two i.p. injections of 5 × 10^6 tumor cells were also given, at biweekly intervals, at the end of this period. The spleens of these immunized pigs (or, for controls, unimmunized strain 2 guinea pigs) were excised and frozen. RNA was extracted and dissolved in Earle's balanced salt solution to a concentration of approximately 500 µg/ml. Some RNA solutions were treated with ribonuclease at 20 µg/ml for 30 min at 37 C. All RNA solutions were made 0.35 M with respect to sucrose prior to use. Suspensions of normal, nonimmune strain 2 spleen cells, prepared as previously described (29), were incubated in the various RNA preparations for 20 min at 37 C and then washed. In the course of these experiments, normal strain 2 spleen cells were incubated with the following experimental and control RNA preparations: 1) RNA from the spleens of strain 2 pigs immunized with MCA-A (MCA-A RNA); 2) RNA from the spleens of strain 2 pigs immunized with MCA-25 (MCA-25 RNA); 3) RNA from the spleens of unimmunized strain 2 pigs (normal strain 2 RNA) 4) MCA-A RNA treated with ribonuclease (MCA-A RNA-ribonuclease). One-quarter ml aliquots (containing 10^7 cells) of the RNA-incubated spleen cells were then dropped on confluent monolayers of MCA-A, MCA-25 or normal strain 2 lung epithelium, and inspected after 48 hr of incubation at 37 C. The flasks were then shaken, the spleen cell droplets floated off, and the monolayers washed and inspected. Clear, acellular, macroscopic zones of lysis, or plaques, within the tumor cell monolayers and corresponding to the areas covered by the spleen cells were taken as evidence of immune cytolysis, as described previously (29). In the absence of immune cytolysis, the tumor cell monolayer remained intact.

Mediation of immunity to tumor isografts in rats by syngeneic RNA. A benzpyrene-induced sarcoma designated BP-1R induced and carried in inbred, female Fisher 344 rats, was used in early transplant generations. It had previously been shown to possess tumor-specific transplantation antigens (P. J. Deckers and Y. H. Pilch, unpublished data). Fisher rats were immunized by excising growing tumor isografts, and then boosted at weekly intervals with three s.c. injections of 10^5 viable BP-1R cells. All these inocula of viable tumor cells were rejected. One week after the last injection of tumor cells, the rats were sacrificed and their spleens excised. RNA was extracted in the usual manner and dissolved in Earle's balanced salt solution to a concentration of approximately 500 µg/ml. Suspensions of normal Fisher spleen cells were incubated in this RNA for 20 min at 37 C at a concentration of 10^7 to 10^8 cells/ml and then washed. Normal Fisher rats were then injected i.v. with 5×10^7 to 5×10^8 of these RNA-incubated spleen cells daily for three days. Twenty-four hours after the final injection of spleen cells, each rat received a s.c. challenge inoculum of 3.5×10^4 viable BP-1R cells. A control group of rats was treated with Fisher spleen cells incubated with RNA extracted from the spleens of unimmunized Fisher rats. Another control group of animals received no spleen cells at all. All animals were observed for tumor development. Tumors were measured at biweekly intervals and tumor volumes calculated by the formula $V = 0.4 \, ab^2$, where 'a' is the major axis of the tumor and 'b' the minor axis (30).

Mediation of immunity to tumor isografts in rats by the direct, systemic administration of xenogeneic RNA. The tumor-host system used in these studies was the BP-1R sarcoma in Fisher 344 rats. Groups of Hartley guinea pigs were immunized as described above with BP-1R tumor cells. RNA was extracted from their lymph nodes and spleens and designated "immune" heterologous RNA. A control RNA preparation was extracted from the nodes and spleens of unimmunized guinea pigs and was designated nonspecific heterologous RNA. Each RNA preparation was then dissolved (800 µg/ml) in Earle's balanced salt solution to which a potent ribonuclease inhibitor, sodium dextran sulfate, mol wt 77,000, had been added to a final concentration of 10 mg/ml. These RNA-dextran sulfate mixtures were then administered (as four 0.25 ml doses injected into each footpad) to groups of normal Fisher rats every other day for ten days. On the first day each rat also received a s.c. challenge inoculum of 10^4 viable BP-1R cells. Control animals received footpad injections of dextran sulfate alone or no treatment at all.

RESULTS

Mediation of immunity to tumor isografts in mice by xenogeneic RNA. The results of these experiments are presented in Tables 1 to 5. The data in Table 1 demonstrate: 1) the marked inhibition in the development of tumor isografts mediated by syngeneic spleen cells preincubated with BP-4 RNA; 2) the abrogation of this response when the active BP-4 RNA preparation was treated with ribonuclease prior to incubation with spleen cells; 3) the failure of normal C3H tissue RNA to mediate this response; 4) the ineffectiveness of nonspecific guinea pig lymphoid RNA (Freund's adjuvant RNA) in this system; 5) the fact that i.p. injections of syngeneic spleen cells alone were without effect.

The results shown in Table 2 show: 1) the reproducible immunity to tumor isografts mediated by BP-4 RNA; 2) the failure of treatment of the BP-4 RNA with deoxyribonuclease to inactivate the preparation; 3) confirmation of the failure of normal C3H tissue to effect a response.

The data in Table 3 show that: 1) once again, BP-4 RNA proved effective in mediating immunity to BP-4 tumor isografts, and 2) treatment of the BP-4 RNA preparation with pronase did not remove activity.

TABLE 1. *Incidence of tumor development in C3H mice following s.c. injection of 10^4 BP-4 tumor cells. Mice received two i.p. injections of 5 to 10 × 10^7 spleen cells treated as indicated*

Treatment of spleen cells[a]	No. mice in group	Final tumor incidence[b]	
		No.	%
BP-4 RNA	25	4/25	(16)[f]
BP-4 RNA (ribonuclease)[c]	29	18/29	(62)
Normal C3H tissue RNA	25	13/25	(52)
Freund's adjuvant RNA	27	18/25	(67)
None[d]	25	14/25	(56)
Challenge control[e]	30	21/30	(70)

[a] Syngeneic spleen cells were incubated with RNA extracted from the lymphoid organs of Hartley guinea pigs immunized with the designated materials.
[b] Cumulative incidence of tumor development expressed as number of mice with tumors/number of mice in experimental group.
[c] BP-4 RNA treated with ribonuclease prior to incubation with spleen cells.
[d] Normal syngeneic spleen cells not incubated with RNA.
[e] These mice received 10^4 tumor cells only. No spleen cells were administered.
[f] $P < 0.025$ when compared with recipients of spleen cells incubated with normal C3H tissue RNA; $P < 0.01$ when compared with all other groups (by χ^2 with Yates' correction).

TABLE 3. *Incidence of tumor development in C3H mice following s.c. injection of 10^4 BP-4 tumor cells. Mice received two i.p. injections of 5 to 10 × 10^7 spleen cells treated as indicated*

Treatment of spleen cells[a]	No. mice in group	Final tumor incidence[b]	
		No.	%
BP-4 RNA	26	16/26	(62)[f]
BP-4 RNA (pronase)[c]	20	10/20	(50)[f]
None[d]	31	29/31	(94)
Challenge control[e]	33	33/33	(100)

[a] Syngeneic spleen cells were incubated with RNA extracted from the lymphoid organs of Hartley guinea pigs immunized with the designated materials.
[b] Cumulative incidence of tumor development expressed as number of mice with tumors/number of mice in experimental group.
[c] BP-4 RNA treated with pronase prior to incubation with spleen cells.
[d] Normal syngeneic spleen cells not incubated with RNA.
[e] These mice received 10^4 BP-4 tumor cells only. No spleen cells were administered.
[f] $P < 0.01$ when compared with recipients of normal spleen cells and with challenge controls.

TABLE 2. *Incidence of tumor development in C3H mice following s.c. injection of 10^4 BP-4 tumor cells. Mice received two i.p. injections of 5 to 10 × 10^7 spleen cells treated as indicated*

Treatment of spleen cells[a]	No. mice in group	Final tumor incidence[b]	
		No.	%
BP-4 RNA	20	10/20	(50)[e]
BP-4 RNA (deoxyribonuclease)[c]	25	5/25	(20)[f]
Normal C3H tissue RNA	22	19/22	(86)
Challenge control[d]	27	26/27	(96)

[a] Syngeneic spleen cells were incubated with RNA extracted from the lymphoid organs of Hartley guinea pigs immunized with the designated materials.
[b] Cumulative incidence of tumor development expressed as number of mice with tumors/number of mice in experimental group.
[c] BP-4 RNA treated with deoxyribonuclease prior to incubation with spleen cells.
[d] Mice received 10^4 BP-4 tumor cells only. No spleen cells were administered.
[e] $P < 0.05$ when compared with recipients of spleen cells incubated with normal C3H tissue RNA and with challenge controls.
[f] $P < 0.001$ when compared with recipients of spleen cells incubated with normal C3H tissue RNA and with challenge controls.

TABLE 4. *Incidence of tumor development in C3H mice following s.c. injection of 10^4 BP-4 tumor cells or 10^4 BP-1 cells. Mice received two i.p. injections of 5 to 10 × 10^7 spleen cells treated as indicated*

Treatment of spleen cells[a]	Tumor used for challenge	No. mice in group	Final tumor incidence[b]	
			No.	%
BP-4 RNA	BP-4	16	6/16	(38)[e]
BP-4 RNA	BP-1	14	12/14	(86)
Challenge control[c]	BP-4	34	34/34	(100)
Challenge control[d]	BP-1	25	25/25	(100)

[a] Syngeneic spleen cells were incubated with RNA extracted from the lymphoid organs of Hartley guinea pigs immunized with the designated materials.
[b] Cumulative incidence of tumor development expressed as number of mice with tumors/number of mice in experimental group.
[c] Mice received 10^4 BP-4 tumor cells only. No spleen cells were administered.
[d] Mice received 5 × 10^3 PB-1 tumor cells only. No spleen cells were administered.
[e] $P < 0.025$ when compared with recipients of spleen cells incubated with BP-4 RNA and challenged with BP-1 tumor cells and with BP-4 challenge controls.

TABLE 5. *Incidence of tumor development in C3H mice following s.c. injection of 0.5 × 10⁴ BP-1 cells or 10⁴ BP-4 cells. Mice received two i.p. injections of 5 to 10 × 10⁷ spleen cells treated as indicated*

Treatment of spleen cells[a]	Tumor used for challenge	No. mice in group	Final tumor incidence[b] No.	%
BP-1 RNA	BP-1	18	9/18	(50)[e]
BP-1 RNA	BP-4	21	19/21	(90)
Challenge control[c]	BP-1	25	22/25	(88)
Challenge control[d]	BP-4	27	26/27	(97)

[a] Syngeneic spleen cells were incubated with RNA extracted from the lymphoid organs of Hartley guinea pigs immunized with the designated materials.
[b] Incidence of tumor development expressed as number of mice with tumors/number of mice in experimental group.
[c] Mice received 0.5 × 10⁴ BP-1 tumor cells. No spleen cells administered to this group.
[d] Mice received 10⁴ BP-4 tumor cells. No spleen cells administered to this group.
[e] $P < 0.025$ when compared with all other groups.

The data presented in Tables 4 and 5 provide evidence of the specificity of these responses for the particular tumor used to immunize the guinea pigs from whose lymphoid organs the "immune" RNA was extracted. From Table 4 it is evident that, while BP-4 RNA was effective in mediating immunity to isografts of BP-4, it was inactive against isografts of BP-1. From Table 5 one may discern that BP-1 RNA transferred immunity to BP-1 isografts, but had no effect on isografts of BP-4.

Induction of immune cytolysis in vitro *with syngeneic RNA.* As can be seen in Table 6, zones of lysis, or plaques, were formed in MCA-A monolayers only three times in 45 tests by normal, nonimmune strain 2 spleen cells. However, 36 plaques were formed in 40 tests with strain 2 spleen cells treated with

TABLE 6. *Plaques formed on monolayers of strain 2 guinea pig liposarcoma MCA-A at 48 hr by spleen cells incubated with RNA*

Groups	No. of plaques formed/ total no. of tests
Strain 2 spleen cells incubated with RNA extracted from the lymphoid organs of strain 2 guinea pigs:	
Immunized with liposarcoma MCA-A (MCA-A RNA)	36/40[b]
Immunized with liposarcoma MCA-A—ribonuclease treated (MCA-A RNA-ribonuclease)[a]	3/15
Unimmunized (normal strain 2 RNA)	10/49
Normal, untreated strain 2 spleen cells (no RNA)	3/45

[a] These RNA preparations treated with ribonuclease prior to incubation with spleen cells.
[b] $P < 0.01$ by χ^2 with Yates' correction when compared to every other group.

TABLE 7. *Plaques formed on strain 2 guinea pig tumor monolayers at 48 hr by spleen cells incubated with RNA*

Groups	No. of plaques formed/ total no. of tests MCA-A monolayers	MCA-25 monolayers
Strain 2 spleen cells incubated with RNA extracted from the lymphoid organs of strain 2 guinea pigs:		
Immunized with liposarcoma MCA-A (MCA-A RNA)	57/65	12/51[a]
Immunized with osteosarcoma MCA-25 (MCA-25 RNA)	3/15[b]	16/18
Unimmunized (normal strain 2 RNA)	10/65	0/12

[a] $P < 0.01$ by χ^2 with Yates' correction when compared with identical cells dropped on MCA-A monolayers. No significant differences when compared with cells incubated with RNA from unimmunized guinea pigs dropped on MCA-A monolayers.
[b] $P < 0.01$ when compared with identical cells dropped on MCA-25 monolayers. No significant difference when compared with cells incubated with RNA from unimmunized guinea pigs dropped on MCA-25 monolayers.

TABLE 8.   *Plaques formed on monolayers of strain 2 guinea pig lung epithelial cells at 48 hr*
by strain 2 spleen cells incubated with RNA

Groups	No. of plaques formed/ total no. of tests
Strain 2 spleen cells incubated with RNA extracted from the lymphoid organs of strain 2 guinea pigs:	
Immunized with liposarcoma MCA-A (MCA-A RNA)	0/15
Immunized with osteosarcoma MCA-25 (MCA-25 RNA)	0/14
Unimmunized (normal strain 2 RNA)	0/13

MCA-A RNA. When this MCA-A RNA preparation was treated with ribonuclease, the activity was largely abolished as evidenced by the formation of only three plaques in 15 tests. RNA from the lymphoid organs in unimmunized strain 2 guinea pigs (normal strain 2 RNA) was ineffective—only 10 plaques in 49 tests.

The specificity of this reaction is demonstrated in the results given in Table 7. Strain 2 spleen cells preincubated in MCA-A RNA induced zones of immune cytolysis in approximately 90% of tests on MCA-A monolayers but in only 23% of tests on MCA-25 monolayers. Likewise, spleen cells incubated in MCA-25 RNA produced areas of lysis in 16 of 18 tests on MCA-25 monolayers but in only three of 15 tests on MCA-A monolayers.

The data shown in Table 8 demonstrate that none of the immune RNA preparations mediated plaque formation on monolayers of normal strain 2 lung epithelial cells.

Mediation of immunity to tumor isografts in rats by syngeneic RNA. The results of this experiment are depicted graphically in Fig. 1, where the mean tumor volumes for each experimental group are plotted against the time in days from the day of injection of the challenge tumor cell inoculum. It can be seen that the mean tumor volumes in the animals treated with syngeneic spleens cells preincubated with RNA extracted from the spleens of unimmunized Fisher rats (nonspecific syngeneic RNA) did not differ significantly from the mean tumor volumes of challenge control

animals. However, animals treated with syngeneic spleen cells incubated with RNA extracted from the spleen of rats immunized with BP-1R ("BP-1 immune" syngeneic RNA) evidenced a marked decrease in mean tumor volume ($P < 0.01$ by Student's "t" test when compared with both control groups). However, the final cumulative tumor incidence in all three groups eventually reached 90 to 100%—11 of 12 in the challenge control group, 12 of 12 in the nonspecific syngeneic

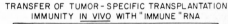

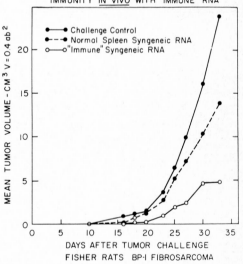

FIG. 1.   Mean tumor volumes in groups of female Fisher 344 rats inoculated s.c. with 1×10^5 viable BP-1R tumor cells. With the exception of the challenge control group all rats received daily i.v. injections for 3 days of 1 to 5×10^8 syngeneic spleen cells preincubated with the indicated RNA preparations.

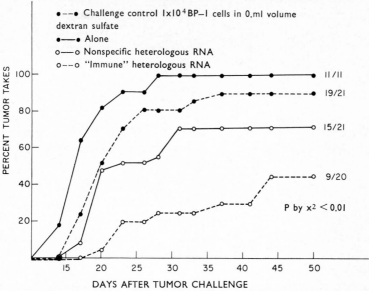

TRANSFER OF TUMOR IMMUNITY BY DIRECT FOOTPAD
INJECTIONS OF HETEROLOGOUS "IMMUNE" RNA

•――• Challenge control 1×10^4 BP–I cells in 0.ml volume
dextran sulfate
•――• Alone
o――o Nonspecific heterologous RNA
o――o "Immune" heterologous RNA

PERCENT TUMOR TAKES

11/11
19/21
15/21
9/20

P by $x^2 < 0.01$

DAYS AFTER TUMOR CHALLENGE

Sixth generation benz-a-pyrene-induced fibrosarcoma in syngeneic F–S44/N female rats

FIG. 2.   Cumulative tumor incidence in female Fisher 344 rats inoculated subcutaneously with 1×10^4 viable BP-1R tumor cells. With the exception of the
challenge control group all rats received injections of dextran sulfate with or
without RNA, as indicated, in each footpad every second day for 10 days.

RNA group, and 9 of 10 in the "BP-1 immune" RNA group.

*Mediation of immunity to tumor isografts in
rats by the direct, systemic administration of
xenogeneic RNA.* The results of this experiment are shown in Fig. 2. Here the cumulative
tumor incidence, expressed as percent tumor
takes, is plotted against time in days following
the injection of the challenge tumor cell inoculum. It is apparent that while treatment
with dextran sulfate alone, or with RNA from
unimmunized guinea pigs (nonspecific heterologous RNA) in dextran sulfate did not
effect the incidence of development of BP-1R
tumor isografts, treatment by footpad injections of BP-1R "immune" RNA in dextran
sulfate markedly inhibited the growth of the
isografts of BP-1R.

DISCUSSION

These data demonstrate that immunity to tu-

mor isografts in inbred mice can be mediated
by syngeneic spleen cells preincubated with
RNA extracted from the lymphoid organs of
guinea pigs immunized with the specific tumor
that is to be treated. Normal, nonimmune
spleen cells appeared to be converted to specific immunoreactive status during this brief,
in vitro incubation with "immune" RNA.
This immunity was manifested when such
RNA-incubated spleen cells were injected into
syngeneic mice. This response was specific for
the particular tumor used to immunize the
guinea pig from whose lymphoid organs the
"immune" RNA was prepared. Thus, spleen
cells incubated with BP-4 RNA inhibited isografts of BP-4, but not isografts of the syngeneic but antigenically different tumor BP-1.
Injection of spleen cells incubated with BP-1
RNA inhibited the growth of BP-1 isografts,
but not BP-4 isografts. Nonspecific factors
associated with guinea pig RNA probably do

not account for the immunoreactivity acquired by normal spleen cells following incubation with "immune" RNA, since RNA from guinea pigs immunized with Freund's adjuvant only was ineffective. Likewise, injections of untreated syngeneic spleen cells (not incubated with RNA) did not inhibit the growth of tumor isografts. Mice treated in this manner had cumulative tumor incidences which did not differ significantly from that of challenge control animals. Most important is the finding that RNA from the lymphoid organs of guinea pigs immunized with normal C3H tissues failed to mediate an antitumor response. This, together with the finding of the specificity of the "immune" RNA for the immunizing tumor, strongly suggests that the immunity expressed by the spleen cells preincubated with BP-4 RNA was directed primarily against tumor-specific transplantation antigens.

The guinea pigs immunized with mouse tumor cells were sensitized to a broad spectrum of murine transplantation antigens as well as to the tumor specific-transplantation antigens present on the tumor cells. Yet immunization with tumor cells appeared to be necessary in order for the "immune" RNA to mediate an antitumor immune response. RNA extracted from the lymphoid organs of guinea pigs immunized with normal C3H mouse tissues failed to induce C3H spleen cells to mediate an antitumor immune response against a C3H tumor. Certainly, our BP-4 RNA preparations must have contained "immune" RNA to C3H transplantation antigens as well as to BP-4 tumor-specific transplantation antigens. The C3H spleen cells incubated with BP-4 RNA were induced to mediate an anti-BP-4 immune response. Were they also sensitized to C3H transplantation antigens? If so, this would constitute immunization against "self" which, in the case of sensitization to transplantation antigens, might manifest itself by a graft-vs.-host

(GVH) reaction. Because of this possibility, experiments were designed to look for evidence of a GVH reaction in C3H mice receiving i.p. injections of syngeneic spleen cells preincubated with BP-4 RNA. This was performed in adult C3H mice (since the tumor isograft experiments had been performed in adult mice) and in neonatal C3H mice which, it was hoped, would provide a much more sensitive host for the detection of a GVH reaction mediated by BP-4 RNA. No evidence of a GVH response was found in either the neonatal or the adult animals (Ramming and Pilch, in preparation). This finding suggests that, at least within our system, recognition of self occurred at the level of interaction between the "immune" RNA and the lymphoid cell. "Immune" RNA to C3H transplantation antigens may have been recognized as self by the C3H lymphoid cells, and consequently no immune response to C3H transplantation antigens was initiated. However, "immune" RNA to BP-4 tumor-specific transplantation antigens were not recognized as self by the C3H spleen cells, and an antitumor immune response to these antigens was elicited.

One or more species of RNA was shown to be the active principle in the BP-4 RNA extracts since treatment of immunologically active BP-4 RNA preparations with ribonuclease prior to incubation with spleen cells completely abolished the response, whereas treatment of the same RNA preparations with deoxyribonuclease or with pronase did not effect their activity.

Because of certain obvious difficulties in the interpretation of results obtained in a xenogeneic model, an entirely syngeneic system was sought wherein the tumor, RNA donor, and normal lymphoid cells would all be from members of a single inbred strain of animals. The MCA-A and MCA-25 tumors in inbred strain 2 guinea pigs provided such a syngeneic tumor-host system. In these experiments, the transfer of immunity to tumor-specific antigens by "immune" RNA was clearly demonstrated.

Strain 2 spleen cells preincubated with MCA-A immune RNA prepared from the spleens of strain 2 guinea pigs (syngeneic with MCA-A) previously immunized with MCA-A mediated immune cytolysis of MCA-A target cells in monolayers. This cytolysis was not due to nonspecific effects of guinea pig spleen RNA, since RNA prepared from unimmunized strain 2 guinea pigs did not produce significant numbers of plaques. Nor was the plaque formation due to nonspecific interactions between normal strain 2 spleen cells and the tumor cells, as untreated spleen cells failed to cause significant plaque formation. Again, ribonuclease treatment of the active preparations abrogated the response, suggesting that RNA was the active moiety. In this system, as in the xenogeneic BP-4 RNA system, specificity of the immunologically active RNA preparations for the immunizing tumor was demonstrated. MCA-A RNA mediated immune cytolysis of MCA-A cells but not MCA-25 cells while MCA-25 RNA caused cytolysis of MCA-25 cells but not MCA-A cells. Moreover, neither MCA-A RNA nor MCA-25 RNA produced cytolysis of normal strain 2 lung epithelial cells.

It then seemed necessary to study syngeneic antitumor "immune" RNA *in vivo* within a syngeneic tumor-host system. Would such "immune" RNA preparations, made following immunization to tumor specific transplantation antigens only, mediate tumor growth retardation or transplantation resistance *in vivo*? If this were accomplished, the transfer of immunity to tumor-specific transplantation antigens by "immune" RNA would be confirmed.

For this purpose, the BP-1R tumor-host system in Fisher 344 rats was utilized. In this experiment, although BP-1R isografts eventually grew in all rats treated with syngeneic

spleen cells preincubated with BP-1R RNA, marked retardation of tumor growth was observed in the treated animals and survival was significantly prolonged. Since syngeneic spleen cells incubated with RNA extracted from the spleens of unimmunized Fisher rats was ineffective, this response was shown not to be due to nonspecific effects of rat lymphoid RNA.

In considering how best to achieve a transfer of immunity *in vivo* by the direct, systemic administration of "immune" RNA, our attention was drawn to the problem of the possible degradation of "immune" RNA by plasma and interstitial ribonucleases. Alexander et al. (22) did not administer their "immune" RNA preparations i.v. because of the high levels of ribonuclease in blood. They therefore administered the RNA by footpad injection. Moreover, these authors reported that the RNA preparations used in their successful experiments had been far from pure, containing considerable DNA as well as some protein—a "DNA-protein gel." When purer RNA extracts were prepared, containing only 10% DNA and providing nonviscous solutions quite unlike the gel-like suspensions obtained by their original method, no antitumor effect was noted. They postulated that the presence of DNA, particularly in a gel form, might protect the RNA from degradation by the ribonucleases in interstitial tissue.

We therefore elected to administer "immune" RNA in a solution containing ribonuclease inhibitor. Ribonuclease is known to be reversibly inhibited by polyanions or "macroanions," macromolecules with strong fixed negative charges distributed over their surface (31, 32). One such polyanion, available commercially in good degrees of purity and in preparations of varying molecular weight, is sodium dextran sulfate. This compound has been shown to be a potent inhibitor of ribonuclease (32, 33). Previous studies in our laboratory had shown that sodium dextran sulfate of mol wt 25,000 and 47,000 was a poor to fair inhibitor of ribonuclease, but that dextran sulfate of mol wt 77,000, 2.75×10^5, 5.0×10^5 and 2.0×10^6 was an excellent ribonuclease inhibitor (Y. H. Pilch and K. P. Ramming, unpublished data). Because of its lower toxicity, dextran sulfate, mol wt 77,000, was utilized in our experiments.

RNA extracted from the lymph nodes and spleens of guinea pigs immunized with BP-1R tumor cells was dissolved in a medium containing dextran sulfate and injected into the footpads of Fisher rats. Animals treated in this manner displayed significant immunity to transplants of the BP-1R tumor. Dextran sulfate alone did not decrease the incidence of tumor isograft growth, thereby evincing no nonspecific antitumor effect. Moreover, RNA from the nodes and spleens of unimmunized guinea pigs when administered in dextran sulfate did not effect an antitumor response.

In these early experiments, the systemic administration of "immune" RNA without dextran sulfate was not studied. Therefore, we cannot say that dextran sulfate (or another ribonuclease inhibitor) is truly necessary for the successful systemic administration of "immune" RNA. Indeed, Londner et al. (24) and Kennedy et al. (25) have published preliminary reports of the transfer of immunity to tumors by direct injection of "immune" RNA preparations without ribonuclease inhibitor. Experiments designed to study the value of adding ribonuclease inhibitors to preparations of "immune" RNA used for systemic administration are currently underway in our laboratory.

The mechanism by which preparations of "immune" RNA effect transfer of immunoreactivity remains controversial. We consider it unlikely that the activity of such RNA preparations is due to the transfer of antigen per se, present as contaminants in the RNA extracts. The rodent transplantation antigens (34, 35), as well as the tumor specific transplantation antigens (28, 36) solubilized and partially characterized to date, have been found to have the chemical properties of proteins. Our RNA preparations contained significant amounts of protein, part of which might consist of tumor or transplantation antigens or both. However, such protein antigens would almost certainly be denatured and inactivated by phenol treatment during the RNA extraction procedure. Moreover, in experiments reported elsewhere (29), strain 2 guinea pig spleen cells were incubated with extracts of the MCA-A tumor, known to contain solubilized tumor specific transplantation antigens, at a protein concentration 50 to 100 times the protein content of our RNA preparations. When spleen cells so treated were tested for cytolytic effect on monolayers of MCA-A cells, no plaque formation was observed, suggesting that the immune cytolysis mediated by MCA-A RNA was not due to simple contamination of the RNA preparations with tumor antigens. In addition, treatment of the active RNA preparations with pronase did not effect their activity, suggesting that the active moiety was not a protein. However, protein antigens complexed to RNA might be resistant to pronase degradation. Indeed, reasoning teleologically, one might speculate that one of the "purposes" of complexing antigenic moieties to RNA might be to protect them from digestion by intercellular and intracellular proteolytic enzymes.

We believe instead that "immune" RNA may act either by means of highly immunogenic complexes of a unique species of RNA with antigen or antigenic determinants (the theory of RNA-antigen complexes or "super antigen"), or due to the presence of true informational RNA moieties which are incorporated by normal lymphoid cells and then code for a specific immune response. Perhaps, both mechanisms are operative in varying degrees, depending on the particular set of experimental circumstances.

The authors wish to thank Mrs. Anne Koons, Mr. George Jenkins and Mrs. Roxane Hume for their expert technical assistance.

REFERENCES

1. FISHMAN, M. Antibody formation in vitro. *J. exp. Med.* **114**: 837, 1961.
2. FISHMAN, M. and ADLER, F. L. Antibody formation initiated *in vitro*. II. Antibody synthesis in X-irradiated recipients of diffusion chambers containing nucleic acid derived from macrophages incubated with antigen. *J. exp. Med.* **117**: 595, 1963.
3. COHEN, E. P. and PARKS, J. J. Antibody production by nonimmune spleen cells incubated with RNA from immunized mice. *Science* **144**: 1012, 1964.
4. COHEN, E. P., NEWCOMB, R. W. and CROSBY, L. K. Conversion of non-immune spleen cells to antibody-producing cells by RNA: strain specificity of the response. *J. Immunol.* **95**: 583, 1965.
5. COHEN, E. P. Conversion of nonimmune cells into antibody producing cells by RNA. *Nature (Lond.)* **213**: 462, 1967.
6. FRIEDMAN, H. P. Antibody plaque formation by normal spleen cells maintained in tissue culture following *in vitro* incubation with immune RNA. *Science* **146**: 934, 1964.
7. CAMPBELL, D. H. and GARVEY, J. S. Nature of retained antigen and its role in immune mechanisms. *Advanc. Immunol.* **3**: 261, 1963.
8. BELL, C. and DRAY, S. Conversion of nonimmune spleen cells by ribonucleic acid of lymphoid cells from an immunized rabbit to produce IgM antibody of foreign light chain allotype. *J. Immunol.* **103**: 1196, 1969.
9. ADLER, F. L., FISHMAN, M. J. and DRAY, S. Antibody formation initiated *in vitro*. III. Antibody formation and allotypic specificity directed by ribonucleic acid from peritoneal exudate cells. *J. Immunol.* **97**: 554, 1966.
10. ASKONAS, B. A. and RHODES, J. M. Immunogenicity of antigen containing ribonucleic acid preparations from macrophages. *Nature (Lond.)* **205**: 470, 1965.
11. FRIEDMAN, H. P., STAVITSKY, A. B. and SOLOMON, J. M. Induction *in vitro* of antibodies to phage T2-antigens in the RNA extract employed. *Science* **149**: 1106, 1965.
12. GOTTLIEB, A. A., GLISIN, V. R. and DOTY, P. Studies on macrophage RNA involved in antibody production. *Proc. nat. Acad. Sci. (Wash.)* **57**: 1849, 1967.
13. GOTTLIEB, A. A. The antigen RNA complex, in: Plescia, O. J., and Braun, W., (Eds.) "Nucleic acids in immunology." New York, Springer-Verlag, 1968, p. 471.
14. GOTTLIEB, A. A. Studies on the binding of soluble antigens to a unique ribonucleoprotein fraction of macrophage RNA. *Biochemistry* **8**: 2111, 1969.
15. FISHMAN, M., and ADLER, F. L. The role of

macrophage RNA in the immune response. *Cold Spr. Harb. Symp. quant. Biol.* **32**: 343, 1967.
16. MANNICK, J. A. and EGDAHL, R. H. Transfer of heightened immunity to skin homografts by lymphoid RNA. *J. clin. Invest.* **43**: 2166, 1964.
17. SABBADINI, E. and SEHON, A. H. Acceleration of allograft rejection induced by RNA from sensitized donors. *Int. Arch. Allergy* **32**: 55, 1967.
18. RAMMING, K. P. and PILCH, Y. H. Transfer of transplantation immunity by ribonucleic acid. *Transplantation* **7**: 296, 1969.
19. WILSON, D. B. and WECKER, E. E. Quantitative studies on the behavior of sensitized lymphoid cells *in vitro*. III. Conversion of "normal" lymphoid cells to an immunologically active status with RNA derived from isologous lymphoid tissues of specifically immunized rats. *J. Immunol.* **47**: 512, 1966.
20. BONDEVIK, H. and MANNICK, J. A. RNA-mediated transfer of lymphocyte vs. target cell activity. *Proc. Soc. exp. Biol. (N.Y.)* **129**: 264, 1968.
21. ALEXANDER, P., DELORME, E. J., HAMILTON, L. D. G. and HALL, J. G. Effect of nucleic acids from immune lymphocytes on rat sarcomata. *Nature (Lond.)* **213**: 569, 1967.
22. ALEXANDER, P., DELORME, E. J., HAMILTON, L. D. G. and HALL, J. G. Stimulation of antitumor activity of the host with RNA from immune lymphocytes, in: Plescia, O. J. and Braun, W. (Eds.), "Nucleic acids in immunology." New York, Springer-Verlag, 1968, p. 527.
23. RIGBY, P. G. Prolongation of survival of tumor-bearing animals by transfer of "immune" RNA with DEAE dextran. *Nature (Lond.)* **221**: 968, 1969.
24. LONDNER, M. V., MORINI, J. C., FONT, M. T. and RABASA, S. L. RNA-induced immunity against a rat sarcoma. *Experientia (Basel)* **24**: 598, 1968.
25. KENNEDY, C. T. C., CATER, D. B. and HARTVEIT, F. Protection of C3H mice against BP8 tumor by RNA extracted from lymph-nodes and spleens of specifically sensitized mice. *Acta path. microbiol. scand.* **77**: 796, 1969.
26. PILCH, Y. H. and RAMMING, K. P. Transfer of tumor immunity with ribonucleic acid. *Cancer (Phila.)* (in press).
27. RAMMING, K. P. and PILCH, Y. H. Mediation of immunity to tumor isografts in mice by heterologous ribonucleic acid. *Science* **168**: 492, 1970.
28. HOLMES, E. C., KAHAN, B. D. and MORTON, D. L. Soluble tumor specific transplantation antigens from methylcholanthrene-induced guinea pig sarcomas. *Cancer (Phila.)* **25**: 373, 1970.
29. RAMMING, K. P. and PILCH, Y. H. Transfer of tumor specific immunity with RNA: Induction of immune cytolysis *in vitro*. *J. nat. Cancer Inst.* (in press).
30. ATTIA, M. A. M. and WEISS, D. W. Immunology of spontaneous mammary carcinomas in mice. V. Acquired tumor resistance and enhancement in strain A mice infected with mammary tumor virus. *Cancer Res.* **26**: 1787, 1966.
31. MORA, P. T. and YOUNG, B. G. Reversible inhibition of enzymes by interaction with synthetic polysaccharide macroanions. *Arch. Biochem. Biophys.* **82**: 6, 1959.

32. FELLIG, J. and WILEY, C. E. The inhibition of pancreatic ribonuclease by anionic polymers. *Arch. Biochem.* **85**: 313, 1959.

33. BACH, M. K. The inhibition of deoxyribonucleotidyl transferase DNAase and RNAase by sodium poly ethenesulfonic acid. Effect of the molecular weight of the inhibitor. *Biochim. Biophys. Acta. (Amst.)* **91**: 619, 1964.

34. KAHAN, B. D. and REISFELD, R. A. Advances in the chemistry of transplantation antigens. *Transplant. Proc.* **1**: 483, 1969.

35. KAHAN, B. D. and REISFELD, R. A. Electrophoretic purification of a water soluble guinea pig transplantation antigen. *Proc. nat. Acad. Sci. (Wash.)* **58**: 1430, 1967.

36. OETTGEN, H. F., OLD, L. J., MCLEAN, L. P. and CARSWELL, E. A. Delayed hypersensitivity and transplantation immunity elicited by soluble antigens of chemically induced tumors in inbred guinea pigs. *Nature (Lond.)* **220**: 295, 1968.